Second Edition

Handbook of Eczema

for Dermatologists

Editors

Kabir Sardana MD, DNB, MNAMS

Professor
Department of Dermatology and STDs
PGIMER, Dr Ram Manohar Lohia Hospital
New Delhi

Ananta Khurana MD, DNB, MNAMS

Associate Professor
Department of Dermatology and STDs
PGIMER, Dr Ram Manohar Lohia Hospital
New Delhi

Assistant Editor

Seema Rani MD

Associate Professor
Department of Dermatology and STDs
PGIMER, Dr Ram Manohar Lohia Hospital
New Delhi

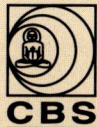

CBS

CBS Publishers & Distributors Pvt Ltd

New Delhi • Bengaluru • Chennai • Kochi • Kolkata • Mumbai
Hyderabad • Jharkhand • Nagpur • Patna • Pune • Uttarakhand

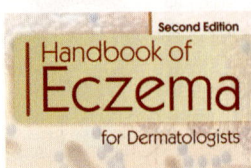

ISBN: 978-93-87085-94-7

Copyright © Editors and Publisher

Second Edition: 2018
First Edition: 2017

Published by Satish Kumar Jain and Produced by Varun Jain for

CBS Publishers & Distributors Pvt Ltd
4819/XI Prahlad Street, 24 Ansari Road, Daryaganj, New Delhi 110 002, India.
Ph: 23289259, 23266861, 23266867   Fax: 011-23243014   Website: www.cbspd.com
e-mail: delhi@cbspd.com; cbspubs@airtelmail.in.

Corporate Office: 204 FIE, Industrial Area, Patparganj, Delhi 110 092
Ph: 4934 4934   Fax: 4934 4935   e-mail: publishing@cbspd.com; publicity@cbspd.com

Branches

- **Bengaluru:** Seema House 2975, 17th Cross, K.R. Road, Banasankari 2nd Stage, Bengaluru 560 070, Karnataka
  Ph: +91-80-26771678/79   Fax: +91-80-26771680   e-mail: bangalore@cbspd.com
- **Chennai:** 7, Subbaraya Street, Shenoy Nagar, Chennai 600 030, Tamil Nadu
  Ph: +91-44-26680620, 26681266   Fax: +91-44-42032115   e-mail: chennai@cbspd.com
- **Kochi:** Ashana House, No. 39/1904, AM Thomas Road, Valanjambalam, Ernakulam 682 016, Kochi, Kerala
  Ph: +91-484-4059061-65   Fax: +91-484-4059065   e-mail: kochi@cbspd.com
- **Kolkata:** 6/B, Ground Floor, Rameswar Shaw Road, Kolkata-700 014, West Bengal
  Ph: +91-33-22891126, 22891127, 22891128   e-mail: kolkata@cbspd.com
- **Mumbai:** 83-C, Dr E Moses Road, Worli, Mumbai-400018, Maharashtra
  Ph: +91-22-24902340/41   Fax: +91-22-24902342   e-mail: mumbai@cbspd.com

Representatives

- **Hyderabad** 0-9885175004   • **Jharkhand** 0-9811541605   • **Nagpur** 0-9021734563
- **Patna** 0-9334159340   • **Pune** 0-9623451994   • **Uttarakhand** 0-9716462459

Printed in Buluji Art, India

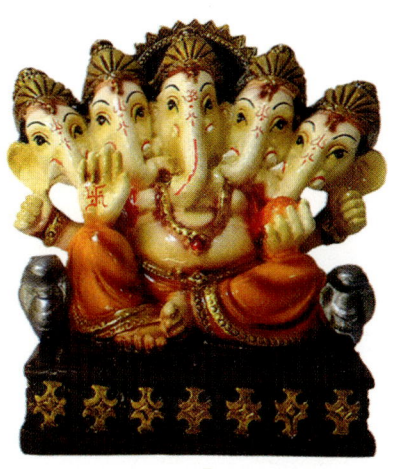

वक्रतुण्ड महाकाय सूर्यकोटि समप्रभ।
निर्विघ्नं कुरु मे देव सर्वकार्येषु सर्वदा॥

I meditate on Sri Ganesha
Who has a Curved Trunk, Large Body,
and
Who has the Brilliance of a Million Suns,
O Lord
Please make all my Works Free of Obstacles, Always

Contributors

Aastha Gupta MD
Senior Resident
Department of Dermatology and STDs
PGIMER, Dr Ram Manohar Lohia Hospital
New Delhi

Abir Saraswat MD, DNB, MNAMS
Consultant Dermatologist
Indushree Skin Clinic
Lucknow

AK Bajaj MD
3/6 Panna Lal Road
Allahabad-211 002, India Tel: 91-532-2256461

Ananta Khurana MD, DNB, MNAMS
Associate Professor
Department of Dermatology and STDs
PGIMER, Dr Ram Manohar Lohia Hospital
New Delhi

Aniket Bhole DNB
Secondary DNB, Hindu Rao Hospital, Delhi

Asit Mittal MD
Professor and Senior Consultant
RNT Medical College and attached Hospitals
Udaipur (Rajasthan)

Chia-Chun Ang MBBS (Singapore), MRCP (UK), MMed (Int Med),
FAMS (Dermatology)
Consultant Dermatologist, Changi General Hospital,
Singapore

Deepshikha Khanna MD (Dermatology)
Consultant (Specialist), Dermatology
Lal Bahadur Shastri Hospital, Mayur Vihar
Khichripur, Delhi 110091

Kabir Sardana MD, DNB, MNAMS
Professor
Department of Dermatology and STDs
PGIMER, Dr Ram Manohar Lohia Hospital
New Delhi

Khushbu Mahajan MD
Assistant Professor, North Delhi Municipal Corporation
Medical College and Hindu Rao Hospital, Delhi

Konchok Dorjay MD
Senior Resident
Department of Dermatology and STDs
PGIMER, Dr Ram Manohar Lohia Hospital
New Delhi

PK Srivastava MD
Consultant Dermatologist
Mansi Skin and Allergy Clinic
George Town, Allahabad

Pooja Arora Mrig MD, DNB, MNAMS
Assistant Professor
PGIMER and RML Hospital
Delhi

Sanjay Ghosh MD
Professor, Department of Dermatology
MGM Medical College and LSK Hospital
Kishanganj, India

Saurav Kundu MD
Assistant Professor, Department of Dermatology
MGM Medical College and LSK Hospital
Kishanganj, India

Seema Rani MD
Associate Professor
Department of Dermatology and STDs
PGIMER, Dr Ram Manohar Lohia Hospital
New Delhi

Shivani Bansal MD, DNB
Max Hospital
Panchsheel
Delhi

Soumya Agarwal MD
Senior Resident, Department of Dermatology
Lady Hardinge Medical College and SSKH
Delhi

Taru Garg MD
Professor, Department of Dermatology
Lady Hardinge Medical College and SSKH
Delhi

Wai-Kwong Cheong MBBS (Singapore), MRCP (UK), FRCP
(Edinburgh), FAMS (Dermatology)
Consultant Dermatologist, Specialist, Skin Clinic and
Associates, Singapore

Foreword

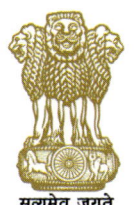

Government of India
Department of Dermatology
Post Graduate Institute of
Medical Education and Research,
Dr Ram Manohar Lohia Hospital
New Delhi

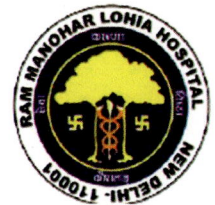

It gives me great pleasure to write the Foreword of this unique handbook on a topic rarely covered in this form targeting dermatologists. It is heartening to note that the book is dedicated to the South Asian population where the manifestations and causes may be different from the Caucasian skin.

Dr Kabir Sardana, who is a Professor in the Department of Dermatology at Dr RML Hospital, is an alumnus of Maulana Azad Medical College, where he has spent a large part of his academic career. He has an impressive academic record with over 130 indexed publications and 9 books to his credit. He is an excellent teacher and orator and is an asset for postgraduates in this institution.

This handbook has the added advantage of succinctly covering the salient forms of eczema and enabling a quick summary of treatment of the commonly encountered disorders. The contributors who have varied interests have exhibited their academic skills which are reflected in the text.

I am sure the book will be a handy and useful addition to practitioners, postgraduates and dermatologists alike.

I wish Dr Sardana best of luck for this endeavour.

RK Gautam
Professor
Dr RML Hospital, New Delhi

Foreword

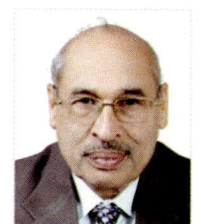

It is a matter of pleasure for me to write the Foreword for this comprehensive handbook on eczema written by authorities in the field. Medicine is a dynamic science which is evolving at a fast pace. Despite massive explosion of online information, a monograph that has been vetted by experts becomes indispensable. The lucid and comprehensive description of the various chapters makes it a pleasurable reading. This book will definitely instill confidence in the minds of dermatologists to manage a wide range of eczemas with the utmost ease.

AK Bajaj
Former Professor, Department of Dermatology, MLN Medical College
Allahabad
Past President, IADVL, CODFI
President, Skin Allergy Research Society
Chairman, IADVL Academy of Dermatology (2008–2009)

Preface to the Second Edition

Eczema is probably one of the most commonly seen skin disorders but is not given its due worth in most standard textbooks and conferences. Although there are other entities vying for conference deliberations, we believe eczematous disorders are the most significant mimickers in dermatological practice, owing to their sheer volume in our daily clinics. It is said that, "better than diagnosing rare cases rarely, it is better to treat common disorders well" and that is the basis of this book on eczema, arguably the commonest disorder in dermatology.

This edition is an expansion of the previous edition, which was largely aimed at dermatologists. In the present edition, we have covered the various entities in greater detail with focus remaining on the management part. Atopic eczema and hand eczema generate maximum interest of all eczemas and have been comprehensively covered. A separate chapter is dedicated to regional manifestations of contact dermatitis to give the reader a concise and updated review of the same at one place. Parthenium dermatitis, the "scourge of India", is separately covered in detail. Newer concepts have been added in the section on prurigo nodularis, pompholyx, photoallergic eczemas and airborne contact dermatitis. The part on erythroderma has been expanded with greater emphasis on establishing a diagnosis and on treatment recommendations. A chapter on miscellaneous eczemas has been added covering some interesting and commonly overlooked entities. The treatment section in all chapters is detailed and a stepwise approach is presented wherever possible. Schematic diagrams have been incorporated at many places all through the book, for better understanding of concepts and giving the reader easily visualized 'at a glance' information. Flowcharts, tables and boxes are included to summarise the points in text and for easy readability and comprehension. Numerous photographs covering varying manifestations are presented in each section. We thank Dr AK Bajaj for significant contributions in this regard.

A book is worth its contributors and we are fortunate to have contributors who have special interest in their respective topics. **Dr Seema Rani** has rewritten the chapter on airborne contact dermatitis, a major problem in India. **Dr Taru Garg** and **Dr Seema Rani** have reworked the chapter on allergic contact dermatitis. We have added a detailed chapter on regional causes of contact dermatitis with the able help of **Dr AK Bajaj**. **Dr Abir Saraswat** has reviewed the chapter on non-eczematous contact dermatitis. **Dr Deepshikha Khanna** had worked for many years in an exclusive pediatric dermatology set up and contributes on diaper dermatitis. **Dr Konchok Dorjay** whose thesis was on hand eczema has helped us rework the chapter on hand eczema, a issue in India, where the majority of housewives who are exposed to ever strong detergents promoted by the media and are consequentially plagued by this problem. We have redone the chapter on atopic dermatitis with newer therapies and cutting edge biological targets in atopic dermatitis. **Dr Wai-Kwong Cheong** has done extensive work on seborrheic eczema, a condition that is common in the humid environment that is seen both in India and Singapore. **Dr Ananta Khurana** has added relevant data to this chapter. **Dr Asit Mittal** who has a special interest in pruritus has reviewed and edited the chapter on prurigo nodularis. Of course, our own department's team of **Dr Ananta Khurana**, **Dr Seema Rani**, **Dr Aastha** and **Konchok Dorjay** have added substantially throughout the book.

This book is not aimed to be a treatise and thus we have purposely left out the verbose pathogenesis and focused on the clinical approach and management concept of this dermatological series that has been supported by CBS Publishers. I am again amazed at the endless capacity of my co-editor Dr Ananta Khurana who has edited, supplanted and spliced portions of the text to make it compact and readable in record time!

Now a brief on **how to use this book.** For the busy practitioner a Therapeutic table of content can help focus on the treatment aspects of the various disorders where as far as possible treatments are graded as first, second and third line. For others the chapters can be referred to, and they would also possibly go backwards from the therapy pages!

A big thanks to CBS Publishers & Distributors, Mr SK Jain CMD and Mr YN Arjuna Senior Vice President—Publishing, Editorial and Publicity and their team, Mrs Ritu Chawla Assistant General Manager—Production, Mr Sanjay Chauhan, Mr Vikrant Sharma and Mr Ananda Mohanty; and Mr SK Verma and Mr Sunil Dutt, apart from the great support staff at their easily accessible office.

Lastly the previous edition of this book, for practitioners and foreworded by **Dr RP Gupta** and **Dr RK Gautam** came at a particularly trying time for me. Herein in hindsight I paraphrase two deep thoughts. It is said that Buddha's primordial thought has been that "the truth of life is suffering". Truly it is necessary to suffer and suffer deeply. As once you walk this path (unlike those who just talk this path) and reach the end of your human efforts, you remember God. And it is said deeper the pain, more intensely you remember God. And believe me God sends people, family and friends to help you out of the trickiest of problems, if you have faith in him. And then one realizes the purpose of life, which as Shri Raman Maharishi said is "to remember and be grateful to God". So a big thanks to the triumvirate—God sent—who helped me realise this truth! I hope you do not go through this though …

Happy reading!

Kabir Sardana

Preface to the First Edition

Eczema is probably one of the most commonly seen skin disorders but there is probably just one book dedicated to it on the Fast Fact Series. In Asian skin the manifestations and causes are different than in the West. The aim of this book was to succinctly cover the major types of eczema focusing on Indian and Asian skin.

A book is worth its contributors and I am fortunate to have contributors who have special interest in their respective topics. **Dr Sanjay Ghosh** has extensive experience in airborne contact dermatitis, a major problem in India. **Dr Taru Garg** has done work on allergic contact dermatitis which in India is massive problem as the number of allergens outmaneuver the tools and I daresay the clinicians to identify them. **Dr Deepshikha Khanna** had worked for many years in an exclusive pediatric dermatology set up and contributes on diaper dermatitis. **Dr Pooja Arora Mrig** has interest in a difficult and recurring problem of hand eczema, a issue in India, where the majority of housewives who are exposed to ever strong detergents promoted by the media and are consequentially plagued by this problem. **Dr Khushbu Mahajan** has an interest in atopic dermatitis, a condition that in the humid weather of the country is still largely a manageable disorder. **Dr Wai-Kwong Cheong** has done extensive work on seborrheic eczema, a condition that is common in the humid environment that is seen both In India and Singapore. Lastly **Dr Shivani Bansal** has done justice to the other topics that encompass the commonly seen eczematous disorders.

The book is not aimed to be a treatise and thus we have purposely left out the verbose pathogenesis and focused on the clinical approach and management concept of this dermatological series that had been supported by CBS Publishers.

A big thanks to CBS Publishers & Distributors, Mr SK Jain CMD and Mr YN Arjuna Senior Vice President—Publishing, Editorial and Publicity and their team, Mrs Ritu Chawla Assistant General Manager—Production, Mr Sanjay Chauhan, Mr Vikrant Sharma and Mr Ananda Mohanty; and Mr SK Verma and Mr Sunil Dutt, apart from the great support staff at their easily accessible office.

Happy reading!

Kabir Sardana

Contents

Therapeutic Index

Introduction

Kabir Sardana, Ananta Khurana

Eczema remains the most common skin condition seen by family physicians and dermatologists. While being a disparate group of diseases, they have some common features including the presence of itch and in the acute stages, edema (spongiosis) in the epidermis. In early disease, the stratum corneum remains intact, so the eczema appears as a red smooth edematous plaque. With worsening disease, the edema becomes more severe, tense blisters appear. If less severe or if the eczema becomes chronic, scaling and epithelial disruption occurs, giving chronic eczema the characteristic appearance. All these are phases of the reaction pattern and are known as eczema. The word eczema comes from the Greek for 'boiling'—a reference to the tiny vesicles (bubbles) that are often seen in the early acute stages of the disorder, but less often in its later chronic stages. The histological findings of eczema are depicted in Fig. 1.1. *Dermatitis* means inflammation of the skin and is, therefore, strictly speaking, a broader term than eczema—which is just one of several possible types of skin inflammation.

Though various classifications exist, we will stick to the time-honoured, division into exogenous and endogenous types (Table 1.1).

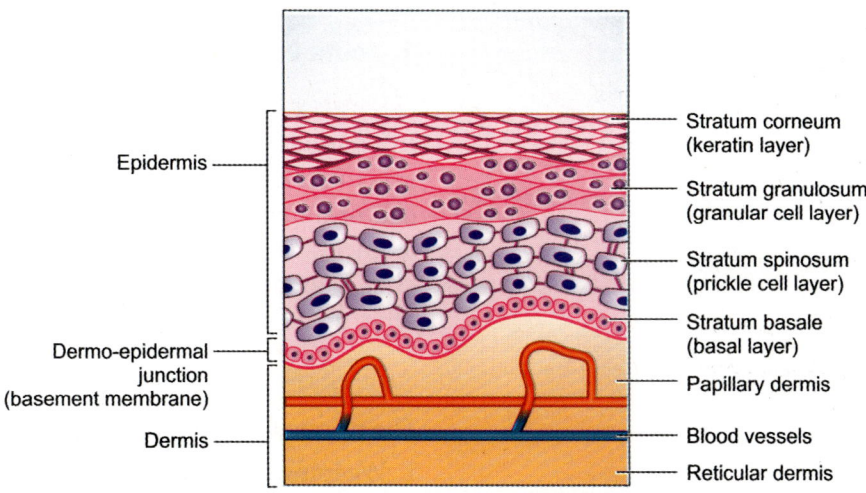

Fig. 1.1a: A depiction of the normal histology of the skin

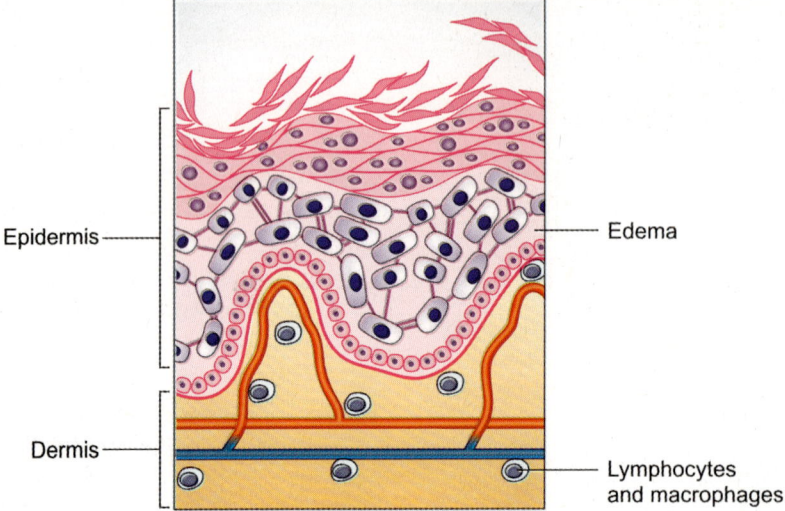

Fig. 1.1b: A depiction of the histology of eczematous skin; edema develops between the keratinocytes (spongiosis), the epidermis is thickened (acanthosis) and there are inflammatory cells in the dermis

Table 1.1: Classification of eczema

Exogenous eczemas
- ABCD
- Allergic contact eczema
- Dermatophytide
- Eczematous polymorphic light eruption
- Infective eczema
- Irritant eczema
- Photoallergic eczema
- Post-traumatic eczema

Endogenous eczema
- Asteatotic eczema
- Atopic eczema
- Chronic superficial scaly dermatitis
- Discoid eczema
- Eczematous drug eruptions
- Exudative discoid and lichenoid chronic dermatosis
- Eyelid eczema
- Hand eczema
- Juvenile plantar dermatosis
- Lichen simplex chronicus
- Pityriasis alba
- Prurigonodularis
- Seborrheic eczema
- Venous eczema

In this book, we will discuss the common types of eczema and the rare variants will be left to specialized dermatology textbooks.

STAGES OF ECZEMA

There are three stages of eczema: Acute, subacute, and chronic. An eczematous disease may start at any stage and evolve into another. We will give detail of the various types and their treatment, though there would be variations for specific types of eczematous disorders.

1. Acute Eczema

Etiology

Inflammation is caused by contact with specific allergens such as Rhus (poison ivy, oak, or sumac) and chemicals. In the id reaction, a reaction occurs at a distant site during or after a fungal infection, stasis dermatitis, or other acute inflammatory processes (Fig. 1.2).

Clinical Findings

The classic features are:

1. Weeping and crusting
2. Blistering—usually with vesicles

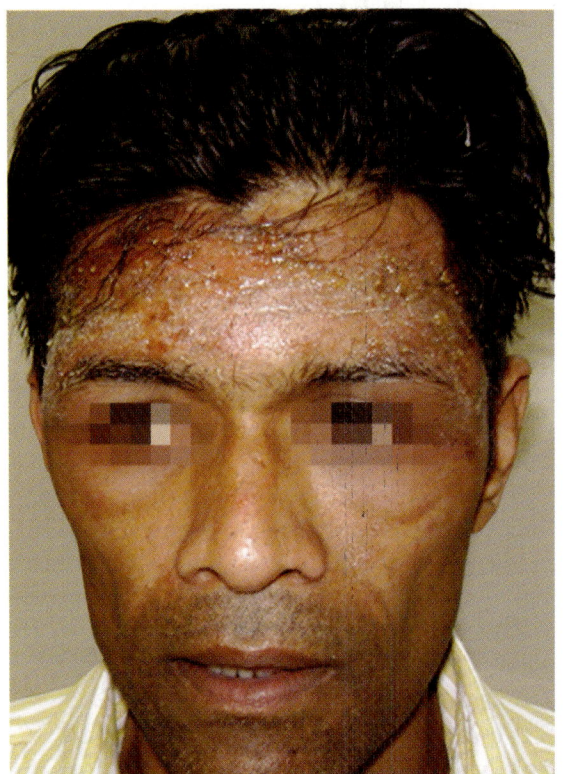

Fig. 1.2: A case of acute eczema in a patient consequent to allergic contact dermatitis to hair dye

3. Redness, papules and swelling—usually with an ill-defined border; and
4. Scaling.

There is frequently intense itching and heat and hot water can accentuate the symptoms. The condition can persist for a week or more and can evolve into a subacute stage before resolving.

Treatment

1. *Cool, wet dressings.* The evaporative cooling produced by wet compresses causes vasoconstriction and rapidly suppresses inflammation and itching. Either Burow's solution or normal saline can be used. A clean cotton cloth is soaked in cool water, folded several times, and placed directly over the affected areas. Evaporative cooling produces vasoconstriction and decreases serum production. Wet compresses should **not** be held in place and covered with towels or plastic wrap because this prevents evaporation. The wet cloth macerates vesicles and, when removed, mechanically debrides the area and prevents serum and crust from accumulating. Wet compresses should be *removed* after 30 minutes and replaced with a freshly soaked cloth.

2. *Oral corticosteroids.* Oral corticosteroids, such as prednisone, are useful for controlling intense or widespread inflammation and may be used in addition to wet dressings. A course of 20 mg dose twice or once a day for 7 to 14 days is enough in most cases though in some cases up to 21 days of therapy may be needed. Topical corticosteroids are of a little use in the acute stage because the cream does not penetrate through the vesicles.

3. *Antihistamines.* Antihistamines relieve itching and provide enough sedation so patients can sleep.

4. *Antibiotics.* The use of oral antibiotics may greatly hasten resolution of the disease, if signs of superficial secondary infection are present. Cephalexin and dicloxacillin are effective.

2. Subacute Eczema

There is erythema and scaling with an indistinct border (Fig. 1.3). The symptoms vary from no itching to intense itching.

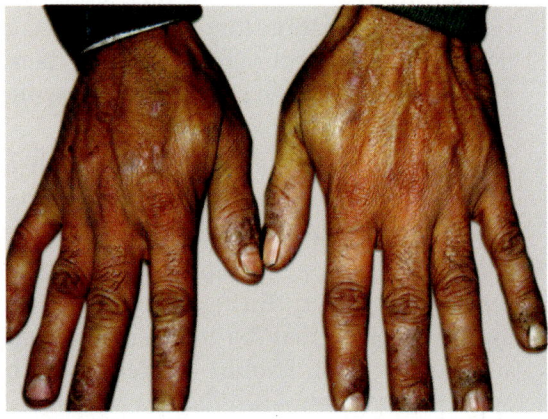

Fig. 1.3: A case of contact dermatitis to cement a prototype of subacute eczema

Subacute eczematous inflammation may be the initial stage or it may follow acute inflammation. If the inciting agent is withdrawn, the condition often resolves but excessive drying created from washing or continued use of wet dressings causes cracking and fissures (Fig. 1.3).

Treatment

It is important to discontinue wet dressings when acute inflammation evolves into subacute inflammation. Excess drying creates cracking and fissures, which predispose to infection.

1. *Topical corticosteroids.* These agents are the treatment of choice.
2. *Topical macrolide immune suppressants.* Tacrolimus ointment and pimecrolimus cream have been used for atopic dermatitis, allergic contact dermatitis, and irritant contact dermatitis and are approved for use in children 2 years or older. Response to these agents is slower than the response to topical steroids.
3. *Lubrication.* This is a simple but essential part of therapy. Inflamed skin becomes dry and is more susceptible to further irritation and inflammation. Resolved dry areas may easily relapse into subacute eczema, if proper lubrication is neglected. They can be applied a few hours *after* topical steroids and should be continued for days or weeks after the inflammation has cleared. Frequent application (one to four times a day) should be encouraged and using them after the skin has been patted dry following a shower seals in moisture.
4. *Mild soaps.* Frequent washing with a drying soap, can be avoided by using superfatted soaps.
5. *Antibiotics.* Eczematous plaques that remain bright red during treatment with topical steroids may be infected. Infected subacute eczema should be treated with appropriate systemic antibiotics, which are usually those active against staphylococci. Systemic antibiotics are more effective than topical antibiotics or antibiotic–steroid combination creams.

3. Chronic Eczema

Chronic eczematous inflammation may be caused by irritation of subacute inflammation, or it may appear as lichen simplex chronicus (Fig. 1.4). Chronic eczematous inflammation is a clinicopathologic entity and does not indicate simply any long-lasting stage of eczema. If scratching is not controlled, subacute eczematous inflammation can be modified and converted to chronic eczematous inflammation.

There is moderate to intense itching. Scratching sometimes becomes violent, leading to excoriation and digging, and ceases only when pain has replaced the itch. Patients with chronic inflammation scratch while asleep. They are:

1. Less vesicular and exudative.
2. More scaly, pigmented and thickened.
3. More likely to show lichenification—a dry leathery thickened state, with increased skin markings, secondary to repeated scratching or rubbing.
4. More likely to fissure.

Treatment

Chronic eczematous inflammation is resistant to treatment and requires potent steroid therapy.

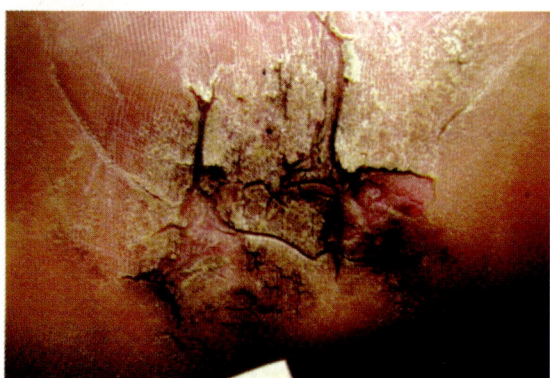

Fig. 1.4: A case of hyperkeratotic eczema, a prototype of chronic eczema

Intralesional injection. Intralesional injection is a very effective mode of therapy. Lesions that have been present for years may completely resolve after one injection or a short series of injections. The medicine is delivered with a 27- or 30-gauge needle, and the entire plaque is infiltrated until it blanches white. Resistant plaques require additional injections given at 3- to 4-week intervals.

Bibliography

1. Eczema, in. Sardana k, Mahajan S, Garg VK. Diagnosis and Management of Skin Disorders: An Evidence-Based Approach, 1/e.: Lippincott Williams and Wilkins, 2012 (reprint 2015).

2. Fast Facts: Eczema and Contact Dermatitis By John Berth-Jones, Eunice Tan and Howard I Malbach Published 2004.

3. Thieme Clinical Companions Dermatology. Sterry, Dermatology© 2006 Thieme.

Irritant Eczema

Kabir Sardana

IRRITANT CONTACT DERMATITIS (ICD)

Exogenous eczemas can be irritant or allergic. They are diagnosed predominantly on the distribution, which suggests contact with a precipitating factor. Irritant eczemas are a result of agents that produce keratinocyte damage without immunological memory.

Allergic contact dermatitis (ACD) is a delayed (type IV) hypersensitivity reaction, mediated by T cells and requiring prior sensitization, while irritant contact dermatitis (ICD) has a non-immunologic mechanism, thus not requiring sensitization. Clinical distinction of the two processes is often challenging, as morphology and histopathology of irritant and allergic dermatitis reactions can be virtually indistinguishable. The two processes may, and often do, coexist, thereby further complicating matters.

The morphological spectrum of ICD is broad and frequently impossible to distinguish from ACD and even endogenous (atopic) dermatitis. Chronological descriptions of these processes are often clinically used. Acute, subacute, and chronic dermatitis are terms applicable to allergic and irritant contact dermatitis, as well as atopic dermatitis.

Clinical Classification of Irritant Contact Dermatitis

Irritant contact dermatitis (synonyms: cutaneous irritation, irritant dermatitis) is the biological response of the skin to a variety of external stimuli that induce skin inflammation without the production of specific antibodies. Formerly considered a monomorphous process, it is now understood to be a complex biologic syndrome, with a diverse clinical appearance, pathophysiology, and natural history. The clinical appearance and course of irritant contact dermatitis varies depending on multiple external and internal factors. This diversity in clinical presentation has generated a classification scheme, based on both morphology and mode of onset. The various "genotypes" of ICD and their respective prognoses are tabulated in Box 2.1. Though no longer relevant, a few common regional irritant dermatitides are also described.

Cause

Strong irritants elicit an acute reaction after brief contact and the diagnosis is then usually obvious. Prolonged exposure, sometimes over years, is needed for weak irritants to cause dermatitis, usually of the hands and forearms. *Water*, *detergents*, *chemicals*, *solvents*, *cutting oils* and *abrasive dusts* are common culprits. Other causes include frequent use of soaps and detergents, exposure to organic or alkaline solvents, exposure to an environment with low humidity, or chronic exposure to saliva

Box 2.1: Classification of ICD	
Ten genotypes of ICD	• Acute ICD
	• Delayed acute ICD
	• Irritant reaction
	• Chronic ICD
	• Traumatic ICD
	• Acneiform ICD
	• Non-erythematous (suberythematous) irritation
	• Subjective (sensory) irritation
	• Friction dermatitis
	• Asteatotic irritant eczema
Regional variants	• Lip lick dermatitis
	• Ring dermatitis
	• Wear and tear dermatitis
	• Finger tip dermatitis
	• Diaper dermatitis

(lip lick dermatitis), urine, or feces. There is a wide range of susceptibility with those with very dry skin being especially vulnerable. Past or present atopic dermatitis doubles the risk of irritant hand eczema. Areas where the water is "hard" tend to have a higher prevalence of ICD due to the potential "drying" effect of hard water. The irritant effect of water is an intriguing phenomenon. The overhydration of the skin in wet-work occupations not only enhances the penetration of many irritants but may also release inflammatory mediators and their inhibitors from the stratum corneum, the mechanism of which may lead to a gradual damage of the skin.

Recently, the SLS test has been used in patch testing as a way of differentiating between allergic and irritant reactions. If SLS reacts during patch testing, it is likely that macular, erythematous reactions to patch test samples have an irritant etiology. On the other hand, if the skin does not react to SLS, it is likely that these reactions to allergens during patch testing are allergic in etiology. Although the SLS can be helpful, it is very important to keep

in mind that it is impossible to correlate results with every possible irritant agent.

CLINICAL FEATURES

1. Acute ICD

When exposure is sufficient and the offending agent is potent, classic signs of acute skin irritation are seen. Erythema, edema, inflammation, and vesiculation are typical features, although acute irritation may range from mild erythema through exudative cutaneous inflammation to ulcerative lesions and frank epidermal necrosis, depending on factors such as the chemical and the exposure time. In case of exposure to a liquid agent, a dripping of the liquid is evident as a skin reaction.

In keeping with an exogenous dermatosis, acute ICD usually exhibits an *asymmetrical* distribution and *sharply demarcated borders* (Fig. 2.1). These borders delineate the area of exposure to the offending chemical.

Contact with a potent irritant is often accidental, and an acute ICD is elicited in almost anyone, independent of constitutional susceptibility—in contrast to chronic ICD.

This classic, acutely developing dermatitis usually heals soon after exposure, assuming there is no re-exposure—this is known as the "decrescendo phenomenon." In contrast, ACD usually exhibits a "crescendo phenomenon", i.e. transient worsening of symptoms and signs despite removal of the allergen.

2. Delayed Acute ICD

Some chemicals produce acute irritation in a delayed manner so that inflammation is retarded until 8–24 hours or more after exposure. Except for the delayed onset, the clinical appearance and course resemble those of acute irritant contact dermatitis. This has atypical "crescendo" periodicity and thus is often confused with allergic contact dermatitis; appropriately performed diagnostic patch tests easily separate the two, i.e. the substances implicated in delayed acute ICD would result

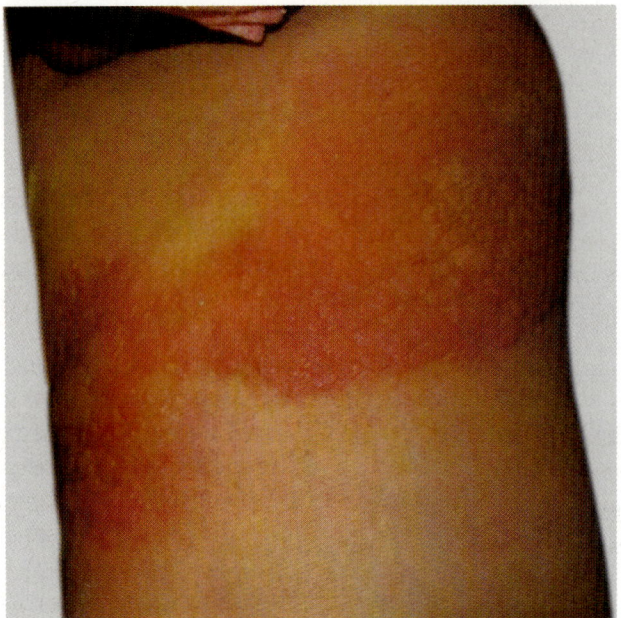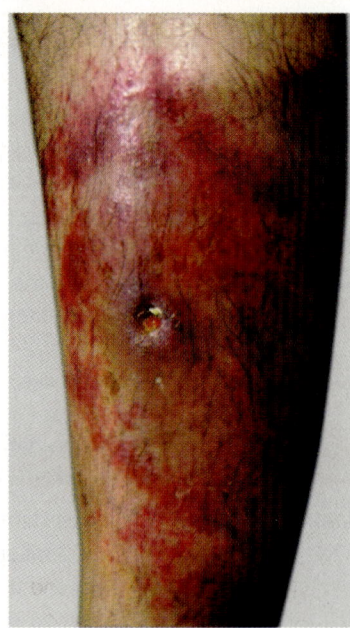

Fig. 2.1a: Acute irritant reaction to betadine

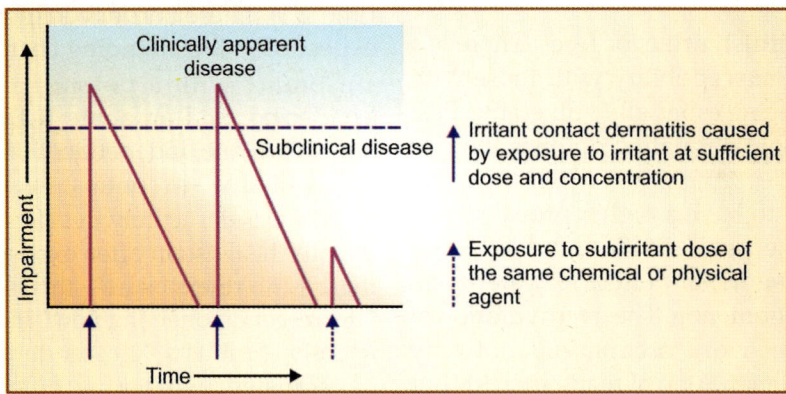

Fig. 2.1b: A depiction of the process of acute ICD

in negative patch test results. In delayed acute ICD, a burning sensation predominates, rather than pruritus. Examples of substances causing delayed irritation are hexanediol and butanediol diacrylates, dithranol (anthralin) (Fig. 2.2a), topical antibiotics (Fig. 2.2b), calcipotriol, and benzalkonium chloride.

3. Irritant Reaction

Individuals extensively exposed to irritants often develop erythematous, chapped skin in the first month of exposure. This irritant reaction may be considered a pre-eczematous expression of acute skin irritation.

The term "irritant reaction" is now increasingly used, if the clinical picture is **monomorphic**, rather than the usual polymorphic appearance of ICD, i.e. only one of the parameters usually seen in ICD are present, e.g. scaling, erythema (Fig. 2.3), vesiculation, pustules, or erosions. This pattern is frequently seen in hairdressers and other wet-workers. Frequently, this condition heals spontaneously, with hardening of the skin.

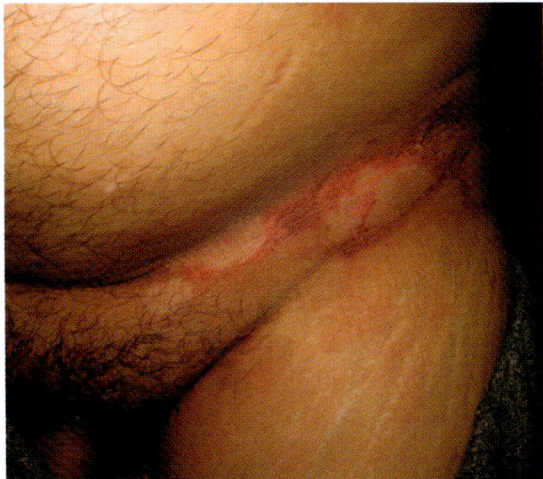

Fig. 2.2a: Delayed irritant reaction to anthralin used for tinea corporis

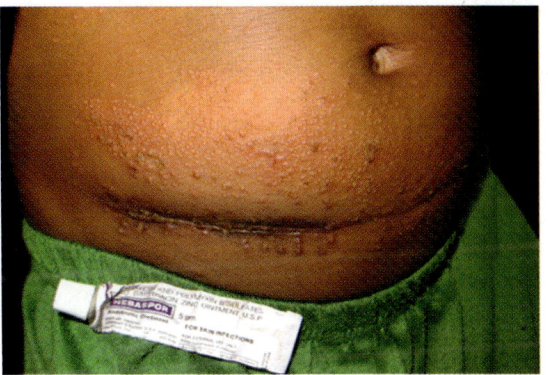

Fig. 2.2b: Delayed irritant reaction to topical triple combination antiseptic cream

However, repeated irritant reactions can sometimes lead to contact dermatitis, usually with good prognosis. Compounds that cause irritant reactions are typically mild irritants, such as detergents, soaps, and water (Fig. 2.3).

4. Cumulative ICD

(*Synonyms:* Cumulative ICD, traumiterative dermatitis, wear and tear dermatitis).

Chronic ICD is the most common type of ICD and is seen when the eczema becomes chronic (more than **6 weeks** has been suggested as an arbitrary threshold period). In chronic ICD, the frequency of exposure is too high in relation to the skin recovery time.

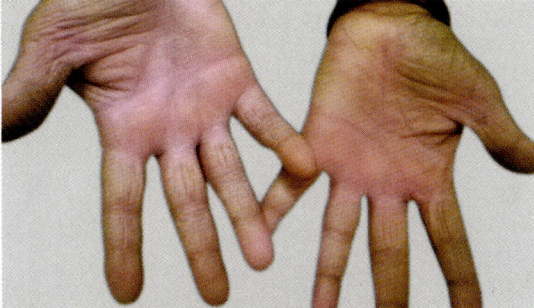

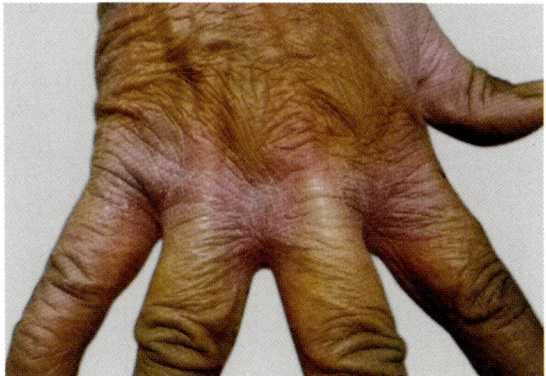

Fig. 2.3: This lady used to wash her hands repeatedly apart from using harsh detergents. The clinical picture is of a "monomorphic" erythema on the palms and web space—irritant eczema

This is caused by repeated exposure to an allergen and most frequently affects the dorsal aspect of the hand, finger webs, face and eyelids (Figs 2.4 to 2.7). Most cases are seen in housewives where it is called "housewives dermatitis or dish pan hands or detergent hands". Other occupations affected include mothers with young children (e.g. from changing diapers), individuals whose jobs require repeated wetting and drying (e.g. surgeons, dentists, dishwashers, bartenders, fishermen), industrial workers whose jobs require contact with chemicals (e.g. cutting oils), and patients with the atopic diathesis.

Pathogenesis: The stratum corneum is the protective envelope that prevents exogenous material from entering the skin and prevents body water from escaping. The stratum corneum of the palms is thicker than that of the backs of the hands and is more resistant

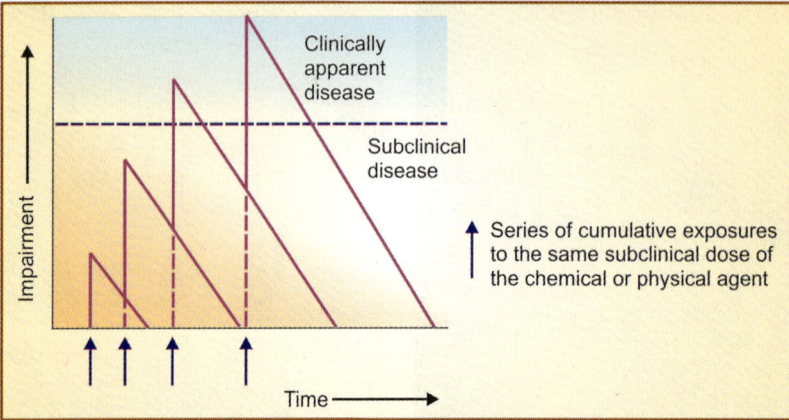

Fig. 2.4a: A depiction of the process of cumulative ICD

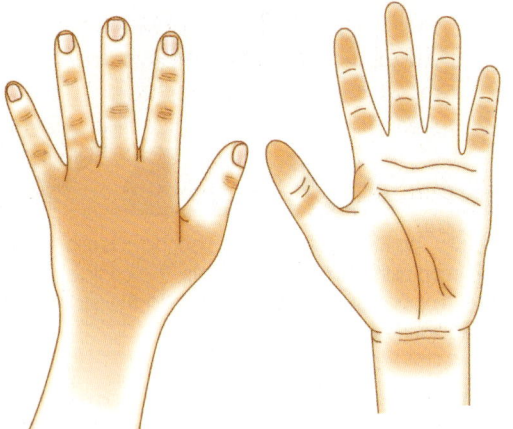

Fig. 2.4b: Typical distribution of irritant contact dermatitis on the hands

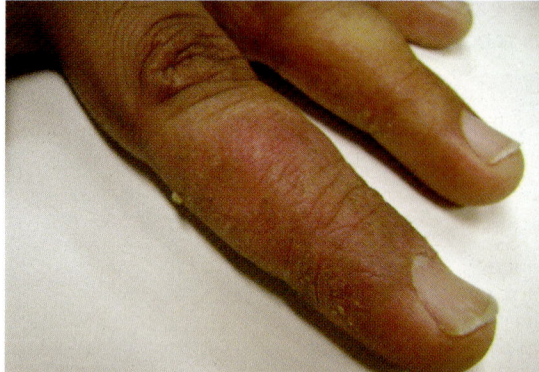

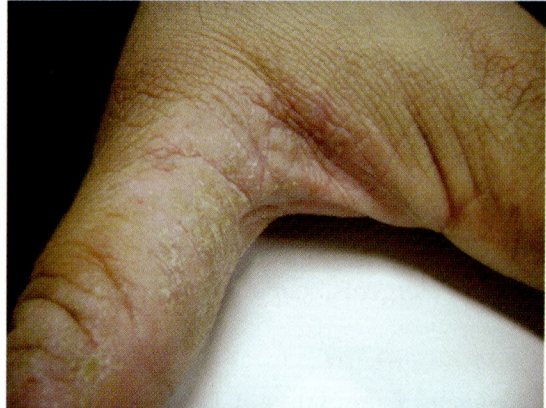

Fig. 2.6: Cumulative ICD involving the fingers

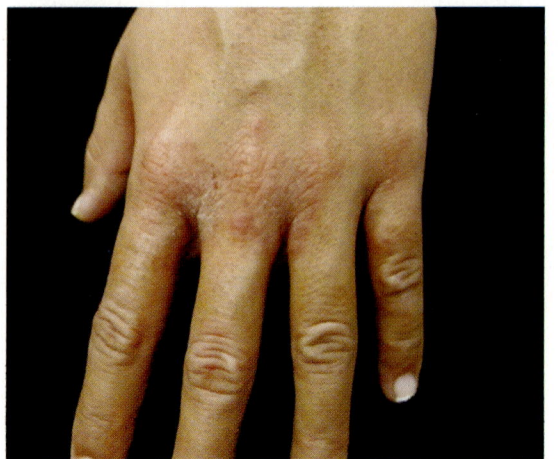

Fig. 2.5: Affliction of the dorsum of hands (cumulative ICD)

to irritation. The pH of this surface layer is slightly acidic. Environmental factors or elements that change any component of the stratum corneum interfere with its protective function and expose the skin to irritants. These

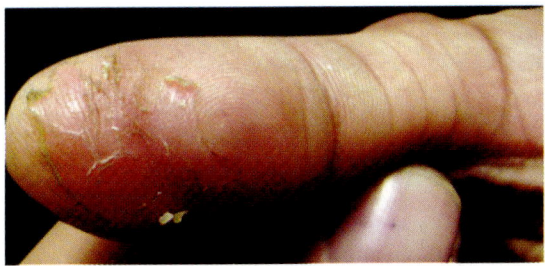

Fig. 2.7: A case of cumulative ICD in a housewife localized on the fingertips, primarily due to a combination of detergent use and cutting vegetables

include hard water, cold winter air, hot water, harsh soaps and low humidity. This repeated insult leads to a higher predisposition to developing eczema.

Clinical findings. Dryness and chapping is the initial change, followed by painful cracks and fissures. The backs of the hands become red, swollen, and tender (Fig. 2.5). The palmar surface, especially that of the fingers, becomes red and continues to be dry and cracked (Figs 2.6 and 2.7).

Differential diagnosis. The differentiation of cumulative irritant contact dermatitis from another dermatitic process or an eczematous lesion of the skin is a challenge.

a. *Atopic dermatitis* often occurs on the hands in young adults and is provoked and aggravated in occupations with a high exposure to water and irritants, such as hairdressing, cleaning, and housekeeping. It is often difficult to weigh the individual role of irritants and atopic constitution. In many cases, it is the atopic disorder of the skin that is primarily responsible for the development of a cumulative irritant contact dermatitis.

b. *Psoriasis* of the hands can *imitate* eczema or an irritant contact dermatitis. Careful examination of the whole skin to look for minor signs of psoriasis is important. In the follow-up of these patients, psoriasis may develop in other areas. Sometimes a combination of atopy and psoriasis occurs on the hands with itchy vesicles. Some of these patients experience a sudden aggravation of the dermatitis after exposure to water.

c. *Tinea of the hands* may simulate a dry palmar dermatitis. Unilateral localization and involvement of the nails are important clues to diagnose tinea.

d. Prolonged exposure to organic solvents may cause scaly, hyperkeratotic skin on the palmar side of the hands, which has to be differentiated from the *hyperkeratotic palmar eczema* (tylotic eczema). Irritants and allergens may complicate hyperkeratotic eczema, another endogenous dermatosis with features of psoriasis and eczema.

e. The differentiation between a cumulative irritant and an allergic contact dermatitis is a great challenge and not often possible (Fig. 2.8). In general, an allergic contact dermatitis is more polymorphic, with an unsharp demarcation, with a tendency for spreading, and with occasional localizations at the wrist, the forearm, and the face, especially on the eyelids. The course is often relapsing, with improvement during weekends and holidays. In the work environment, only one or a few persons are affected, and a relevant positive patch test makes the diagnosis definitive.

Especially in the case of fingertip dermatitis and eczema, it is impossible to differentiate an allergic contact dermatitis from a cumulative irritant contact dermatitis or psoriasis. Long-standing cases of allergic contact dermatitis with a lichenoid character (nickel and chromate allergies) may change in character from eczematous to more psoriasis-like.

Treatment. The simplest method is by prevention of allergen and the use of an emulsion cleanser (e.g. cetaphil lotion) can lead to a marked decrease in dryness and eczema.

Barrier-protectant creams. Loss of skin barrier function by mechanical or chemical insults

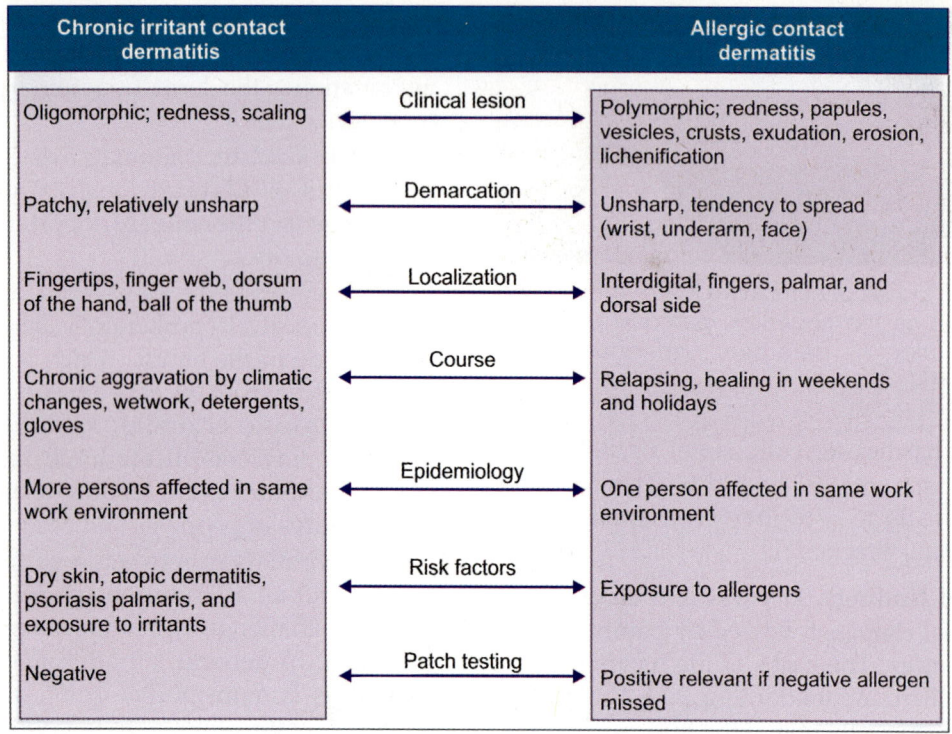

Fig. 2.8: A depiction of the differences between chronic ICD and ACD

Chronic irritant contact dermatitis		Allergic contact dermatitis
Oligomorphic; redness, scaling	Clinical lesion	Polymorphic; redness, papules, vesicles, crusts, exudation, erosion, lichenification
Patchy, relatively unsharp	Demarcation	Unsharp, tendency to spread (wrist, underarm, face)
Fingertips, finger web, dorsum of the hand, ball of the thumb	Localization	Interdigital, fingers, palmar, and dorsal side
Chronic aggravation by climatic changes, wetwork, detergents, gloves	Course	Relapsing, healing in weekends and holidays
More persons affected in same work environment	Epidemiology	One person affected in same work environment
Dry skin, atopic dermatitis, psoriasis palmaris, and exposure to irritants	Risk factors	Exposure to allergens
Negative	Patch testing	Positive relevant if negative allergen missed

Table 2.1: A list of common methods to avoid recurrence of hand eczema

a. Wash hands as infrequently as possible. Ideally, soap should be avoided and hands simply washed in lukewarm water.

b. Shampooing must be done with rubber gloves or by someone else.

c. Avoid direct contact with household cleaners and detergents. Wear cotton, plastic, or rubber gloves when doing housework. A sensible option is to use cotton gloves under rubber gloves.

d. Do not touch or do not do anything that causes burning or itching (e.g. contact with wool; wet diapers; peeling potatoes or handling fresh fruits, vegetables, and raw meat).

e. Wear rubber gloves when irritants are encountered. Rubber gloves alone are not sufficient because the lining collects sweat, scales, and debris and can become more irritating than those objects to be avoided. Dermal white cotton gloves should be worn next to the skin under unlined rubber gloves. Several pairs of cotton gloves should be purchased so they can be changed frequently. Ensure the rubber gloves fit comfortably over the white cotton gloves.

may result in water loss and hand eczema. Barrier creams applied at least twice a day on all exposed areas protect the skin and are formulated to be either water-repellent or oil-repellent. The water-repellent types offer little protection against oils or solvents.

The inflammation is similar to principles of treating subacute eczema. Lubrication and avoidance of further irritation help to prevent recurrence (Table 2.2). For details see the Chapter 15 (Hand Eczema).

5. Traumatic Irritant Contact Dermatitis

Traumatic ICD develops after acute skin trauma, such as burns, lacerations, or acute ICD. The skin does not completely heal, but erythema, vesicles, papules, and scaling appear at the site of injury. The clinical course later resembles discoid (nummular) dermatitis. It may be compounded by a concurrent allergen exposure. The healing period is generally prolonged.

Often these patients are considered to have factitial dermatitis because of a healing phase followed by exacerbation. Although factitial aspects may occur in some patients, this peculiar form of irritation appears to be a disease sui generis. Its chronicity and recalcitrance to therapy provides a challenge to both patient and physician.

6. Acneiform Irritant Contact Dermatitis

(*Synonyms:* Pustular ICD, follicular ICD)

Certain exogenous substances have the capacity to elicit an acneiform eruption, and even allergic reactions may sometimes be pustular or follicular. Acneiform ICD should always be considered in the differential diagnosis of an adult with acneiform lesions. The pustules are usually sterile and transient.

In occupational exposure, only a minority of subjects develop pustular or acneiform dermatitis. Thus, the development of this type of ICD appears to be dependent on both constitutional and chemical factors.

Chloracne is an industrial disease caused by exposure to chlorinated aromatic hydrocarbons, in particular chlorinated dioxins, which are the most potent acnegenic agents. Many of the chloracnegens are also hepatotoxic—therefore, this is a disease of medical importance. Acneiform ICD may also develop from exposure to *metals, mineral oils, greases, tar, asphalt, cutting oils, and metal working fluids.*

Acne cosmetica represents acneiform ICD caused by cosmetics. This is one of the commonest causes of persistent or new onset acne in females (>25 years of age). The irony is that when you are young you have acne but no money to buy cosmetics but when you get old, you have money to buy cosmetics and well you again get acne! Many cosmetics,

fractions, and modifications of lanolins are comedogenic, as are emulsifiers such as butyl stearate, isopropyl myristate and sodium lauryl sulfate (Fulton JE Jr).

Acne cosmetica is easiest to diagnose in women who have never experienced acne until after use of a particular cosmetic or skin care product. The main culprits are:

- Skin care, cosmetic, or hair care products
- Mineral oils
- Moisturisers and sunscreens

The ingredients that cause it are extensive but the common causes are listed in **Box 2.2**.

A simple thumb rule to identify a good moistures is what I call the 'transparency rule' (**Fig. 2.9**). A transparent gel-based moisturizer almost never causes acne. In a landmark study by Mills and Kligman, 14 of 29 proprietary sunscreen formulations, including suntan promoters, were found to be comedogenic when applied to the external ear canal of albino rabbits. Ultraviolet exposures enhanced the comedogenic effect. The vehicles, rather than the UV-absorbing compounds, seemed to be responsible. Accordingly, 'sunscreen acne' may be a subtype of acne cosmetica. Remember the active ingredient of a sunscreen is lipophilc, hence all sunscreen bases are also oil based! Phenylbenzimidazole sulfonic acid is water soluble and used in products formulated to feel lighter and less oily, such as daily-use cosmetic moisturizers. Thus, an ideal sunscreen is either mat based or gel

Box 2.2: Ingredients of creams, sunscreens and moisturizers that are potent acnegenic agents

1. Cocoa butter
2. Oil
3. Isopropyl myristate
4. Sodium lauryl sulfate
5. Mineral oil/paraffin
6. Olive oil/peanut oil
7. Petrolatum
8. Sunflower oil
9. Jojoba oil

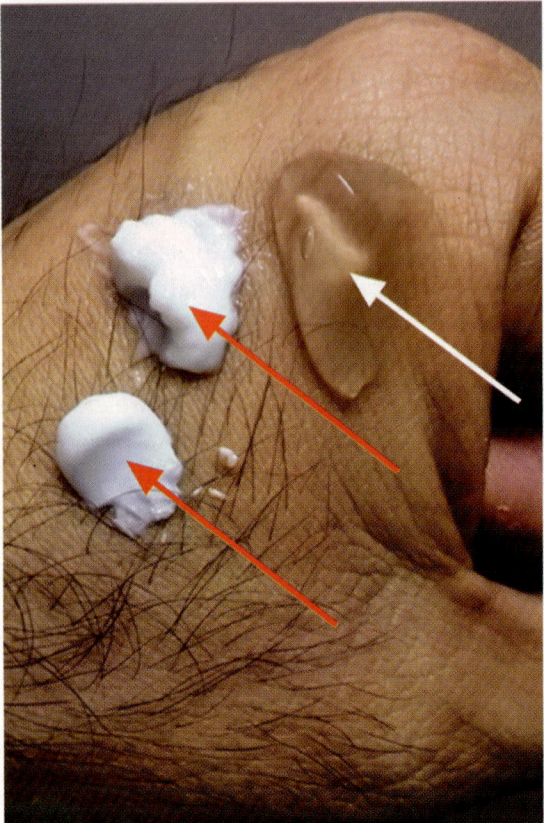

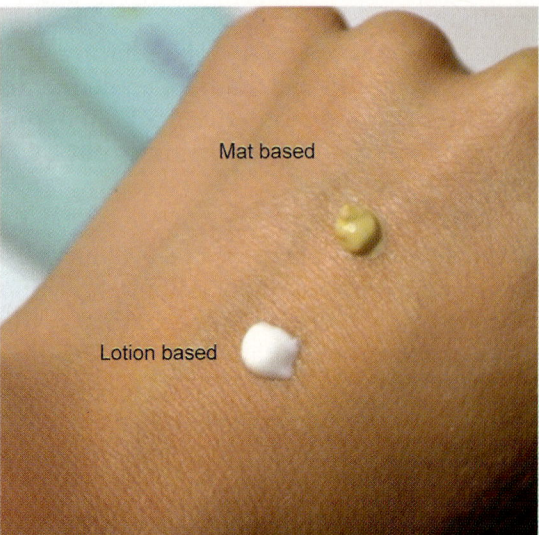

Mat based

Lotion based

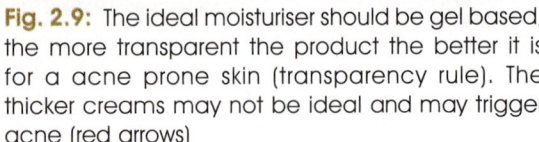

Fig. 2.9: The ideal moisturiser should be gel based, the more transparent the product the better it is for a acne prone skin (transparency rule). The thicker creams may not be ideal and may trigger acne (red arrows)

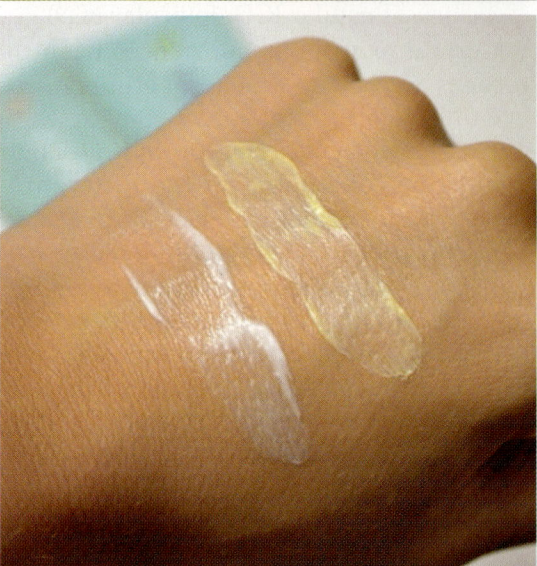

Fig. 2.10: The ideal sunscreen for acne prone skin should be transparent gel based, a close second is the mat-based sunscreen. The cream- and lotion-based sunscreens are not ideal for acne prone skin. Most chemical sunscreen ingredients are oils soluble in the oil phase of emulsion systems, accounting in part for the heavy, greasy esthetic properties of many of these products

based (Fig. 2.10). Replacement of a cream-based mositurizer to a gel-based moisturizer can achieve near miraculous result, in patients who notice sudden onset acne with no other discernable cause (Fig. 2.11).

7. Nonerythematous or Suberythematous Irritation

In the early stages of skin irritation, subtle skin damage may occur without visible inflammation. As a correlate of nonvisible irritation, objectively registered alterations in the damaged epidermis have been reported via cutaneous bioengineering techniques (O Berardesca E, Maibach HI). It is customary in Japan to screen new chemicals, cosmetics and textiles for subtle signs of stratum corneum damage, employing replicas of stratum corneum (the Kawai method; Kawai, 1971). A similar technique, squamometry or corneosur-fametry has now been refined to detect subtle

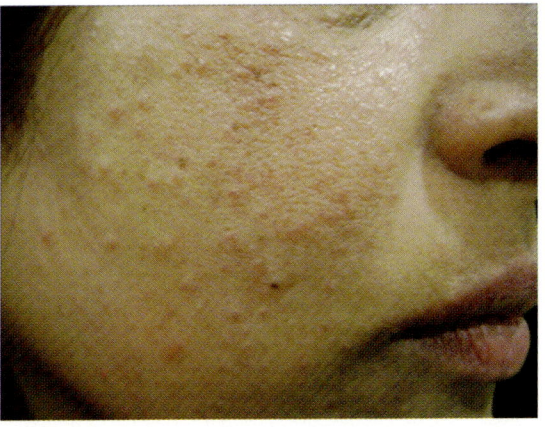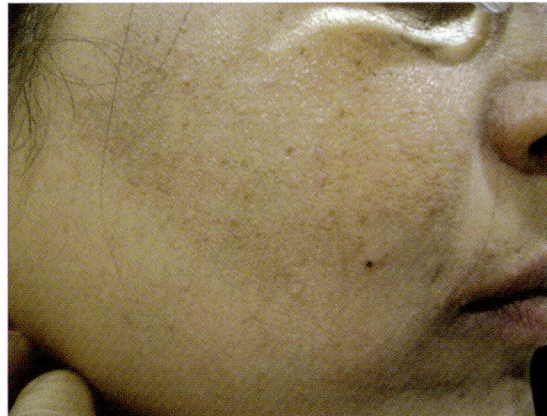

Fig. 2.11: This patient had sudden onset acne 2 weeks after use of OTC deep moisturizer touted as a antiaging cream. Note the follicular pattern of acne. Change to a gel-based moisturizer leads to a profoundly happy outcome!

subclinical alterations in the stratum corneum caused by application of mild irritants (Charbonnier V).

8. Subjective or Sensory Irritation

Some individuals ("stingers") experience itching, stinging, burning, or tingling sensations on contact with certain chemicals (Lammintausta K), despite a distinct lack of objective signs on clinical examination. Despite the lack of clinical manifestations, the subjective sensations are reproducible, typically occurring within seconds to minutes following exposure; this type of irritation is known as subjective or sensory irritation. Lactic acid is a model for this nonvisible cutaneous irritation. Although subjective irritation may have a neural component, recent studies suggest that cutaneous vasculature may be more responsive in "stingers" than nonstingers (Berardesca E). At least 10% of women complain of stinging with certain facial products; thus, further work is needed to develop a strategy to overcome this type of discomfort.

9. Friction Dermatitis

True friction dermatitis is the development of ICD in response to low-grade friction—this is seen clinically as erythema, scaling, fissuring,

and itching surrounding the area of frictional contact. The syndrome has been characterized by Susten.

Repeated friction of low intensity is known to induce callus formation (hyperkeratosis and acanthosis), hardening of the skin, hyperpigmentation and friction blisters in normal skin. In atopic people, lichenification and lichen simplex chronicus may ensue as a result of friction. All of the above may be considered as adaptive phenomena to friction and should not be confused with friction dermatitis.

Cases of occupational friction dermatitis in the literature are seldom documented, but most often reported in association with paper work (Bennike NH).

10. Asteatotic Irritant Eczema

Asteatotic eczema (synonyms: asteatotic dermatitis, exsiccation eczematid, eczema craquele), is a variant of ICD seen in elderly individuals, as a result of worsening xerosis, particularly during dry winter months. Clinically, the skin is dry (xerotic), with loss of smoothness, ichthyosiform scale and cracking of the superficial epidermal layers, often associated with eczematous changes. Environmental insults, such as low humidity, low temperatures and very high doses of ultraviolet radiation (UVR) (>3 or 4 MEDs) can accelerate this process. In an occupational setting, this is sometimes combined with repeated exposure to wet work, chemical insults, and friction, cumulating in perturbation of the skin barrier (*see* Chapter 12).

REGIONAL IRRITANT DERMATITIS

1. Lip Lick Dermatitis

This is a common variant seen in children and is consequent to licking of the lips. It is usually periorificial in distribution (Fig. 2.12) and is usually complicated by secondary infection and contact allergy due to the use of topical medicaments.

2. Ring Dermatitis

This is seen in females after marriage as a patch of eczema that begins around the wedding ring (Fig. 2.13). This is due to three factors, trapping of detergent under the ring, friction and trauma. The eczema patch frequently extends beyond the involved finger to involve the middle finger and adjacent palm.

Removing the ring while working is one of the simplest ways to avoid this type of eczema.

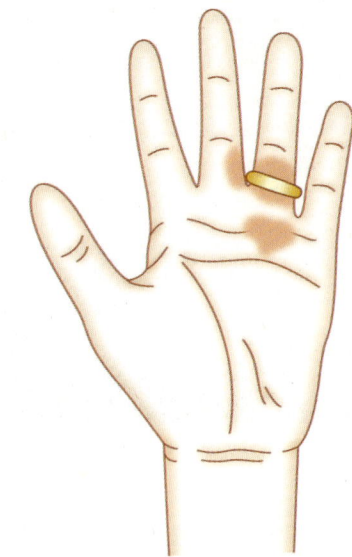

Fig. 2.13a: Ring dermatitis

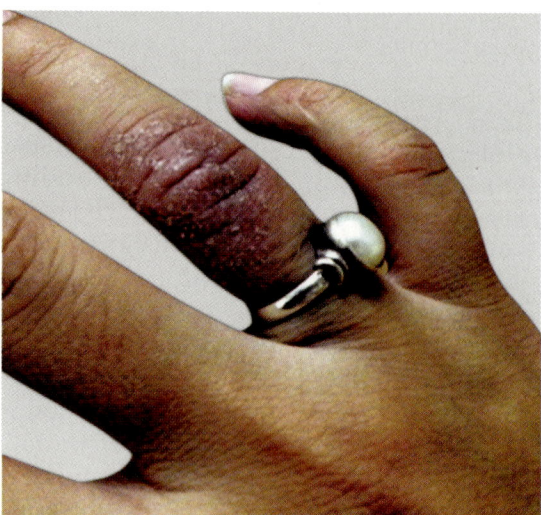

Fig. 2.13b: A case of ring eczema in a newly married patient due to the use of detergents

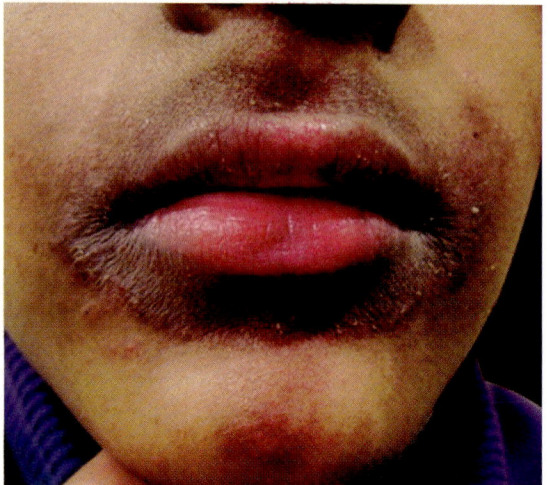

Fig. 2.12: A case of lip lick dermatitis in a school going child aggravated due to exam stress

3. Wear and Tear Dermatitis

Again this is seen in housewives and cleaners and is characterized by sharply demarcated areas of thick scaling or hyperkeratosis on the palms (and frequently on the soles) (Fig. 2.14). The condition may be confused with psoriasis, but there is a little or none of the redness and none of the scaling or nail changes typical of psoriasis. The condition is more common in middle-aged and elderly persons and in men.

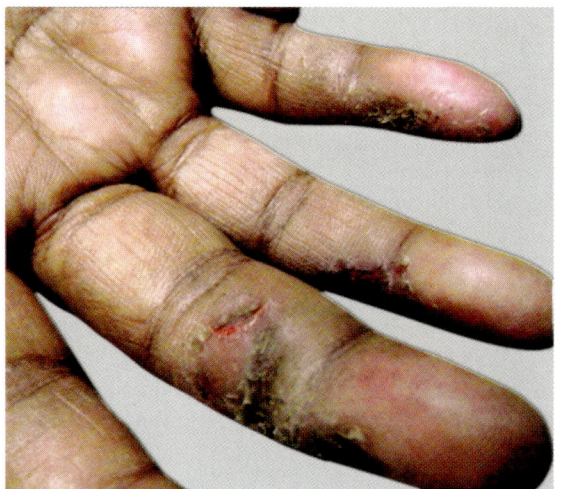

Fig. 2.14: Chronic eczema in a housewife, note the hyperkeratosis and fissuring in the involved areas

4. Fingertip Eczema

This may be due to both allergic contact dermatitis and irritant contact dermatitis. One finger or several fingers may be involved. Initially the skin may be moist and then may become dry, cracked, and scaly and when the skin peels from the fingertips distally, a dry, red, cracked, fissured, tender or painful surface without skin lines is revealed (Fig. 2.15). Once allergy and psoriasis have been ruled out, fingertip eczema should be managed the same way as subacute and chronic eczema—by avoiding irritants and lubricating frequently.

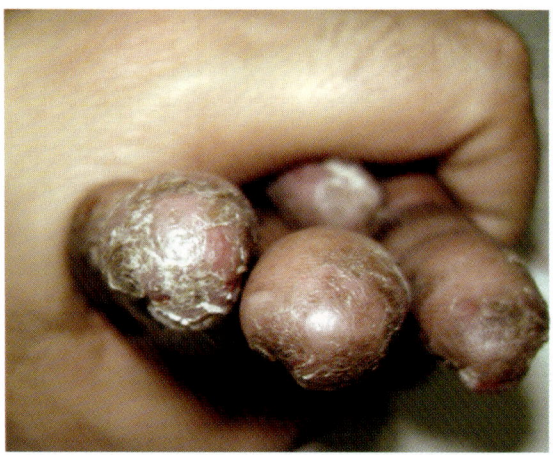

Fig. 2.15: Fingertip eczema

5. Diaper Dermatitis

Though various causes can lead to diaper dermatitis, the most common is the irritant diaper dermatitis which is rare in the neonatal period but is common in the first 18 months of life (also *see* Chapter 8).

Irritant dermatitis is caused by exposure of the skin to feces and/or urine trapped in the diaper as infants are physiologically incontinent. Using absorbent diapers and changing the diaper frequently can limit the occurrence of irritant dermatitis.

The most commonly encountered clinical presentation is erythema of the convex zones. The bright red erythema covers the convex areas of the buttocks (in a W shape) and may spread to the pubis and upper thighs. It can become shiny and erosive with a corroded appearance (Fig. 2.16). Other, rarer forms of irritant dermatitis include: The pseudoverrucous papules form, the papuloerosive form (known as Sevestre and Jacquet erosive dermatitis), the vesicular form (known as Parrot dermatitis), and the nodular form or infantile gluteal granuloma.

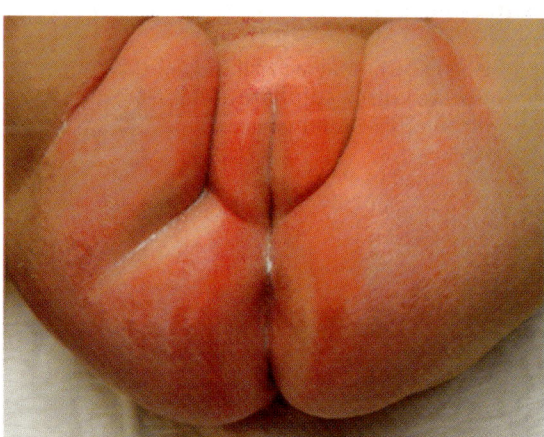

Fig. 2.16: Diaper dermatitis. The most commonly encountered clinical presentation is **erythema of the convex zones**. The bright red erythema covers the convex areas of the buttocks (in a W shape) and may spread to the pubis and upper thighs. It can become shiny and erosive with a corroded appearance (*Courtesy:* Dr Lorette G., France)

Treatment

The first-line treatment, where possible, is to eliminate the cause (e.g. cloth diapers). Parents often feel guilty about diaper dermatitis which leads them to employ over-zealous hygiene measures and multiple topical treatments which ultimately aggravate the irritation. They must be reassured, told to be patient and given clear advice about how to care for the diaper area. The diaper should be changed frequently (>6/day), the area washed with a gentle detergent (soap-free detergent or a cleansing oil) and a barrier cream applied at least twice a day (especially those containing zinc and copper). A short course of topical corticosteroids can be prescribed to treat forms with papular lesions.

If the presence of *C. albicans* is suspected, particularly if there is no improvement after several days, a topical antifungal preparation may be used.

Bibliography

1. Bennike NH, Johansen JD, Menné T. Friction from paper and cardboard causing occupational dermatitis in non-atopic individuals. Contact Dermatitis 2016 May;74(5):307–8.

2. Berardesca E, Maibach HI. Racial differences in sodium lauryl sulphate-induced cutaneous irritation: black and white. Contact Derm 1988; 18:65–70.

3. Berardesca E, Cespa M, Farinelli N, Maibach H. In vivo transcutaneous penetration of nicotinates and sensitive skin. Contact Derm 1991; 25:35–38.

4. Charbonnier V, Morrison BM, Paye M, et al. Open application assay in investigation of subclinical irritant dermatitis induced by sodium lauryl sulfate (SLS) in man: advantage of squamometry. Skin Res Tech 1998; 4:1–7.

5. Eczema, in. Sardana k, Mahajan S, Garg VK. Diagnosis and Management of Skin Disorders: An Evidence-Based Approach, 1/e.: Lippincott Williams and Wilkins, 2012 (reprint 2015).

6. Fast Facts: Eczema and Contact Dermatitis By John Berth-Jones, Eunice Tan and Howard I Malbach Published 2004.

7. Fulton JE Jr, Bradley S, Aqundez A, Black T. Non-comedogenic cosmetics. Cutis 1976 Feb;17(2): 344-5, 349–51.

8. Lammintausta K, Maibach HI, Wilson D. Mechanisms of subjective (sensory) irritation propensity to nonimmunologic contact urticaria and objective irritation in stingers. Dermatosen Beruf Umwelt 1988; 36:45–49.

9. Mills OH Jr, Kligman AM. Comedogenicity of sunscreens. Experimental observations in rabbits. Arch Dermatol 1982 Jun;118(6):417–9.

10. Susten AS. The chronic effects of mechanical trauma to the skin: a review of the literature. Am J Intern Med 1985; 18:281–288.

11. Ten Genotypes of Irritant Contact Dermatitis(in) Ai-Lean Chew· Howard I. Maibach (Eds.) Irritant Dermatitis. © Springer-Verlag Berlin Heidelberg 2006.

12. Thieme Clinical Companions Dermatology. Sterry, Dermatology© 2006 Thieme.

3

Contact Eczema

A. INTRODUCTION AND REGIONAL CAUSES OF CONTACT DERMATITIS

The list of allergens that cause ACD continues in sync with the rapid pace of industrialization and in India the literal "dumping" of allergenic personal care products from the West have made this list grow rapidly. There are over 3,500 environmental contact allergens reported in the literature (Mortz CG). Exposure to a particular allergen can occur for years before developing a delayed hypersensitivity immune response. After sensitization occurs, subsequent exposure to the allergen may result in ACD, even if used in small concentrations (Fig. 3.1) (James WD).

Topical medications are a common cause of contact dermatitis, including antibiotics (58%), corticosteroids (30%), and anesthetics (6%). This is a therapeutic issue as 30% of patients with a medication allergy had a positive patch test to a topical corticosteroid, either the steroid or the vehicle (Spring SA). List of products that are used on a daily basis contains one or more potential allergens (Table 3.1).

Irritant dermatitis is more common in women than men. ICD is also much more common in certain locations on the body, such as the hands and face, as these areas are frequently exposed to irritants. Some of the most commonly implicated irritants include low humidity, heat, metals, paper, tools, fibers/fabrics, plastics, dust, woods, rubber, jewelry, seasonal environment, fiberglass, and hearing aids (Morris-Jones R). In many cases, the mechanisms, such as friction and drying, are just as important in causing ICD as the physical irritant.

Our aim here is not to present a treatise on contact dermatitis but give a regional view of common causes from head to toe (Fig. 3.2). Needless to say more can be learnt from practice, but it is this author's personal view that contact dermatitis is misdiagnosed most of the times, and is the biggest mimicker in dermatology.

SCALP

Although the scalp is commonly exposed to many articles and products containing known allergens, isolated scalp dermatitis due to contact dermatitis is relatively uncommon. This appears to be primarily due to a topographical property innate to the scalp. The thicker scalp skin, with abundant pilosebaceous units and a relative absence of rhytids or crevices, is the ideal barrier against contact dermatitis. In contrast, the eyelids are on the other end of the spectrum, with very thin skin and many folds that retain substances, increasing time exposure and

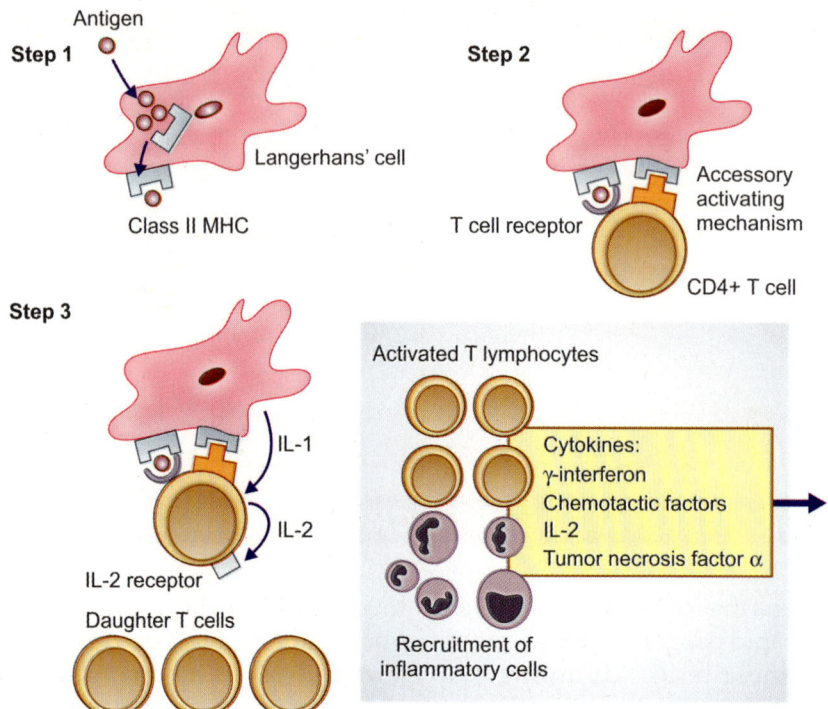

Fig. 3.1: Cell-mediated immune (type IV) reaction. In step 1, the antigen is taken up by antigen-presenting cells (e.g. Langerhans' cells in the skin), processed and bound to class II major histocompatibility complex (MHC). In step 2, these complexes migrate to the paracortical area of the draining lymph node via the afferent lymphatics. The MHC and antigen are recognized by T cell receptors on CD4+ T cells. In step 3, interieukin-1 is released stimulating the release of IL-2 which stimulates T cell expressive IL-2 receptors and helps profilerate T cells. Daughter T cells, including memory cells, are generated. On re-exposure to the same antigen, the memory T cell recognize the antigen after it has been processed in steps 1 and 2. T lymphocytes become activated and secrete cytokines, which include the components of inflammation

Table 3.1: Allergens in commonly used products (arranged alphabetically*)	
Adhesives	Colophony, ethylenediamine dihydrochloride, epoxy resin, p-tert-butylphenol formaldehyde resin, ethyl acrylate, methyl methacrylate
Clothing and textiles	*Dyes:* Disperse blue 106 and 124 (increased amounts found in dark clothing) *Permanent press clothing* (used most often to provide wrinkle resistance in cotton, rayon, and cotton polyester blends, and not often used in wool, nylon, and silk fabrics): Ethylenureamelamine, formaldehyde, dimethylol dihydroxyethyleneurea *Footwear:* Mercaptobenzothiazole (MBT), potassium dichromate, and colophony
Cosmetics and personal care products	*Fragrances and preservatives:* Propylene glycol, phenylenediamine, lanolin alcohol, amidoamine, benzophenone, chloroxylenol, alpha tocopherol, cocamidopropyl betaine, cocamide DEA, ylang-ylang oil, paraben mix, methyldibromo glutaronitrile/phenoxyethanol, iodopropynylbutylcarbamate, 2-bromo-2-nitropropane-1, 3-diol (Bronopol®)
Emollients	*Fragrances and preservatives:* Lanolin (wool alcohol), methylchloroisothiazolinone/ methylisothiazolinone (MCI/MI) in Eucerin®

(Contd.)

Table 3.1: Allergens in commonly used products (arranged alphabetically) *(Contd.)*

Fragrance	Balsam of Peru (Myroxylon Pereirae), ylang-ylang oil, jasmine, Fragrance mix I (cinnamic aldehyde, cinnamyl alcohol, hydroxycitronellal, isoeugenol, eugenol, oak moss absolute, α-amyl cinnamic aldehyde (geraniol), Fragrance mix II (Lyral®, citral, farnesol, citronellol, hexyl cinnamic aldehyde, coumarin)
Hair	*Shampoos:* Quaternium-15, methyldibromo glutaronitrile/phenoxyethanol, cocamidopropyl betaine/amidoamine, imidazolidinyl urea, cocamide DEA, methylchloroisothiazolinone/methylisothiazolinone (MCI/MI), fragrances *Permanent wave solutions:* Glyceryl thioglycolate *Hair dyes:* p-phenylenediamine (PPD), cobalt
Leather	*Tanning solutions:* Potassium dichromate *Leather gloves and watch bands:* p-tert-butylphenol formaldehyde resin
Metals	Nickel, cobalt, sodium gold thiosulfate, potassium dichromate
Nails	*Nail polish:* Tosylamide formaldehyde resin *Artificial nail glue:* Ethyl acrylate, methyl methacrylate
Rubber accelerators and latex	Carba mix, mercaptobenzothiazole (MBT), thiuram mix, mercapto mix, black rubber mix, mixed dialkyl thioureas
Sunscreen	Fragrances and preservatives *Photocontact:* Benzophenone-3/oxybenzone, cinnamic aldehyde
Temporary Tattoos (black henna)	p-Phenylenediamine (PPD)
Topical medications	Fragrances and preservatives *Antibiotics:* Neomycin sulfate, bacitracin *Corticosteroids:* Tixocortol-21-pivalate (Class A), budesonide (Class B), desoximetasone (Class C), and hydrocortisone-17 butyrate (Class D) *Anesthetics, including medications for hemorrhoids, teething, cold sores, canker sores:* Lidocaine, benzocaine *Antihistamines:* Ethylenediamine dihydrochloride *Ophthalmic drops and vaccines:* Thiomersal (preservative) *Antabuse:* Thiuram mix *Vehicles and emulsifiers:* Colophony, lanolin, propylene glycol, sorbitan sesquioleate
Preservatives	Formaldehyde-releasing preservatives: Quaternium-15, formaldehyde, diazolidinyl urea, imidazolidinyl urea, DMDM hydantoin, 2-bromo-2-nitropropane-1,3 diol (Bronopol®), ethylene urea/melamine formaldehyde, dimethylol dihydroxyethyleneurea *Other preservatives:* Methylchloroisothiozolinene, paraben mix, methyldibromoglutaronitril, thiomersal, methyldibromo glutaronitrile/phenoxyethanol, iodopropynyl butylcarbamate, tosylamide formaldehyde resin, phenoxyethanol, benzalkonium chloride, glutaral

*Preservatives are listed separately.

resulting in more severe reactions. For these reasons, contact dermatitis is unlikely to be at the top of the differential diagnosis for isolated scalp dermatitis. Even in cases where an aggressive allergen is present, the scalp is often not affected or only minimally affected, despite significant involvement of the face, ears and/or neck. Potential allergens involved in *scalp* dermatitis include *hair dyes, hair cleansing* products, and **medicaments** (Hillen U) (Table 3.2).

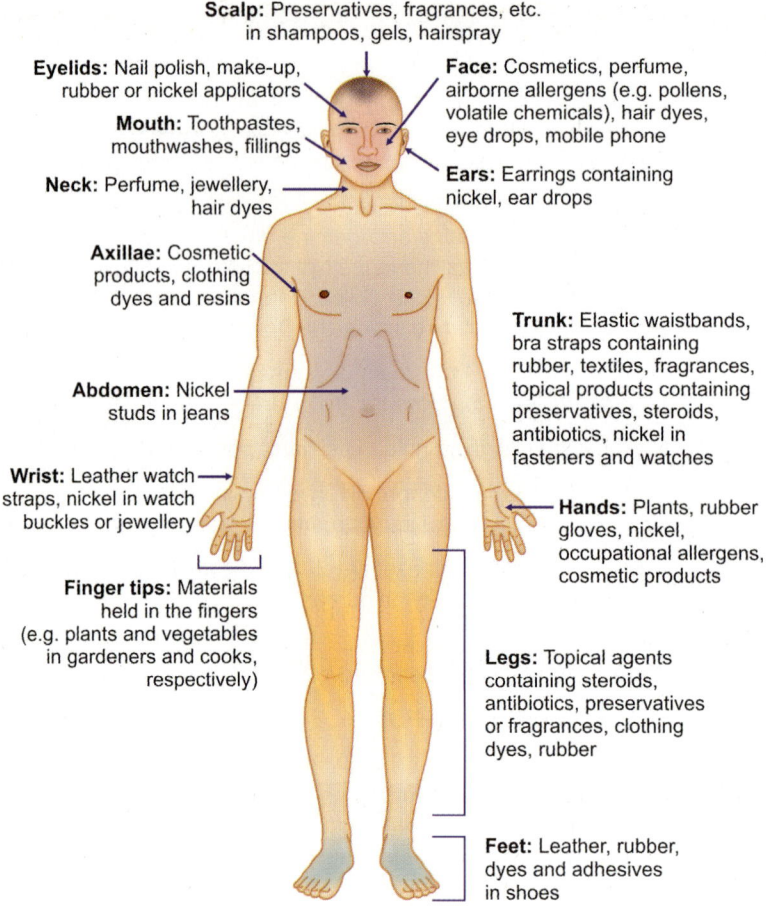

Fig. 3.2: Region-wise causes of contact dermatitis

Object	Allergen	Morphology
Table 3.2: Scalp dermatitis—allergens with morphological patterns		
Bobby pins, hair pins	Nickel	Discrete Corresponds with shape of offending agent
Hair dyes	PPD	Acute edematous dermatitis
Headband, bathing cap, hairnet, hats	Leather or rubber	Linear rash across forehead Encircles head May involve ears
Leave-in styling aids (mousse, gels, pomades, hairspray)	Fragrances, preservatives, acrylates	Chronic dermatitis with episodic flares Hairspray can cause a dermatitis at the temples adjacent to the scalp
Permanent wave solutions	Glyceryl thioglycolate	Acute edematous dermatitis
Wash-out products including shampoos and conditioners	Quaternium-15, methyldibromo glutaronitrile, phenoxyethanol, fragrance, MCI/MI, cocamidopropyl betaine	Rinse-off pattern Patchy distribution
Wigs	Adhesives	Encircles head

The figure labels (Fig. 3.2):

Scalp: Preservatives, fragrances, etc. in shampoos, gels, hairspray

Eyelids: Nail polish, make-up, rubber or nickel applicators

Mouth: Toothpastes, mouthwashes, fillings

Neck: Perfume, jewellery, hair dyes

Axillae: Cosmetic products, clothing dyes and resins

Abdomen: Nickel studs in jeans

Wrist: Leather watch straps, nickel in watch buckles or jewellery

Finger tips: Materials held in the fingers (e.g. plants and vegetables in gardeners and cooks, respectively)

Face: Cosmetics, perfume, airborne allergens (e.g. pollens, volatile chemicals), hair dyes, eye drops, mobile phone

Ears: Earrings containing nickel, ear drops

Trunk: Elastic waistbands, bra straps containing rubber, textiles, fragrances, topical products containing preservatives, steroids, antibiotics, nickel in fasteners and watches

Hands: Plants, rubber gloves, nickel, occupational allergens, cosmetic products

Legs: Topical agents containing steroids, antibiotics, preservatives or fragrances, clothing dyes, rubber

Feet: Leather, rubber, dyes and adhesives in shoes

Some unique morphological patterns and common allergens are described below (Figs 3.3 and 3.4a to f):

1. *Bands of dermatitis* that span the forehead, encircle the head, and/or affect the helices of the ears are suggestive of **head accessories** with leather or rubber parts, such as in hat bands or hat linings (Fig. 3.3). With such distribution, exposure to adhesive tapes used to fix wigs to the scalp should also be considered (Torchia D).

2. Hair allergens involve the face, eyelids, ears, and neck. A high degree of suspicion is critical to the diagnosis. The *rinse-off or drip pattern* sign is a clinically useful clue to suggest a scalp-applied allergen (Fig. 3.4a). This appears as a well-demarcated and relatively linear streaking dermatitis involving the preauricular face and lateral neck. In patients with classic rinse-off pattern of dermatitis, personal hair care products should be considered (Hillen U).

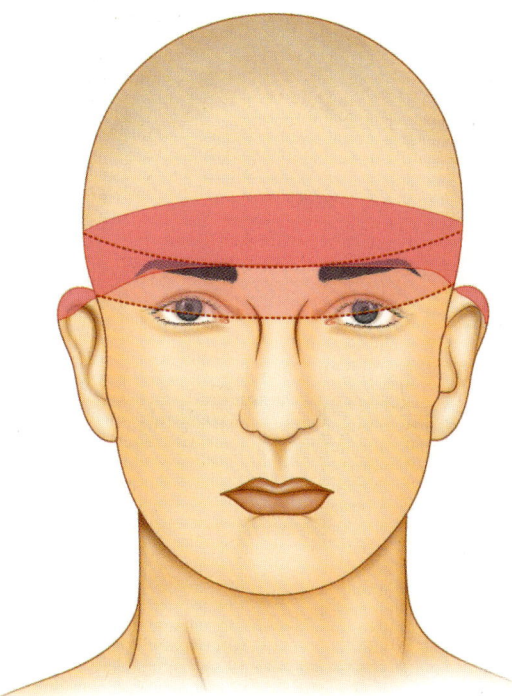

Fig. 3.3: Band of dermatitis affecting the forehead and ears

The most important potential allergens in shampoos and conditioners are fragrances, cocamidopropyl betaine (CAPB), and preservatives including quaternium-15. CAPB is of particular interest and is contained in many shampoos, including those marketed as "no tears" products for infants and young children. Two somewhat unique patterns have been observed with CAPB sensitivity: chronic scalp pruritus and flaking, and a chronic dermatitis with episodic flares (Hillen U).

3. PPD is the common allergen, it is the foremost and there are various patterns (Handa S) and except the acute variant, this is usually misdiagnosed (Fig. 3.4b to f). An option is to use herbal dyes.

4. *Tea tree* oil is another common allergen and can actually cause an aggravation of seborrheic dermatitis. Clinicians should consider this allergen in patients with recalcitrant, worsening, or flaring

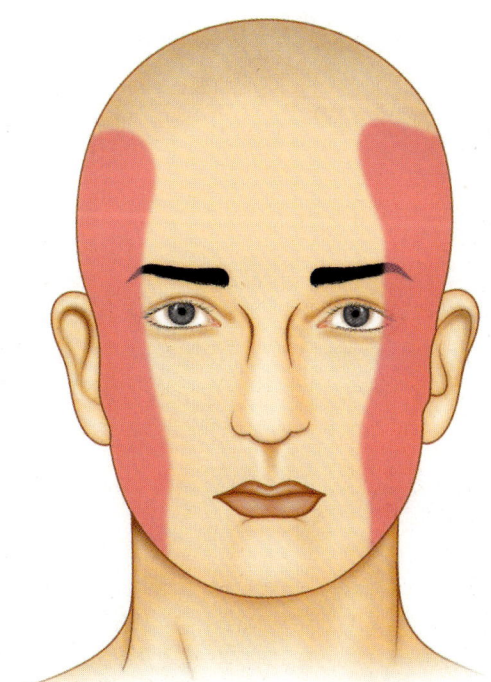

Fig. 3.4a: Rinse-off pattern due to shampoo, conditioner, dyes and other rinse-off products

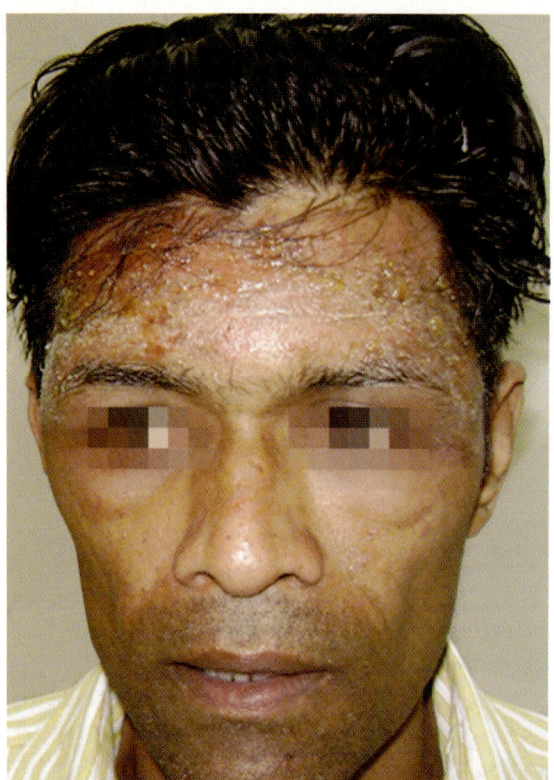

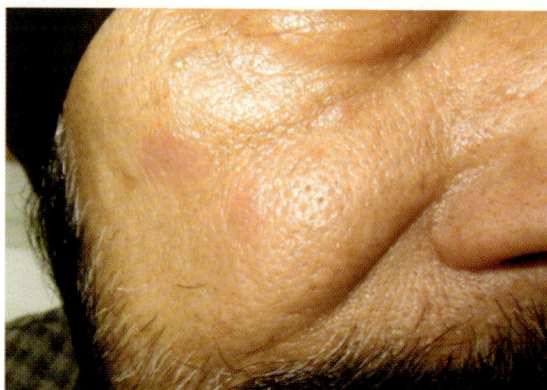

Fig. 3.4c: Cyclically recurring papular rash on the face diagnosed as PMLE

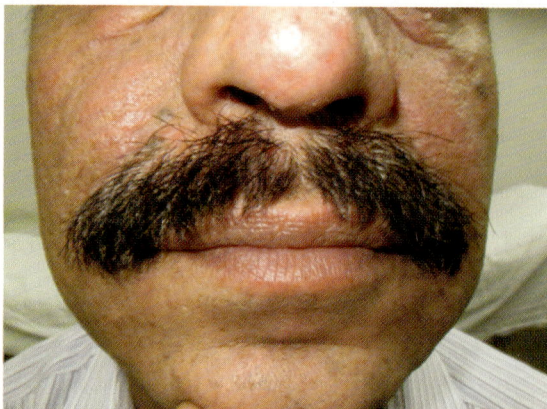

Fig. 3.4d: Papular rash on the face involving the upper lip

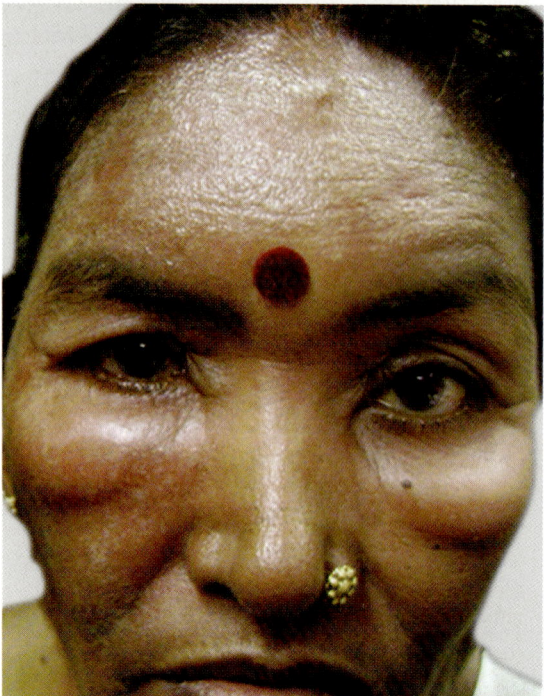

Fig. 3.4b: Acute odematous swelling consequent to PPD

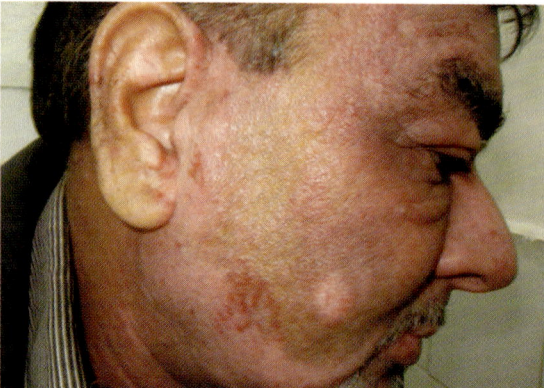

Fig. 3.4e: Diagnosed variably as PMLE, acute phototoxicity, psoriasis, seborrheic dermatitis and then treated by a homeopathy for vitiligo. This patient had diffuse erythema, crusting in some areas and extending to photoprotected sites. The erythema in the scalp was a give away to the diagnosis of PPD allergy

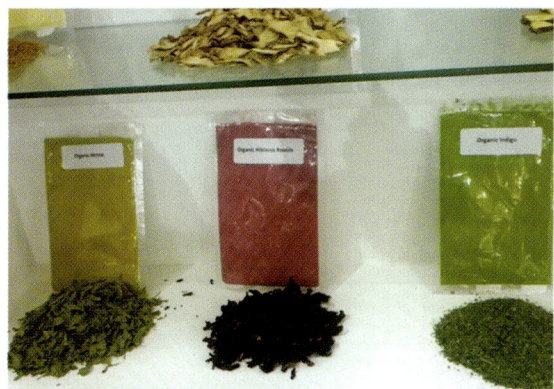

Fig. 3.4f: The fine and proportionate admixture of the three natural herbal extracts (henna, hibiscus and indigo; L-R) helps to make the various shades of herbal hair dyes. (*Source on site*, 19th organic world congress Greater Noida, India—Dr Supriya Mahajan MD)

manufacturers after many patients came with acute erythema on the face on applying the medicine.

5. Minoxidil may be the most frequent cause of scalp dermatitis medicamentosa (Corazza M). Although irritant contact dermatitis is the most frequent reported outcome of topical use of minoxidil, there are reports of allergic contact dermatitis on the scalp. This is common as one uses higher concentration of minoxidil with an increase in the concentration of propylene glycol which may caused ACD. A pustular eruption of the scalp has also been reported (Rodríguez-Martin M).

seborrheic dermatitis or sebopsoriasis. In this setting, asking the patient about the use of "natural" or over-the-counter remedies may lead to the discovery of Melaleuca exposure. A famous antiacne brand in India (clindamycin and aloe vera), shockingly had or may be still has tea tree oil! It was pointed out to the

FACE

Facial contact dermatitis has a fairly well defined group of frequent offending allergens. Using a regional approach helps simplify this list into three main categories—scalp dermatitis, aerosolized allergens, and directly applied facial allergens/irritants (Table 3.3). As scalp dermatitis is discussed (above), we will focus on the other two entities.

Table 3.3: Face dermatitis—allergens with morphological patterns	
Scalp-applied allergens	
Shampoos, conditioners, hair dye	Periphery of the face (pre-auricular, submental, and mandibular region), 'rinse-off' pattern (Fig. 3.4a)
Aeroallergens	
Fragrance, plant allergens, aerosols, animal dander, dust mites, pollen	Facial dermatitis, cutoff at shirtcollar (Fig. 3.5a and b)
Face-applied allergens	
Cell phone (nickel or chromate)	Mid-to-lower cheek of lateral face, unilateral, bilateral if simultaneous use of two cell phones (Fig. 3.14).
Cosmetic products (makeup)	Bilateral, centralized (forehead, cheeks, chin), patchy/diffuse (Fig. 3.6)
Eyewear (eyeglasses, sunglasses)	Bilateral, symmetrical, linear rash, corresponds to shape of eyewear, below eyes on upper cheeks
Leave-in products (lotions, sunscreens)	Bilateral, diffuse distribution
Rubber cosmetic sponge	Patchy distribution, asymmetrical
Scuba diver face masks	Bilateral, symmetrical, corresponds to shape of mask
Wash-out products (soaps)	Bilateral, centralized (forehead, cheeks, chin), patchy/diffuse

Aerosolized Contact Allergens (Aeroallergens)

It is often restricted to animal dander, dust mites, and pollens, which more frequently drive type I hypersensitivity reactions. Aeroallergens include fragrances, plant allergens, and things that become temporarily aerosolized during repair or manufacturing processes. Aeroallergens have been classically reported to present as facial dermatitis with a distinct cutoff along the shirt collar (Fig. 3.5). Aeroallergens are also sometimes contributors to a phototoxic or photoallergic reaction. Sparing under the chin or behind the ears is a clue to photoexacerbation. The **"head-light"** sign, which refers to the presence of facial dermatitis that dramatically *spares* the nose, may be useful clinically to suggest such patients.

Face-applied Allergens

Needless to say females more frequently presented with facial contact dermatitis secondary to cosmetic-associated allergens (Castanedo-Tardan MP). Common sources among both females and males include

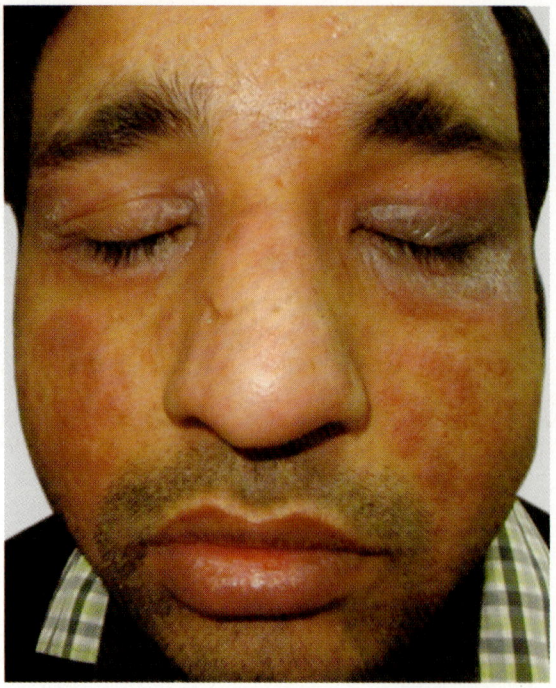

Fig. 3.5b: This patient received antifungals and topical steroids repeatedly with little response. Then sunscreens and HCQS for PMLE. The patient used to drive his bike through a under construction national highway. The "dust" with allergens was trapped in his helmet. A classic of "aeroallergy"

moisturizers, sunscreens, hair products, and *fragrances* (Rietschel RL). In general, cosmetic-related dermatitis favors a bilateral facial distribution. It is often patchy and diffuse. Predilection for the *periphery* of the face involving the pre-auricular, submental, and mandibular region should direct consideration toward *scalp-applied* allergens, such as shampoos, conditioners, and hair dyes, as well as wash-off products such as facial cleansers. A predominantly *central facial distribution* (forehead, cheeks, and chin) suggests makeup, moisturizers, or jewellery (Fig. 3.6).

In India bindi dermatitis (Tewary M, Laxmisha C, Baxter KF, Koh D, Bajaj AK) is common and can be due to thiomersal, colophony, PTBP or nickel (Fig. 3.7). Another condition, pigmented contact dermatitis (Fig. 3.8a and b) is seen commonly in India and can be due to various allergens including

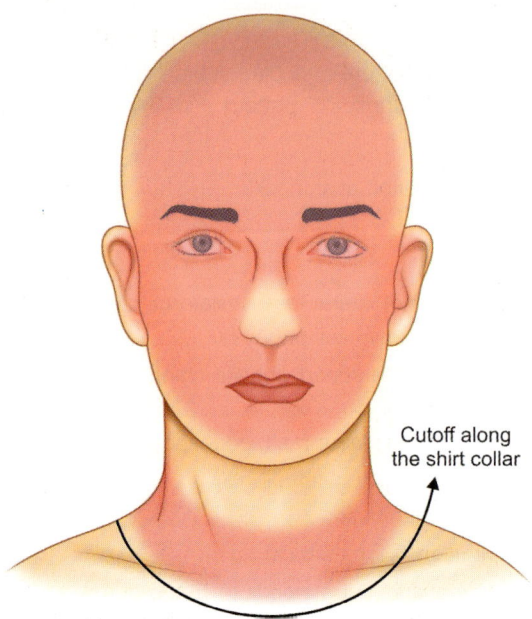

Cutoff along the shirt collar

Fig. 3.5a: A depiction of aeroallergen pattern

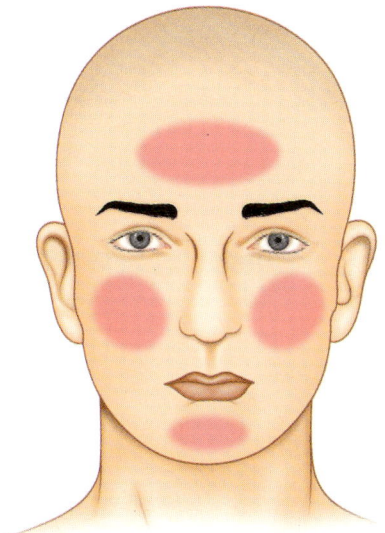

Fig. 3.6: Sites for contact dermatitis of facial products

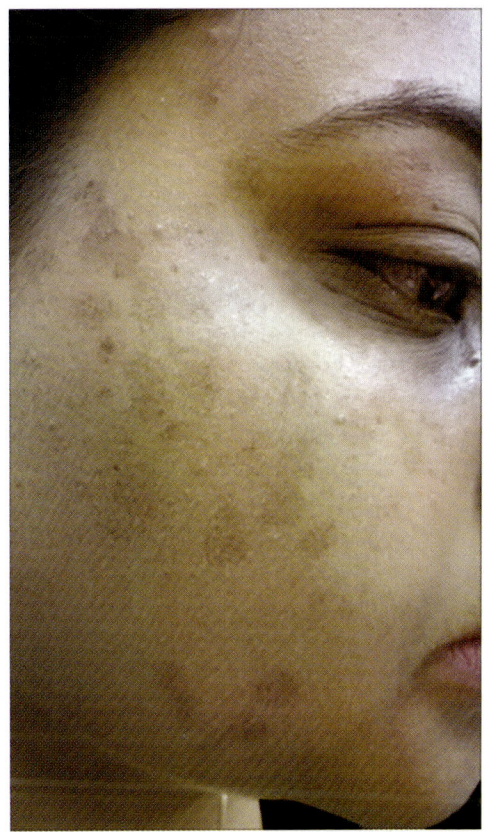

Fig. 3.8a: This patient applied kojic acid for her acne PIH and developed PCD

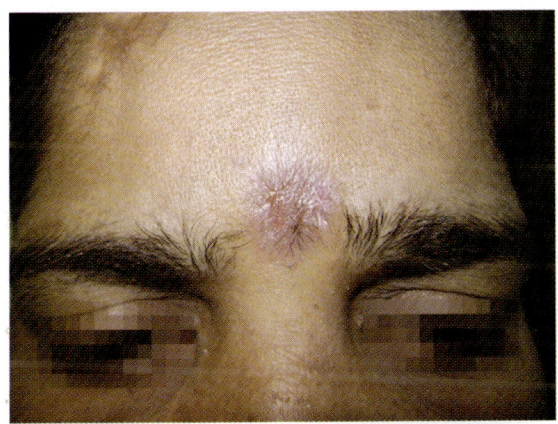

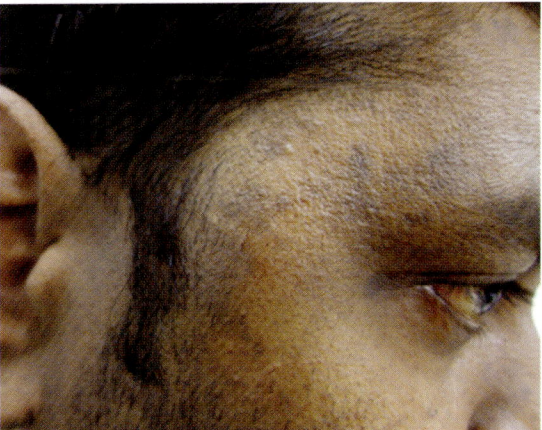

Fig. 3.8b: Another case of PCD due to mustard oil

thimerosal, gallate, PPD, kojic acid, Kum Kum, mustard oil, hair oils with jasmine and ylangylangoil (Nath AK, Kozuka I, García-Gavín J).

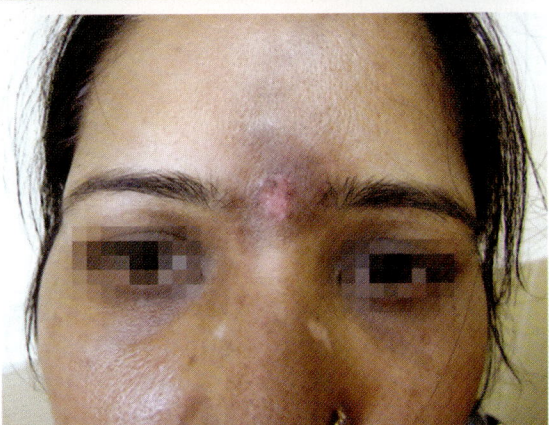

Fig. 3.7: Bindi dermatitis due to PTBP, a compound added to the sticky part of the bindi. The "adhesive" is the culprit

EYELIDS

The eyelids are one of the most sensitive regions and this is as the skin of the eyelids is quite thin (0.55 mm) compared to other sites on the face (2.0 mm), which makes them prone to contact dermatitis (Castanedo-Tardan MP). Also the sphincter function of the orbicularis oculi, due to its accordion-like movement, which enables the upper eyelid to blink, leads to potential allergens becoming trapped and retained between the folded skin when the eye is open.

The eyelid region can be more easily appro-ached by considering categories of allergen exposure. The five major categories are:

a. Scalp-applied allergens (discussed previously)
b. Aeroallergens (discussed previously)
c. Directly contacted allergens
d. Ectopic allergens
e. Inadvertent allergens.

Directly applied allergens include anything directly applied or exposed to the eyelid. This list is nearly endless and includes a myriad of cosmetics, cleansers, and ophthalmic medica-ments. The most common allergens in this category are *fragrances*, *preservatives*, and *nickel* (Rietschel RL, Valsecchi R). Nickel can be found as an ingredient or contaminate in personal care products such as makeup, but it is also found frequently in applicators. These applicators may also be a source of rubber or black dye (p-paraphenylenediamine) exposure. A predominance of the lower eyelids with a "run-off" or "drip" pattern should raise suspicion of ophthalmic solutions (Fig. 3.9a). Ophthalmic medications may contain poten-tially irritating and sensitizing preservatives, such as benzalkonium chloride, thimerosal (merthiolate), chlorobutanol, chlorohexidine, or phenylmercuric nitrite (Fig. 3.9b). Topical medications such as antibiotics and steroids should also be considered.

Bilateral involvement or occasionally unilateral affliction can be seen (Fig. 3.9c) due to swim goggles, binocular or telescope eyepieces, and eye patches.

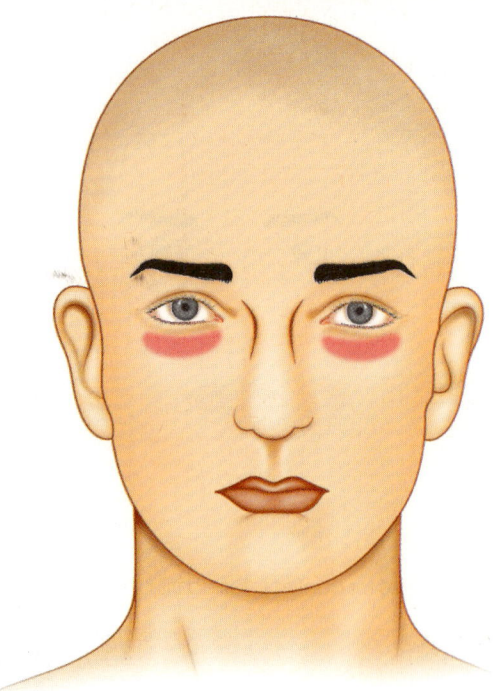

Fig. 3.9a: Lower eyelid dermatitis due to ophthalmic medicaments

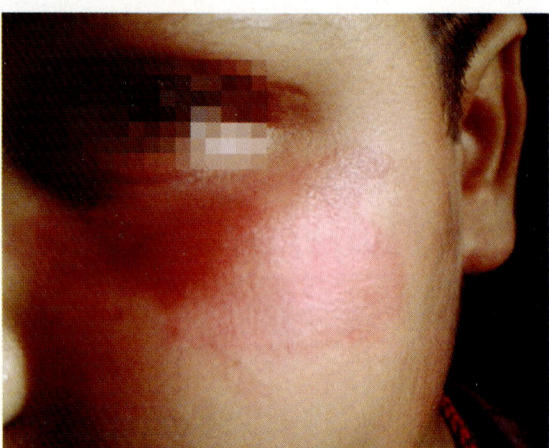

Fig. 3.9b: Allergic reaction to "thiomersal" in eye drops

Ectopic allergens This term is restricted largely when eyelid dermatitis is because of gold (Nedorost S) and refers to the allergen source being removed or at an ectopic site from the dermatitis. Typically, this can be from a gold ring on the finger. The situation may be somewhat perplexing in that patients

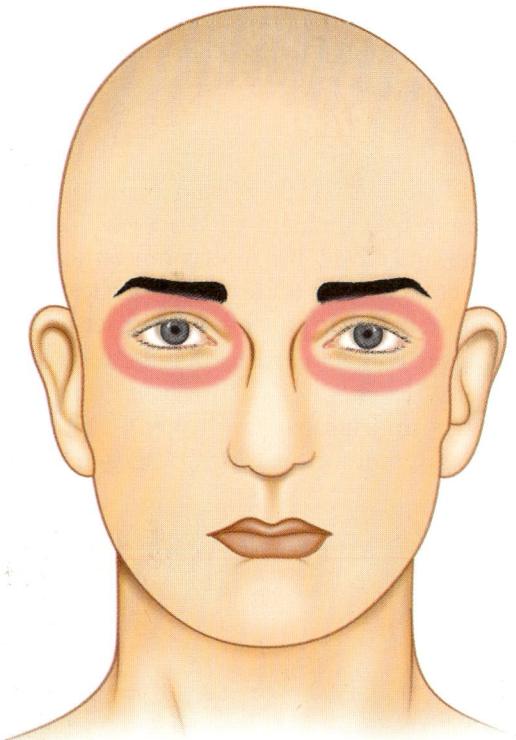

Fig. 3.9c: Annular dermatitis due to goggles, binoculars, and other eyepieces

Toluene sulfonamide formaldehyde resin	5/200	2.5%

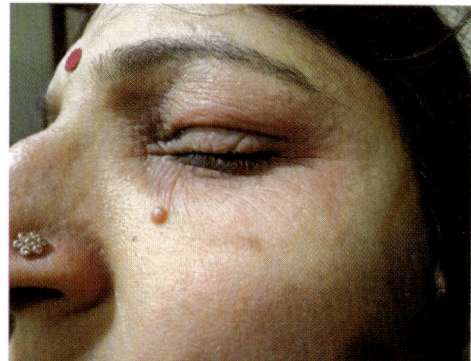

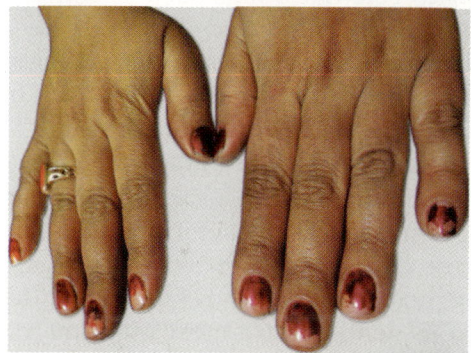

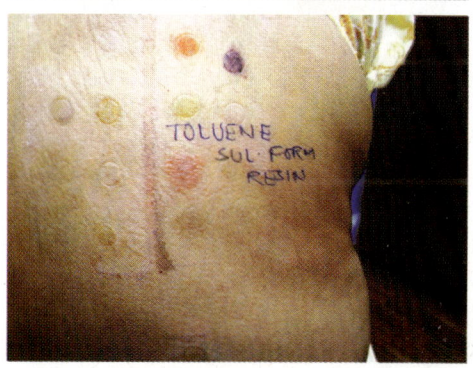

Fig. 3.9d: Inadvertent allergen transfer of nail polish to the eye. Here the allergen was **Toluene sulfonamide formaldehyde**. Alternative options for individuals with allergic contact dermatitis reactions to these ingredients can be avoidance of these procedures or use of products that are "3, 4, 5 free", in which the common allergens *dibutyl phthalate*, *toluene*, and *formaldehyde* are absent (Chou M, Dhingra N, Strugar TL. Contact Sensitization to Allergens in Nail Cosmetics. Dermatitis. 2017 Jul/Aug; 28(4):231–240)
(*Courtesy:* Dr PK Srivastava, Dr AK Bajaj)

frequently do not have a reaction to the allergen on the finger. The explanation for this seems to be that gold is released from the allergen source and transferred to the eyelid in the presence of sweat and abrasive particles such as titanium dioxide, a physical sunscreen and common ingredient in cosmetics.

"Inadvertent" allergens are an easily forgotten but important cause of eyelid dermatitis. The eyelids are frequently rubbed and touched, which leads to transfer of substances from the hands. In this manner, the eyelids may be exposed to a multitude of potential allergens. This type of allergen spread often appears as an *isolated*, *asymmetric upper* eyelid dermatitis. Some common sources include hand sanitizer, hand soap, hand moisturizer, and nail polish (Fig. 3.9d). The thicker skin of the hands is often spared.

MOUTH, LIPS, AND PERIORAL REGION

Oral Cavity

The signs and symptoms of contact dermatitis in the oral cavity are less well defined than those seen with other regions. The classic symptomatology of itching and scaling is often absent. Lichenoid reactions are a particularly important pattern seen involving the oral mucosa. While oral lichen planus is the prototypical example of this pattern, extrinsic agents such as drugs and contactants should not be overlooked as a potential etiology. A biopsy is typically warranted and helps to rule out things such as connective tissue disease, immunobullous disease and malignancy. *Eosinophils* seen on histology are helpful in pointing the diagnosis away from lichen planus and favoring an extrinsic driving force such as a drug or contactant.

The common *sites* affected are the lateral tongue and buccal mucosa. These are the areas in closest proximity to amalgams (fillings) and most prosthetic devices (Schlosser BJ). Metals used in dentistry are most often mercury, nickel, gold, cobalt, palladium, and chromium. Sources of exposure to these metals include dentures, braces, crowns, and fillings (amalgams). Other causes of oral lichenoid contact dermatitis include flavorings (with cinnamon being the classic example) and dental adhesives (acrylates) (Tremblay S). Allergy to acrylates from dental prostheses may also cause tingling or jaw pain (Gawkrodger D).

Oral hygiene products may cause allergic contact dermatitis in either the mucosa of the oral cavity or on the lips (Kind F). Therefore, rashes that involve both the oral cavity and the lips are very suggestive of an allergy to chemicals in mouthwashes, toothpastes, dental floss, and chewing gum. One area of concern is flavorings in toothpastes and oral care products. In general, non-mint-flavored products may be less allergenic. A common offending irritant in these products is sodium lauryl sulfate. In toddlers with skin eruptions in the mucosa of the oral cavity or on the lips, exposure to rubber in pacifiers should also be considered (Lee PW).

Lips

Isolated lip dermatitis is seen commonly to fragrance mix, balsam of Peru (*Myroxylon Pereirae*), and nickel. The most common allergen source are cosmetics (Orton DI). Patch testing is an important step in patients with lip dermatitis.

Allergic contact cheilitis may be the result of allergy to chemicals in *lip balms, lipsticks, lip glosses,* and *sunscreens* (Orton DI) (Fig. 3.9e and f). A common historical allergen in lip

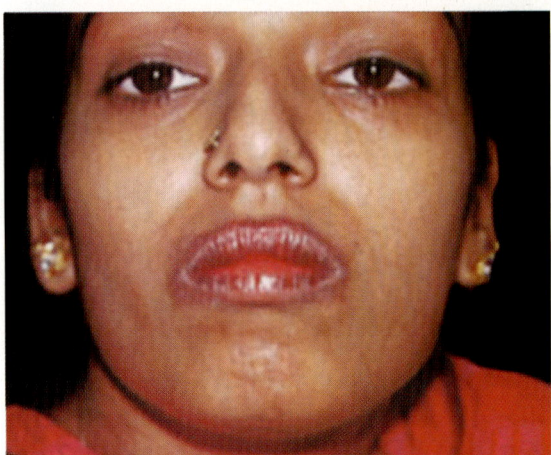

Fig. 3.9e: Allergic cheilitis (*Courtesy*: Dr PK Srivastava, Dr AK Bajaj)

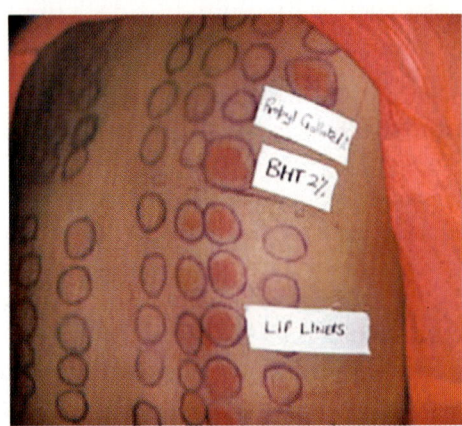

Fig. 3.9f: Patch Test shows positivity to preservative propyl gallate and BHT (*Courtesy*: Dr PK Srivastava, Dr AK Bajaj)

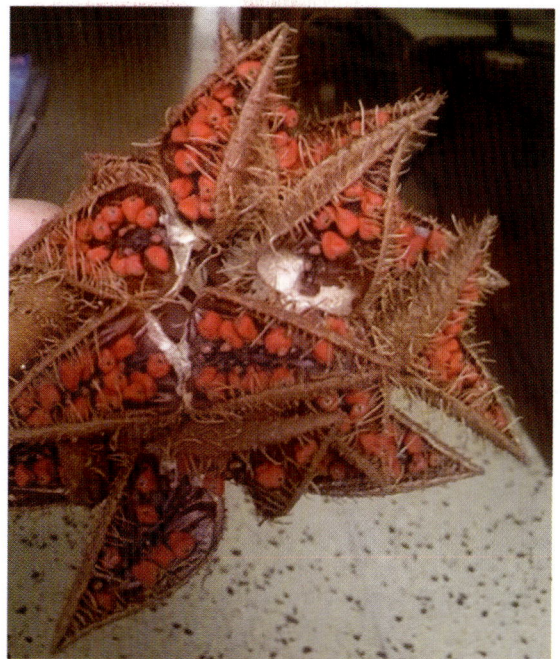

Fig. 3.9g: *Bixa orellana* aka lipstick tree. This tree's fruits can be used as a natural coloring agent in lipsticks, but it gives only a red color! (The tree grows in tropical forests in India, this photograph was taken in Goa by, Dr Supriya Mahajan. MD)

dermatitis. The prototypical presentation is a wife with allergic contact cheilitis to her husband's aftershave.

Perioral

While dental products (mouthwash, toothpaste, dental floss, and chewing gum) and medicaments (neomycin, bacitracin, budesonide, tetracaine) are common allergen sources for isolated allergic contact cheilitis, spillover to the perioral skin can also be seen. This is particularly seen in the case of toothpaste-driven allergic contact dermatitis (Fig. 3.9h). Both the foaming action of the toothpaste and the movement of the brush contribute to the spread of the toothpaste contactants. Clinically, this can be seen as contact dermatitis at the angles of the mouth. Another helpful clue is that the angles are affected in an *asymmetric* fashion, with the side on which the toothbrush is held showing more involvement. This is typically the right side in right-handed individuals.

A summary of the common causes are listed in Table 3.4.

products is *castor oil*, which is used as a solvent for pigments. *Lanolin*, another common component in lip products, is used as an emollient and has induced an allergic response in individuals. *Benzophenone*, a chemical sunscreen found in many lip products and sunscreens, has also been found to be a common allergen.

One almost forgotten simple solution is to crush the seeds of the 'Lipstick tree' which is a natural coloring agent and can be used in lipsticks and lip balms (Fig. 3.9g).

Exposure to metal lipstick casings or the habitual sucking of metallic objects (pen or pencil) can also be the cause of isolated allergic contact cheilitis to nickel. Anything that contacts the lips should also be considered, including a significant other or spouse. The transfer of a contactant inadvertently from one person to another (usually a significant other or spouse) has been referred to as consort contact

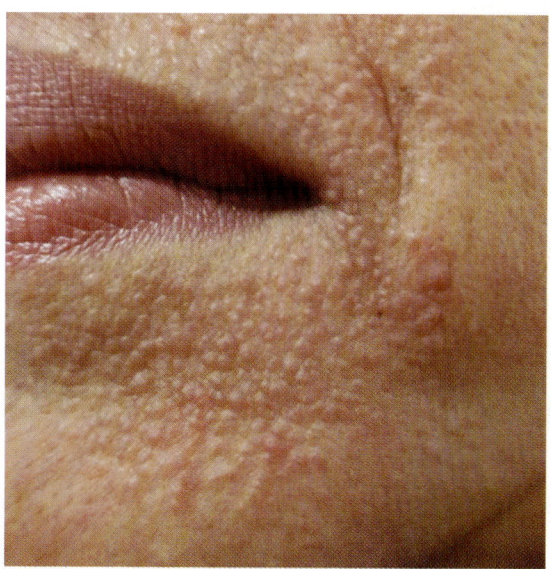

Fig. 3.9h: Perioral dermatitis due to the use of "herbal ayurvedic toothpaste". A proof of the chemical nature of the paste

Product	Allergen	Morphology
Oral cavity		
Dental crowns, fillings/ amalgams, dentures, dental braces	Made most commonly from mercury, nickel, gold, and cobalt (allergens)	Buccal mucosa and lateral tongue Lichenoid
Oral hygiene products	Sodium lauryl sulfate (irritant) in toothpastes and mouthwash Flavoring including cinnamon and mint (irritant)	Can be seen on the lips as well as oral mucosa Patchy distribution Toothpaste may show asymmetric involvement of corners of mouth.
Lips		
Cosmetics	Peppermint oil in lip balm (allergen)	Seen on the upper and lower lips Diffuse distribution
Habitual oral placement of objects	Pencil, pen, necklace containing nickel (allergen); repetitive trauma (irritant)	Seen on the upper and/or lower lips Corresponds with shape of offending product
Musical instrument held outward from the lips	Recorder, trumpet	Seen on the upper and lower lips Corresponds with shape of offending product
Perioral region		
Lip licker dermatitis	Saliva (irritant)	Circumferential irritant

Table 3.4: Perioral and mucosal dermatitis—allergens with morphological patterns

NECK

The neck analogous to the eyelids, has a thin skin and thus is prone to reaction by contact allergens. There are three primary categories that should be considered:

1. Scalp-applied contact allergens with run-off to the neck
2. Aeroallergens
3. Directly applied contact allergens.

A list of allergens is detailed in Table 3.5.

Scalp-applied allergens are given above, as discussed before the pre-auricular face, submandibular chin and lateral neck constitute what is known as the rinse-off pattern, suggesting a scalp-applied allergen that is rinsed off, such as shampoo or oils (Figs 3.4 and 3.10a). Aeroallergens were discussed above and the neck is typically exposed to the same airborne contactants. In the setting of an aeroallergen-driven dermatitis, the neck may offer the greatest clue—a sharply demarcated cutoff at the shirt collar (Fig. 3.5b).

Another classic clue found on the neck is what some refer to as the "atomizer sign" (Jacob SE). This is when there is a focal dermatitis located on the anterior neck in the Adam's apple region (Fig. 3.10b). It is evidence of a focal application of an aerosolized contactant—typically a spray of perfume or cologne. Presence of the atomizer sign is a diagnostic pearl for fragrance-based allergic contact dermatitis.

Directly applied allergens to the neck can be subdivided into two basic types of contactants: (a) *personal care products*, including cosmetics and sunscreen, and (b) personal *articles* such as jewellery and clothing. Castanedo-Tardan MP reviewed the results of patch testing to personal care products. Preservatives were the most common allergen to cause a positive patch test result, followed

Table 3.5: Neck dermatitis—allergens with morphological patterns

Product	Allergen	Morphology
Aeroallergens Fragrance (cologne, perfume)	Balsam of Peru Fragrance mix 1 and 2	Anterior region "Atomizer" sign Patchy distribution
Photoallergen/UV driven Sunscreens	Benzophenones	Facial and neck dermatitis *Sparing* under chin and behind ears
Indirectly contacted allergens Nail polish	Tosylamide formaldehyde resin Acrylates	*Asymmetric*
Directly contacted allergens Dress shirt/coat collar	• Dyes including disperse blue 106 and 124 (increased amounts found in dark clothing) • Permanent press clothing containing ethyleneurea/melamine • Formaldehyde resin	Encircles the *neck* Corresponds with shape of offending product
Jewellery/neck pieces/mobile phones	Nickel	Crescent pattern Anterior neck Corresponds with shape of offending product
Necklace clasp	Nickel	Posterior neck Corresponds with shape of offending product
Violin	Exotic woods, metal components, rubber or varnishes	Left side of the anterior neck (just below the angle of the jaw) Patchy distribution Unilateral distribution "Fiddler's neck"
Zippers	Nickel	Patchy distribution Anterior or posterior neck Corresponds with shape of offending product

by fragrances. Sunscreens are a unique subset of personal care products that deserve particular consideration (Fig. 3.10c). Allergy to the active ingredient in sunscreens appears to be very low (less than 1% of the general population) (Wetter DA). However, sunscreens are a very common cause of photoallergic contact dermatitis. Benzophenones are the major class of photoallergenic sunscreens. The primary clue on exam that suggests photoallergic reaction to sunscreens is the photodistribution pattern.

Photodermatitis may be mistaken for aeroallergen-driven dermatitis. A helpful distinguishing feature is that the region under the *chin* and behind the *earlobes* is typically *spared* in a photoallergic process.

Nail polish can be considered under the category of personal care products and cosmetics. According to a study on allergic

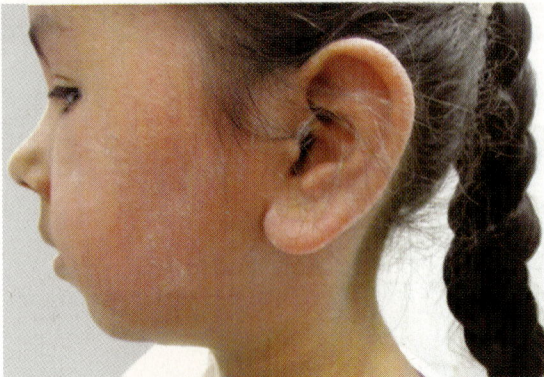

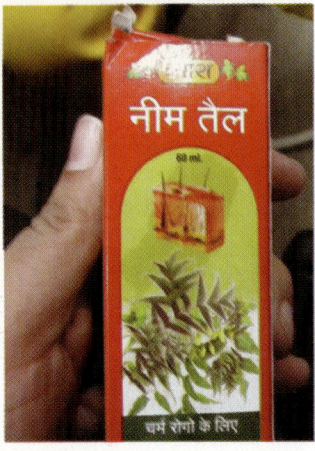

Fig. 3.10a: This girl has intense papular dermatitis on the face and neck due the use of popular "herbal" "ayurvedic" oil with its obviously "chemical" based ingredients

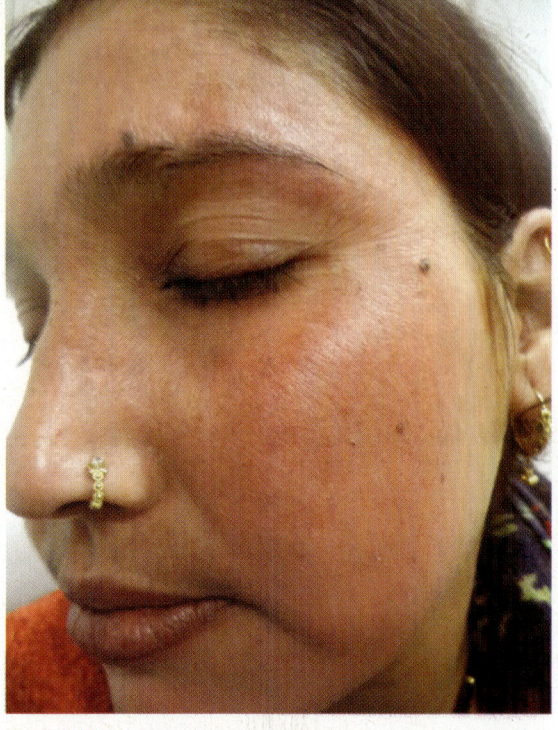

Fig. 3.10c: Allergic contact dermatitis with photo-aggravation to a sunscreen. Note the sharp cut off that determines the common usage pattern of sunscreen (Dr Seema Rani)

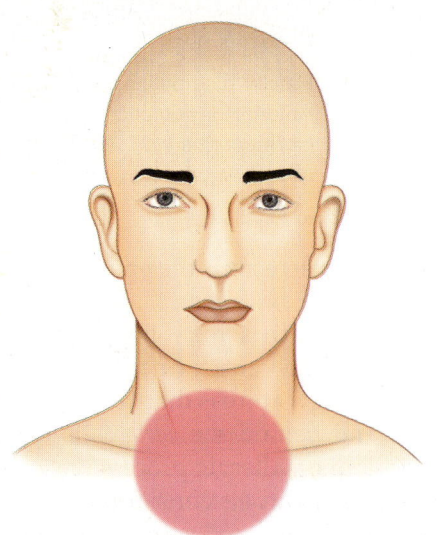

Fig. 3.10b: Atomiser sign

contact dermatitis, the face and neck were the most commonly affected sites for patchy dermatitis secondary to exposure of acrylates in acrylic nails (Lazarov A).

Personal articles include a wide array of items. An allergy to metal in jewellery such as necklaces and earrings (Figs 3.11a and 3.12c), and the neck pieces of stethoscopes, may appear as crescent-shaped rashes on the anterior neck (Castanedo-Tardan MP). Wooden necklaces made from exotic woods may also produce an allergic reaction. A more linear band of dermatitis encircling the neck can be a clue that a patient is reacting to the collar of a dress shirt or coat. This may be an irritant reaction, if the textile is coarse, such as wool, in a patient with an underlying atopic diathesis. The reaction may also be allergic in nature. The allergen may be primary to the article of clothing, such as textile resins and

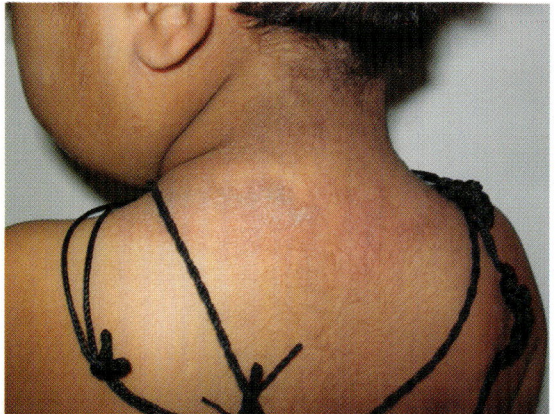

Fig. 3.11a: Allergic reaction to "holy" necklace in a child

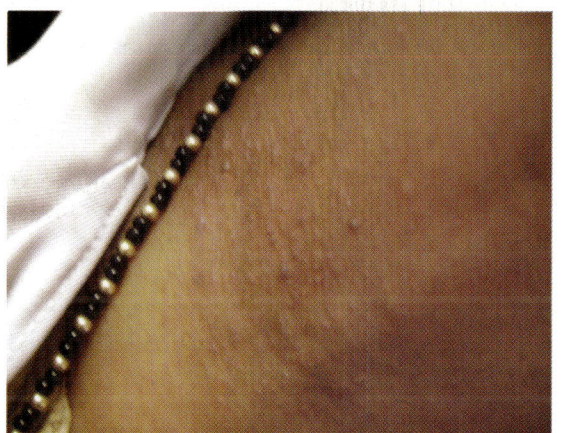

Fig. 3.11b: Allergic reaction to a necklace

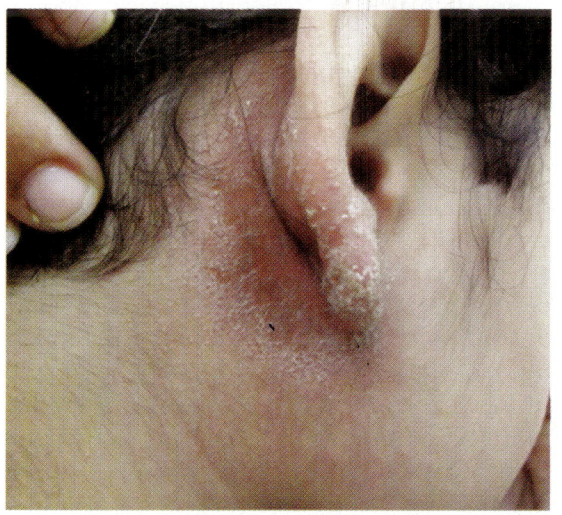

Fig. 3.12a: Allergy to ear drops

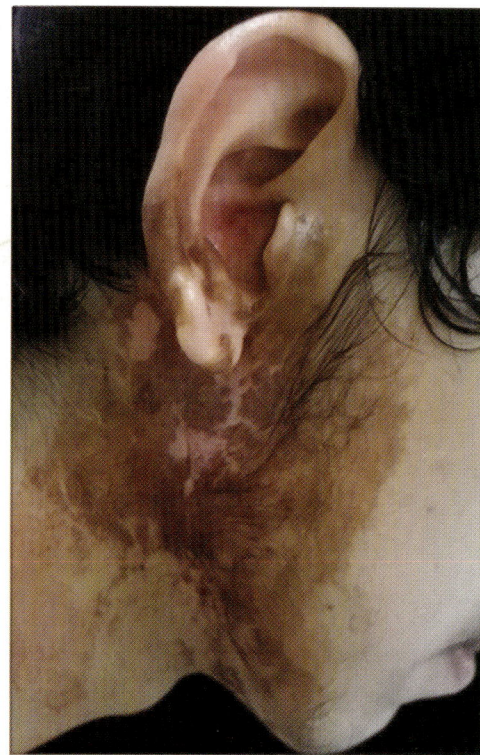

Fig. 3.12b: Allergic reaction to neomycin, a common additive in most ear drops

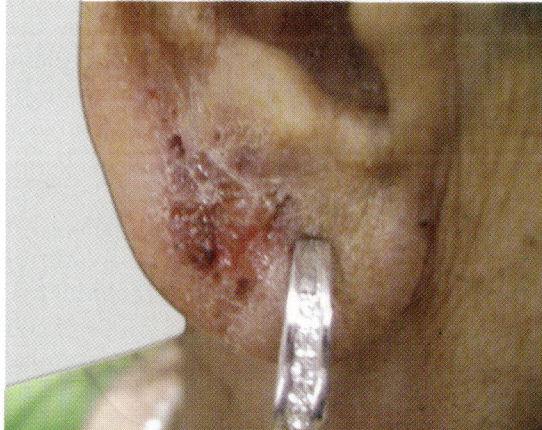

Fig. 3.12c: Artifical jewellery is a frequent cause of earlobe dermatitis

dyes, or it may be a retained allergen. Retained allergens are most often found in articles that are not frequently washed, such as coats, hats, and shoes. These allergens represent an allergen that has become embedded and

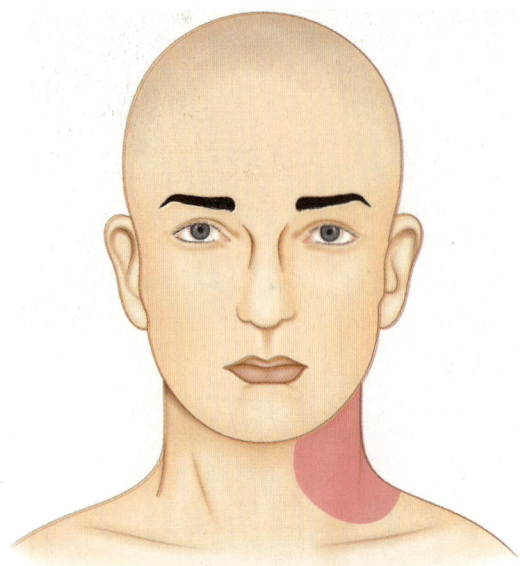

Fig. 3.13: Fiddler's neck

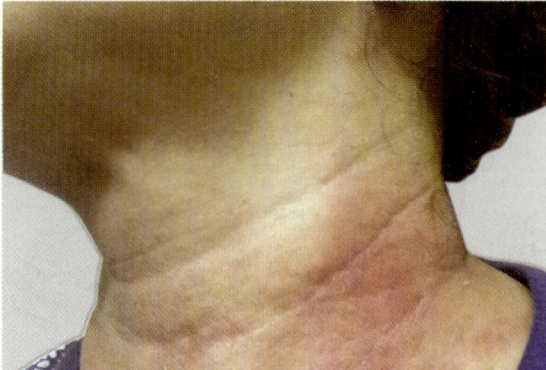

Fig. 3.14a: This patient was diagnosed and failed treatment for Tinea, PMLE , dye dermatitis, ABCD. On close scrutiny the problem began after using a iPhone®. Nickel was the possible allergen. The patient initially was not convinced but after a persistence of the allergen the patient condition resolved on changing the make of the phone

retained within the article of clothing. A final pattern is that of posterior neck dermatitis. This pattern may indicate a reaction to dress labels or necklace clasps (Sheard C).

Musical instruments can also be considered under personal articles known to cause contact dermatitis affecting the neck. A rash on the left side of the anterior neck (just below the angle of the jaw) in an individual who plays the violin or viola is very suggestive of an allergy to something in the string instrument. This has led to the term "fiddler's neck" being used to describe such presentations (Fig. 3.13). These affected individuals often have an allergy to the exotic woods, metal compo-nents, or varnishes on the chin rest (Onder M).

Another common and rising cause is cell phones in which nickel is the implicated cause (Fig. 3.14a).

HANDS

Introduction

The hands are a common site for dermatitis and we will not discuss it in detail as a separate chapter is devoted to this topic. Needless to say, it is a complex region due to the multifactorial nature of hand dermatitis. Both endogenous and exogenous factors play a role in hand dermatitis. The professions traditionally considered high risk for *women* are hair-dressing and healthcare worker, and for *men* manufacturing and construction.

The common allergens include, *gloves,* which affect the thinner skin of the dorsal hand and wrists. Chronic dermatitis of the mid-palm (Fig. 3.15) has been termed the **'palmar grip pattern'**. This distribution suggests an allergen that is grasped in the palm, such as a computer mouse, cell phone, vehicle stick shift, railing, and cane. Metal is another common allergen that can affect the hands. **Contact dermatitis medicamentosa** is also important to consider in the evaluation of hand dermatitis (Fig. 3.14b and c). Many cases of hand dermatitis likely begin as xerosis or in adults with atopic dermatitis manifesting as chronic hand dermatitis. This endogenous barrier disruption then sets the stage for hand dermatitis, which becomes secondarily driven by allergic contact dermatitis to the agents utilized for treatment. In these cases, there are more patients who demonstrate palmar or diffuse involvement than seen with glove dermatitis. Propylene glycol is another important allergen to consider.

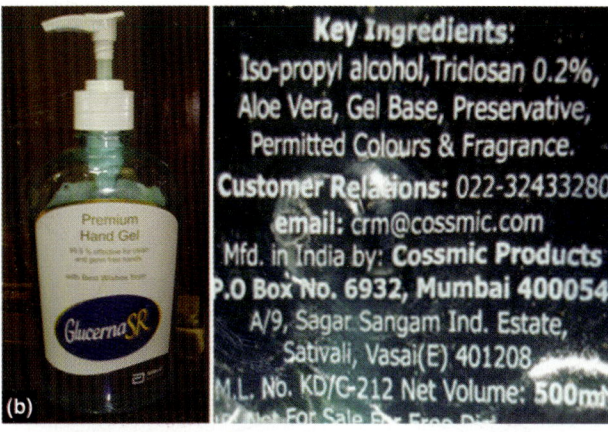

Triclosan 2%	2/200	1.0%

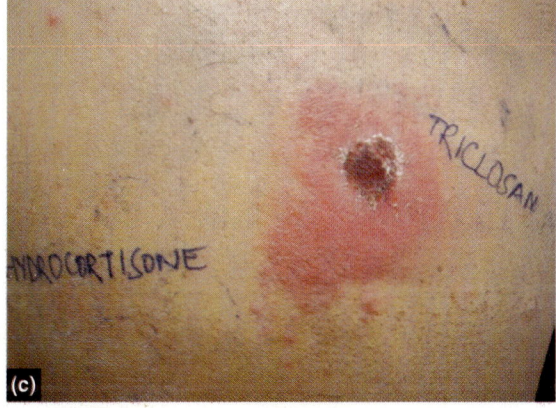

Fig. 3.14b and c: Hand dermatitis in a patient due to Triclosan. A case of contact dermatitis medicamentosa (*Courtesy:* Dr PK Srivastava, Dr AK Bajaj)

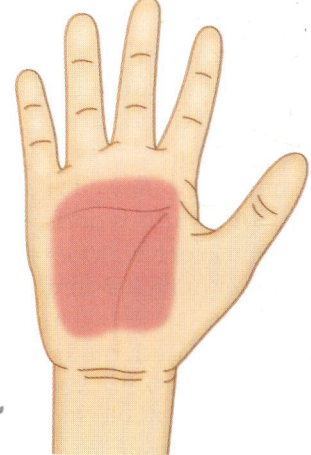

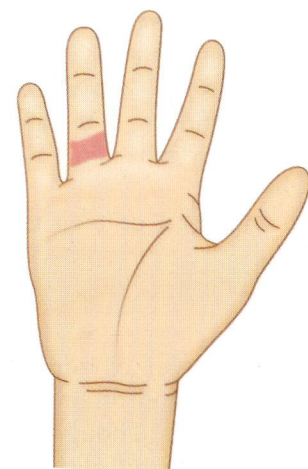

Fig. 3.15: Hand dermatitis displaying palmar grip pattern

Fig. 3.16: Negative image dermatitis due to a metal ring on the fourth finger

Table 3.6: Hand dermatitis—allergens with morphological patterns	
Product/allergen or irritant	Morphology
Rubber	
Gloves (latex and rubber additives)	Patchy distribution Favors **dorsal** hands and wrists
Rubber grip on mechanical pencil/pen	Seen near **distal phalanges** Corresponds with shape of offending product
Topical medicaments	
Topical antibiotics or corticosteroids	Chronic hand dermatitis refractory to treatment or flaring with treatment
Metals	
Escalator railing, metal bed rail	Seen on **palm** of hand Corresponds with shape of offending product
Handheld devices (cell phone, computer mouse, etc.)	Seen on **palm** of hand Corresponds with shape of offending product
Keys, coins, hand-held work tools with metal parts	Corresponds with shape of offending product
Ring	Encircles digit Annular pattern Corresponds with shape of offending product
Scissors, crochet hooks	Seen on fingers that hold instrument Corresponds with shape of offending product
Miscellaneous	
Artificial nails and/or nail polish	Periungal
Smoking pipe (uncommon in India)	Most often affects the thumb, index finger, and middle finger (digits 1–3) Varies according to individual preference for holding the smoking pipe

While systemic ingestion of foods high in nickel has been associated with dyshidrosis, hand dermatitis related to metals is more often due to the handling of metal-containing instruments or wearing metal jewellery (Fig. 3.16).

A list of common causes is listed in Table 3.6.

EXTREMITIES

The upper and lower extremities are in frequent movement and often make contact with the surroundings. Though contact may be brief or prolonged, this allows upper and lower extremities to be susceptible to many sources of irritants and allergens.

Wrists

Linear rashes encircling the wrist are suggestive of a contactant worn around that region for an extended period of time. Jewellery (Fig. 3.17a) and bangles (kara— Fig. 3.17b) are a common source and may elicit a reaction to either metal or exotic woods (Torres F). Individuals who wear watches may have a reaction to leather or nickel-containing straps (Goon AT) (Fig. 3.17c). There may be occupationally related rashes in rubber-sensitive individuals who frequently wear rubber bands around the wrist, such as post office workers. In children, exposure to nickel in identification bracelets would also be considered.

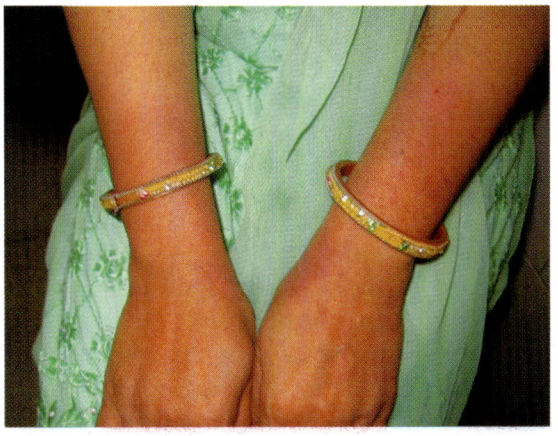
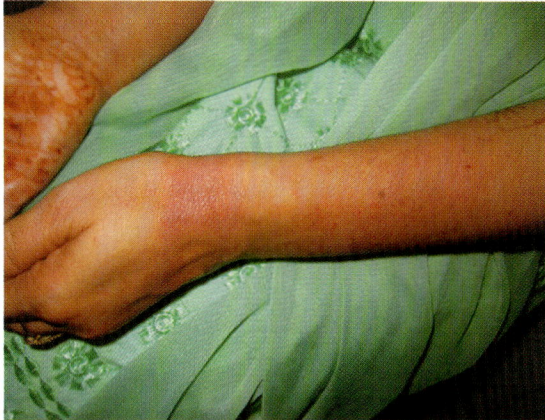

Fig. 3.17a: The new bangles laden with exotic colors, which are potent allergens, cause a dermatitis from the mid-forearm to the medial wrist as the bangles slide down to the wrist from the mid forearm

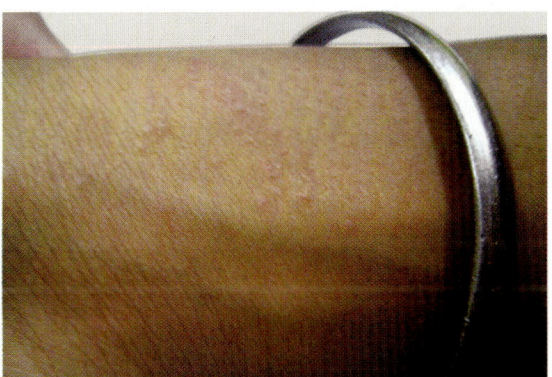

Fig. 3.17b: Nickle-induced bangle allergy

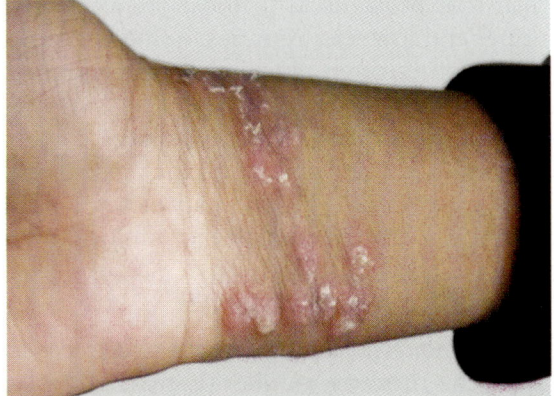

Fig. 3.17c: Papular dermatitis due to the nickel in the strap of an imitation "Omega" watch

Bilateral and symmetrical linear rashes that do not completely encircle the wrists in an individual who works in front of a computer for long periods of time is very suggestive of an irritation or allergic response to keyboard wrist pads and computer wrist rests (Yokota M). Exposure to black leather in workout gloves or the dye in the straps (due to the leather or dye) would also be considered.

Forearms

The forearms often rest upon various surfaces, leaving the forearm susceptible to linear rashes with a patchy distribution limited to the medial junction of the volar and extensor forearm surfaces. This presentation would be suggestive of contact dermatitis from worn-out foam, rubber, metal, or Japanese lacquered wood on certain surfaces of furniture such as chairs, sofas, and desktops. Bilateral involvement of the forearms has been reported due to occupational contact dermatitis from ethylene oxide that was used to sterilize green surgical cotton gowns.

Hypersensitivity to paraphenylenediamine (PPD) and related compounds induced by temporary black henna tattoos has become a serious health problem worldwide (Calogiuri G). Different patterns of sensitization with various clinical aspects are described in literature due to PPD associated to henna tattoo and these manifestations are likely correlated with the immunological and dermatological pathomechanisms involved. To make tattoos,

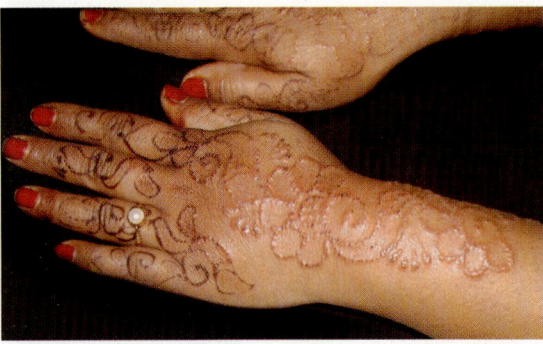

Fig. 3.18a: Black henna dermatitis (Dr AK Bajaj)

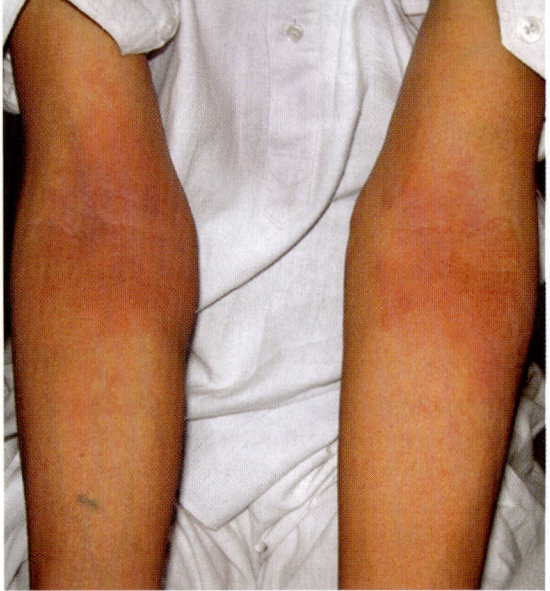

Fig. 3.18b: Intense flexural erythema in a case probably due to "finishers" of a newly bought shirt

darker and long-lasting, PPD has been associated to henna in tattoo drawings mixtures, so obtaining "black henna" (Fig. 3.18a). Occasionally flexures can be affected due to clotting (Fig. 3.18b).

Thighs

Although the thighs are often covered by articles of clothing, rashes may occur from the items within the pockets of the clothes. A nummular or coin-shaped rash on the anterior thigh in individuals who keep these objects in their pants pockets is very suggestive of an allergy to certain metals (e.g. nickel)

in keys and coins. The rashes are often unilateral, but bilateral cases have been reported in individuals who use two cell phones simultaneously.

A bilateral nummular rash on the posterior thighs in school-aged children is very suggestive of an allergy to metal in the bolts in certain types of seats. Individuals who made contact between the back of their legs and the metal chair rungs had linear rashes that spanned horizontally across the posterior region of the legs. This pattern below the calves under these circumstances is very suggestive of an allergy to the metal in the chair rungs.

Individuals with chronic leg ulcers are particularly susceptible to polysensitization to topical drugs and antiseptics used to treat their wounds and the surrounding skin. Positive tests were most frequently to balsam of Peru, fragrance, lanolin, and the lanolin derivative (Amerchol L). The duration of the ulcer influenced the patients' sensitization. Frequency of sensitization was 67.5% within 1 year and 79% within 1–10 years (Barbaud A).

Scattered Arms and Legs

One of the most commonly encountered presentations in the clinical setting is a skin rash that presents as a linear streak on the upper and lower extremities. In these cases, a brief history often reveals a recent camping trip or other outdoor activity. This characteristic linear pattern is typical of allergic contact dermatitis due to poison ivy or poison oak. The arms and leg can also exhibit sofa dermatitis, as explained in the trunk chapter.

Asymmetric Arm Involvement

Photocontact dermatitis occurs when certain allergens produce an allergic reaction upon sun exposure. The left arm is more likely to experience photocontact dermatitis than the right arm, although both may be involved. In North America, the left arm faces the driver's side window, and this sets up the unilateral preference. In India, the reverse is true thus

Table 3.7: Extremities—allergens with morphological patterns	
Product/allergen or irritant	Morphology
Wrists	
Jewellery (bracelets), wrist watches, identification bracelets (children), rubber band	Encircles wrist Linear pattern Corresponds with shape of offending product
Keyboard wrist pads, computer wrist rests	Patchy or linear distribution Corresponds with shape of offending product
Forearms	
Wheelchair, chair arms, desktops (worn-out foam, rubber, metal, Japanese lacquered wood)	Volar forearm Patchy distribution Corresponds with sites contacted by offending product
Thighs	
Coins, keys, matchboxes	Seen in anterior thigh region (pant's pockets) Nummular pattern (coins) Patchy distribution
Metal bolts in seats	Seen in posterior thigh region Nummular pattern Patchy distribution Corresponds with shape of offending product
Metal bar in school chairs (chair rungs)	Seen below the calves Linear or patchy Corresponds with sites contacted by offending product
Arms and legs	
Poison ivy, poison oak	Linear streaky pattern
Furniture (sofa, chairs)	Buttocks, back, dorsal upper thighs, and arms
Fragrances and preservatives (soaps and lotions)	Patchy dermatitis

the right arm is affected. Involvement on the dorsal aspects of the arm with sparing of covered regions is a clue to the diagnosis (Levin N).

A list of the common allergens is given in Table 3.7.

FEET

The feet can be affected by the irritant or allergen, which is absorbed by socks and the surrounding shoes. Wearing shoes is a common cultural practice and occurs almost daily for extended periods of time. Since shoes are not routinely washed and socks may be worn for extended periods of time, this allows prolonged exposure to potential irritants and allergens (Table 3.8).

Like the hand dermatitis involving the thinner dorsal skin is more likely to be contacted in nature. Since sources of contact irritants/allergens causing contact dermatitis of the feet are often more limited, *footwear* and *topical* agents are typically at the top of the differential for contactants (Nedorost S).

Shoe components have been found to be common allergens in both children and adults. Contact dermatitis due to shoewear can be symmetric or asymmetric, typically starting on the dorsal toes and gradually extending to the dorsum of the foot, sparing the interdigital

Table 3.8: Foot dermatitis—allergens with morphological patterns

Allergen	Morphology
Rubber Mercaptobenzothiazole (MBT), thiurams, and p-phenylenediamines	Patchy distribution
Leather Potassium dichromate	Patchy distribution Seen on dorsum of feet Corresponds with shape of offending product
Adhesives P-tert-butylphenol formaldehyde resin (PTBFR), colophony	Patchy distribution
Alta	CSM (Crocein Scarlet M 'brilliant crocein' and para-phenylenediamine (PPD)

folds (Fig. 3.19a and b). Typical allergens in *shoe* contact dermatitis include rubber *accelerators*, leather *tanning* agents, and *adhesives* (Rietschel RL). The most commonly reported rubber-related allergens are the accelerators, including mercaptobenzothiazole (MBT), thiurams, and p-phenylenediamines. More recently, Crocs ™ shoes, which have become very popular among physicians and other hospital staff over the past several years, were identified as a source of allergic contact dermatitis on the feet (Mortz CG). Other major footwear-related allergens are chromates, p-tert-butylphenol formaldehyde resin (PTBFR), colophony, and paraphenylenedia-mine (PPD). Chromates, such as potassium dichromate, are used in the leather tanning process, while PTBFR and colophony are common adhesives found in footwear (Warshaw EM). Dr AK Bajaj (1988) found that majority of the cases were chrome-positive, other causes being plastic material, rubber and rubber chemicals 1, 3-diphenylguanidine and N-cyclohexyl-2-benzothiazolesulfenamide. Patients will need to switch shoe types to avoid allergens, such as avoiding leather shoes, if there is a potassium dichromate allergy.

In India leukoderma (Fig. 3.20) is a common finding, which is also seen by other items

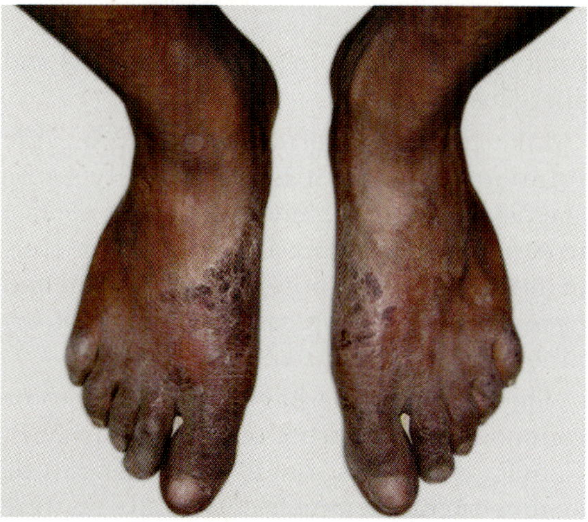

Fig. 3.19a: Symmetrical dermatitis on the dorsum of the foot

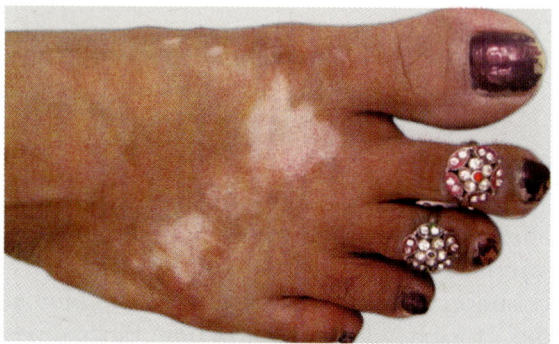

Fig. 3.19b: Contact leucoderma due to rubber chappals

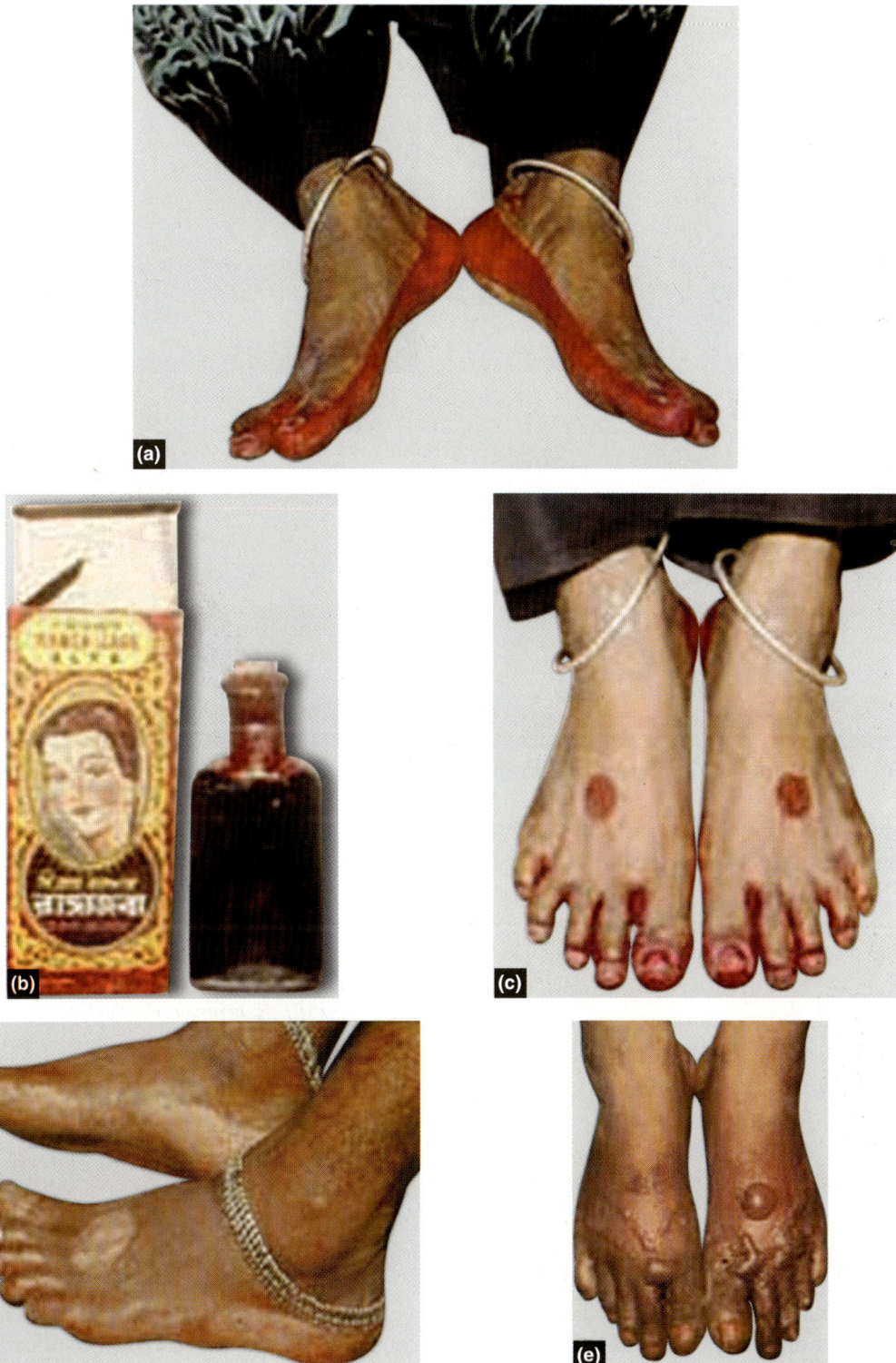

Fig. 3.20a to e: Chemical leukoderma consequent to use of 'alta' in female patients

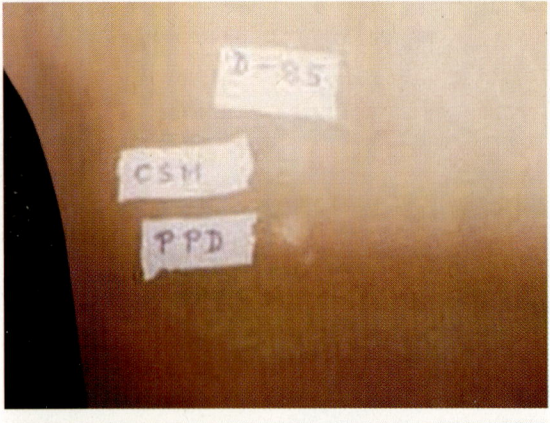
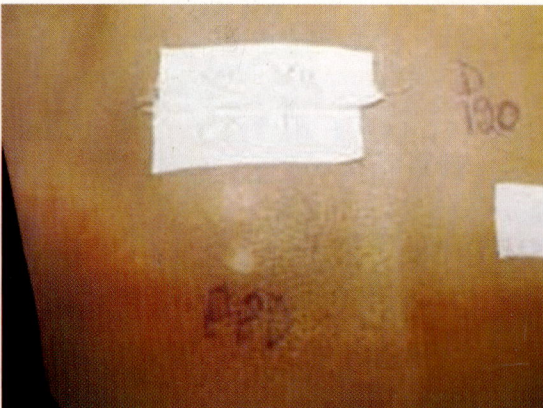
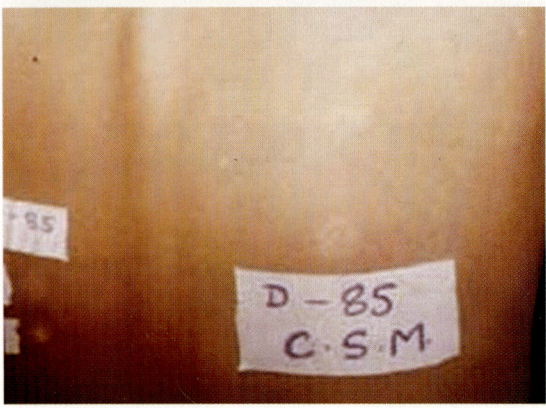
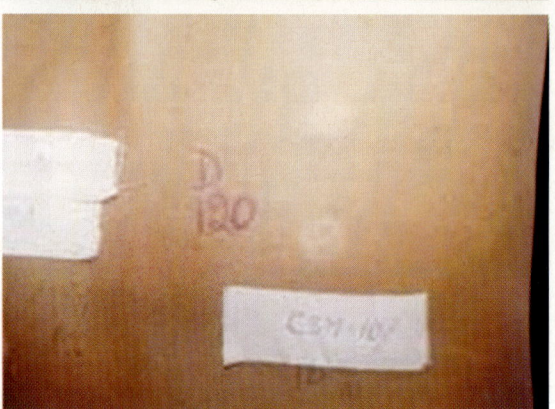

Fig. 3.20f: ACD with chemical leukoderma due to Alta. Postive patch test to both CSM and PPD

including sticker bindis, rain shoes, plastic chappals, hair dye/black henna (kali mehndi), alta, wallets and even mobile plastic covers (Bajaj AK, 2010). Alta has 2 dyes: Crocein Scarlet MOO (CSM) (brilliant crocein) and rhodamine B (tetraethyl rhodamine) which can cause leukoderma (Fig. 3.20b).

In the case of topical antifungals and topical corticosteroids, the patient more often is reacting to the vehicle rather than the active ingredient itself. Expanded patch testing is helpful in determining the precise allergen.

TRUNK

Certain allergens have classical presentations on the trunk (Table 3.9). *Nickel* is one of the most common allergens, and it is often the source of contact dermatitis on the trunk (Wentworth AB). Nickel that exists in belt buckles, buttons on jeans, navel rings, backpack or handbag straps, or clasps of bras will present in a classic distribution with a localized eruption at the site of contact (Fig. 3.21a). It can also present as dermatitis on the buttocks or groin/anterior thighs from putting metal objects such as keys, coins, or cell phones in the pockets. Nickel can also cause a unilateral eruption of the left chest in men from objects (such as a cigarette lighter) kept in the left breast shirt pocket. When an allergy on the trunk due to nickel is identified, it may also be present in other classic locations such as the wrist from a watchband or earlobes or neck from earrings.

An allergy to *deodorants* will also present in a classical distribution in the axilla. The most common allergens present in deodorants are fragrance, propylene glycol, essential oils and biological additives, and parabens (Zirwas MJ).

Table 3.9: Truncal dermatitis—allergens with morphological patterns

Allergen	Morphology
Nickel	
• Belt buckle	• Often localized to site of contact
• Buttons/clasps	• Discrete eczematous patches, vesicles may be present
• Jewellery (necklace, navel ring)	
• Coins/keys	
Clothing	
• Textiles	• Patchy distribution
• Dyes	• Diffuse eczematous dermatitis
• Melamine formaldehyde	
• Resins	
• Detergents/fabric softeners	
• Fragrance	
• Preservatives	
• Dyes	
Personal hygiene product	
• Soaps, moisturizers	• Patchy distribution
• Preservatives	• Diffuse eczematous dermatitis (except in the case of deodorants where the eruption will be localized to the axilla)
• Fragrances/botanicals	
• Deodorants	
• Fragrance	
• Propylene glycol	

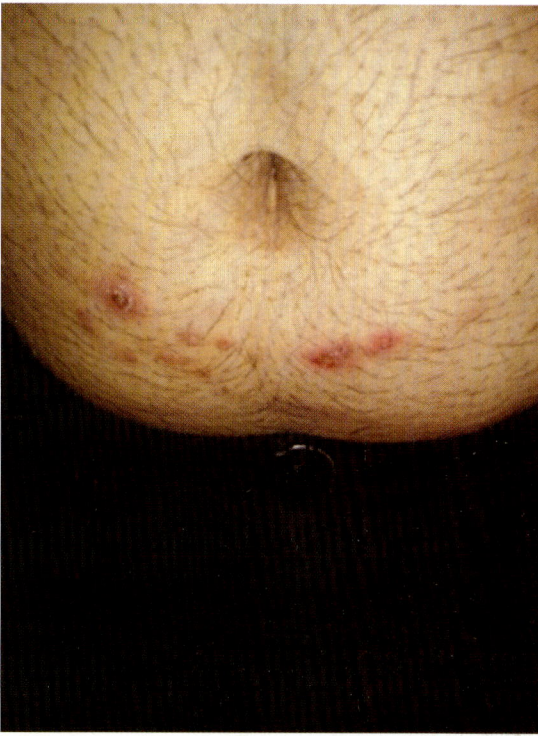

Fig. 3.21a: Recurring rash on the trunk with a marked predilection for the belt line. This rash was triggered by tinned food, including fish and dry fruits. Nickel free diet was advised

Preservatives and fragrances are the most common allergens in personal hygiene products such as soaps and moisturizers, as well as in laundry detergents and fabric softeners (Wetter DA). Here the presentation may be a more *diffuse* eruption with less discrete erythematous papules or eczematous patches and plaques. It may be difficult to distinguish such eruptions from atopic dermatitis or irritant dermatitis.

Clothing is a common source of allergens; aside from the detergent or softener being used for washing, the textiles themselves can be the source. The pattern of distribution with textile contact dermatitis is generally increased in areas of friction and perspiration (Brookstein DS). The dyes used in manufacturing textiles are most frequently responsible (average prevalence was highest for disperse blue 106 and disperse blue 124), however, formaldehyde and resins are also common, especially in instances of occupational textile contact dermatitis. In one study, nearly 6% of patients who underwent patch testing were reactive to p-phenylenediamine, a black dye which is the traditional textile allergen used in the standard series (Wentworth AB).

Contact dermatitis on the back can be related to objects that patients lean against when seated. Hexavalent chromium and azo dyes have been identified as allergens present in leather chair and sofa backs, while Japanese lacquer can be the responsible allergen on wood surfaces.

An outbreak of "sofa dermatitis" was linked to dimethyl fumarate (DMF), a compound found in both leather and fabric

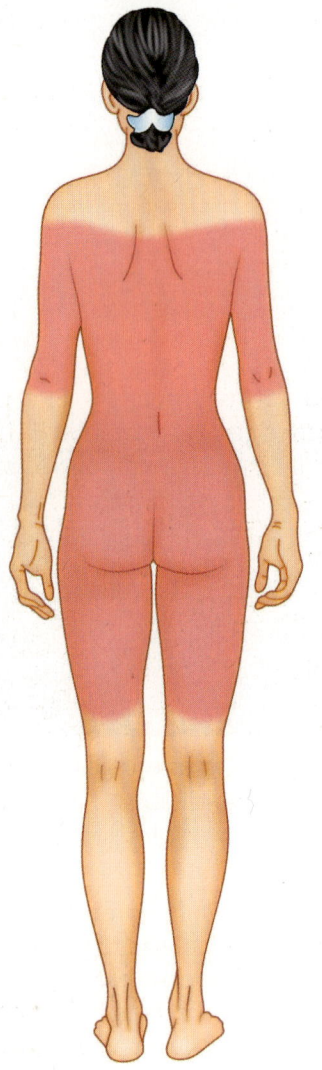

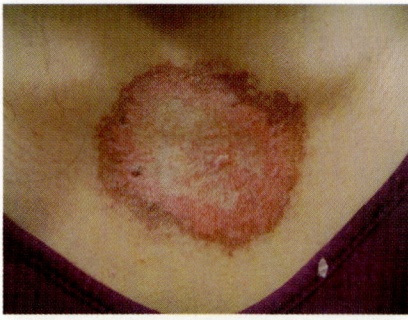

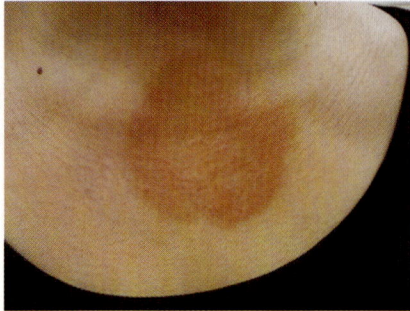

Fig. 3.21b: Pattern of sofa dermatitis

Fig. 3.22: This patient was applying a topical antibiotic cream (Neosporin) with progressive aggravation of her dermatitis. The patient asked to apply mupirocin acid ointment with Vaseline and administered a short course of oral steroids

sofas made by a Chinese manufacturer (Ma XM). This allergen was responsible for contact dermatitis, in some cases severe, of the trunk, buttocks, and lower extremity (Fig. 3.21b). This epidemic of furniture dermatitis was notable in that it led to DMF being selected as the 2011 Allergen of the Year by the American Contact Dermatitis Society (Bruze M).

As is the case some cases are essentially contact medicamentosa. An aggravation of a rash that is normally responsive to a cream, is suggestive of an allergy to the base or the compound (Figs 3.22 and 3.23).

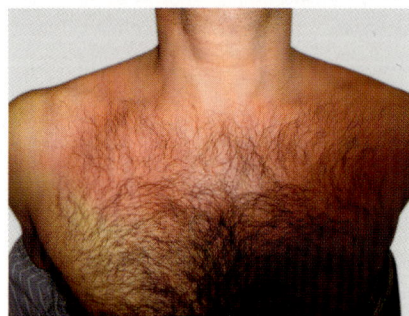

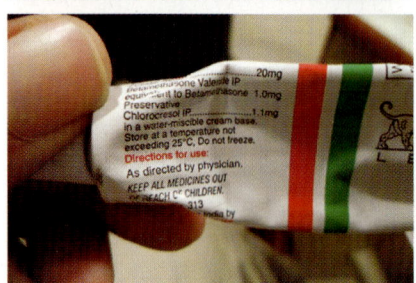

Fig. 3.23: This patient was given a topical steroid for a photoburn but the condition worsened. The steroid cream was changed to an ointment. The cause was "chlorocresol", a preservative added to this topical cream

ANOGENITAL REGION

Similar to the eyelid region, the anogenital region is intrinsically prone to irritation and sensitization. Parallels are seen in the fact that both regions have thin epidermal barriers and show a tendency for irritant/allergen retention. The anogenital region differs from other regions in that there is also a high degree of friction, heat, and moisture.

Similar to other regions, it is important to consider both irritant and allergic contact dermatitis. Barrier creams, management of incontinence, and the removal of any harsh irritants are important aspects in controlling anogenital irritant dermatitis.

Data collected by the North American Contact Dermatitis Group have been reviewed with regard to patients with anogenital dermatitis who were referred for patch testing. Of the 575 patients with anogenital dermatitis who underwent patch testing, 347 had isolated anogenital disease. After patch testing, 73 patients were classified as having isolated allergic anogenital dermatitis. In this group, the most common allergens were cosmetics, medicaments, and corticosteroids (Warshaw EM).

A high index of suspicion is required for the possibility of contact dermatitis medicamentosa in the anogenital region, especially in the setting of a dermatitis that is not responding as expected to conventional therapies. In this setting, particular emphasis should be placed on searching for exposure to topical anesthetics, antibiotics, antiseptics, and preservatives (Table 3.10).

Buttocks

An isolated annular rash on the buttocks and posterior thighs is nearly pathognomonic for contact dermatitis to a component in toilet seats. Exposure to wooden toilet seats and associated varnish, lacquers, and paints has been reported to result in ACD (Litvinov IV). This characteristic pattern of allergic contact dermatitis in the buttocks region is known as "**toilet seat**" dermatitis (Fig. 3.24). Toilet seats can also retain irritants and allergens from cleansers. These include formaldehyde.

Diaper dermatitis affects the area covered by the diaper and is most often irritant in nature. A secondary infection with *Candida* should also be considered. A clue to ACD secondary to diaper components is an eczematous dermatitis that spares the skinfolds and is refractory to conventional therapies for diaper dermatitis. Allergens to consider in this setting include fragrances utilized to provide a pleasant odor to the diaper, coloring dyes, glues, and rubber-related allergens; it is also important to

Allergen	Morphology
Table 3.10: Anogenital dermatitis—allergens with morphological patterns	
Buttocks Toilet seats Referred to as "toilet seat dermatitis"	Seen on buttocks/proximal posterior thighs, annular pattern, corresponds with shape of seat
Diapers Referred to as "allergic contact diaper dermatitis"	Seen in diaper region, spares bottom of skin folds
Perianal Moistened toilet paper (wet wipes)	Patchy distribution
Vulvar Medicaments, condoms, perfumes	Patchy distribution
Penile Medicaments, condom	Patchy distribution along the areas covered by the condom

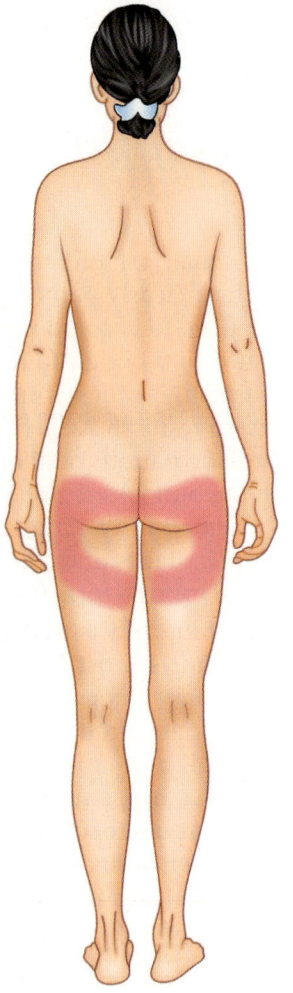

Fig. 3.24: Toilet seat dermatitis

consider wet wipes, which are often used during the diaper-changing process. For dermatitis that favors the hips and lateral buttocks, rubber accelerators such as mercaptobenzothiazole should be considered. This pattern has been referred to as the "Lucky Luke" dermatitis and is a subset of allergic contact diaper dermatitis in which the child is reacting to the elastic bands found in disposable diapers (Roul S).

Perianal Region

With rashes involving the perianal regions, exposure to perfumed and/or colored toilet paper should be considered. Wet wipes has

led to an increase in the number of cases of ACD due to the presence of certain preservatives and fragrances in this consumer product (Zoli V). Another cause is 'caine' allergy (Figs 3.25 to 3.27).

Vulvar Region

The vulvar region is susceptible to the same factors as the general anogenital region. However, estrogen is integral to maintaining the strength and integrity of the vulvar barrier to potential irritants and allergens. Therefore, it is during stages of estrogen deficiency that the barrier is most compromised, thereby leading to susceptibility to both irritant and allergic contact dermatitis. As is always the general rule, the most common type of vulvar contact dermatitis is irritant in nature. Common causes of irritant contact dermatitis include urine, feces, sweat, topical medications, aggressive cleansing, and feminine hygiene products.

Common causes of allergic contact dermatitis include topical medicaments (such as anesthetics, antibiotics, antifungals, antiseptics, and corticosteroids), latex condoms, and perfumes (Schad K).

Reports have also indicated that flavorings and spices may contribute to contact dermatitis in the vulvar region. This presentation is rare but can be seen in a patient who is reacting to

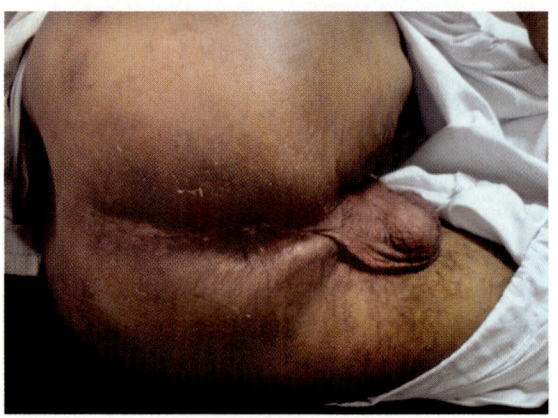

Fig. 3.25: Perianal allergy
(*Courtesy:* Dr PK Srivastava, Dr AK Bajaj)

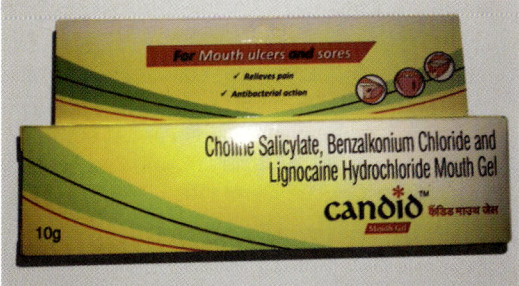

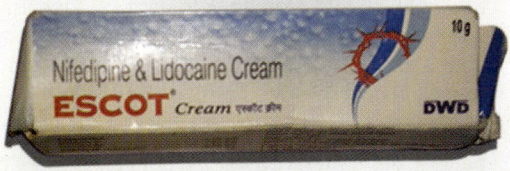

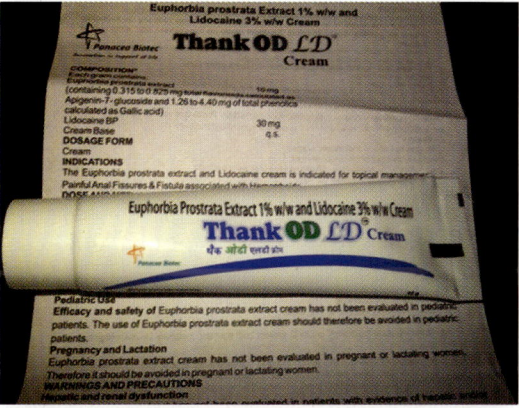

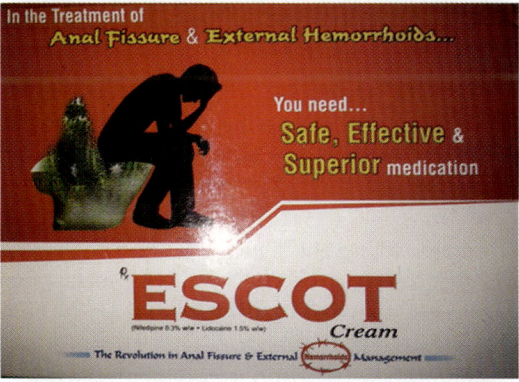

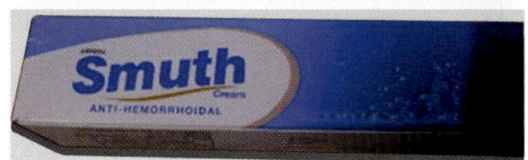

Fig. 3,26: Commonly products used in the perianal region (*Courtesy:* Dr PK Srivastava, Dr AK Bajaj)

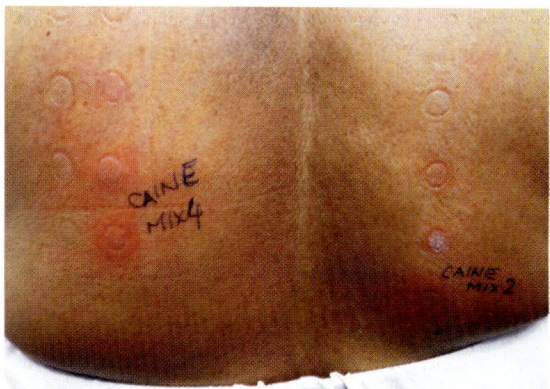

Fig. 3.27: Positive caine mix
(*Courtesy:* Dr PK Srivastava, Dr AK Bajaj)
Almost 70% of allergic reactions to local anesthetics would have been missed if benzocaine had been used as a screening allergen. A study supports the recommendation to replace benzocaine with a caine mix containing cinchocaine in the baseline patch test series. (Brinca A, Cabral R, Gonçalo M. Contact allergy to local anaesthetics-value of patch testing with a caine mix in the baseline series. Contact Dermatitis. 2013 Mar;68(3):156–62.)

allergens that are excreted in the urine and/ or feces. The classic example would be a patient with sensitivity to balsam of Peru, which is a marker not only for fragrance sensitivity but also for flavorings and spices. Therefore, it is important to keep in mind that not only locally applied products may lead to contact dermatitis.

Penile Region

The foreskin may facilitate the retention and absorption of allergens and eventually play a role in the development of ACD. There is some evidence that circumcision may decrease the risk of inflammatory dermatoses of the anogenital area.

Similar to other areas in the anogenital region, a study by NACDG concluded the most common allergens consisted of fragrances, preservatives, medications, vehicles, and corticosteroids. There should be careful inspection for potential contactants. For example, condoms to increase sexual performance may contain benzocaine gel, which is a known potential contact allergen. Reports indicate ACD has resulted from latex proteins, rubber accelerators, and antioxidants in condoms. Related personal products such as lubricants, dyes, creams, and powders may also contain potential allergens.

CONCLUSIONS

It is said that contact dermatitis is a great mimicker. A host of varied manifestations are seen in contact dermatitis and they can mimic many other disorders (Tables 3.1 to 3.10). Though conventionally syphilis and sarcoidosis are considered as the great mimickers, it has been our experience that contact dermatitis is probably much more common. The shift of dermatology to the "trivial" and passing focus on cosmetology has denigrated our intelligence to the art of "superficial" therapy that was once the domain of beauticians. The plethora of OTC products in addition to beautician administered products has added to the array of dermatoses caused by contact allergy.

Ideally, if a dermatologist is able to identify the patterns of contact dermatitis, this correlates largely with the objects used. Simple avoidance can solve the dermatosis. Can anything be more simple than this in dermatological management? Hopefully the regional listing (Tables 3.2 to 3.10) given here will help the clinician focus on the likely causes, as the "eye will only see, if the mind knows".

Bibliography

1. Bajaj AK, Gupta SC, Chatterjee AK, Singh KG. Shoe dermatitis in India. Contact Dermatitis 1988 Nov;19(5):372–5.

2. Bajaj AK, Gupta SC, Chatterjee AK. Contact depigmentation from free para-tertiary-butylphe-nol in bindi adhesive. Contact Dermatitis 1990 Feb;22(2):99–102.

3. Bajaj AK, Pandey RK, Misra K, Chatterji AK, Tiwari A, Basu S. Contact depigmentation caused by an azo dye in alta. Contact Dermatitis 1998 Apr; 38(4):189–93.

4. Bajaj AK, Saraswat A, Srivastav PK. Chemical leucoderma: Indian scenario, prognosis, and treatment. Indian J Dermatol 2010 Jul-Sep;55(3): 250–4.

5. Barbaud A, Collet E, Le Coz CJ, Meaume S, Gillois P. 2009. Contact allergy in chronic leg ulcers: Results of a multicentre study carried out in 423 patients and proposal for an updated series of patch tests. Contact Dermatitis 60(5):279–287.

6. Baxter KF, Wilkinson SM. Contact dermatitis from a nickel-containing bindi. Contact Dermatitis 2002 Jul;47(1):55.

7. Bregnbak D, Johansen JD, Jellesen MS, Zachariae C, Menné T, Thyssen JP. Chromium allergy and dermatitis: prevalence and main findings. Contact Dermatitis 2015 Nov;73(5):261–80.

8. Brookstein DS. Factors associated with textile pattern dermatitis caused by contact allergy to dyes, finishes, foams, and preservatives. Dermatol Clin 2009;2009;27(3):309–322, vi-vii.

9. Bruze M, Zimerson E. Dimethyl fumarate. Dermatitis 2011;22(1):3–7.

10. Calogiuri G, Di Leo E, Butani L, Pizzimenti S, Incorvaia C, Macchia L, Nettis E. Hypersensitivity reactions due to black henna tattoos and their components: are the clinical pictures related to the immune pathomechanism? Clin Mol Allergy 2017 Apr 10;15:8.

11. Castanedo-Tardan MP, Zug KA. Patterns of cosmetic contact allergy. Dermatologic Clinics 2009;27(3):265–230.

12. Castanedo-Tardan MP, Zug KA. Patterns of cosmetic contact allergy. Dermatologic Clinic 2009;27(3):265–230.

13. Clinical Handbook of Contact Dermatitis: Diagnosis and Management by Body Region 1st Edition by Robin Lewallen (Editor),? Adele Clark (Editor)? Steven R. Feldman (Editor). CRC Press, 2015.

14. Corazza M, Borghi A, Ricci M, Sarno O, Virgili A. Patch testing in allergic contact dermatitis from minoxidil. Dermatitis 2010 Jul-Aug;21(4):217–8.

15. García-Gavín J, González-Vilas D, Fernández-Redondo V, Toribio J. Pigmented contact dermatitis due to kojic acid. A paradoxical side effect of a skin lightener. Contact Dermatitis 2010 Jan;62(1):63–4.

16. Gawkrodger D. Investigation of reactions to dental materials. Br J Dermatol 2005;153(3):479–485.

17. Goon AT, Goh CL. Metal allergy in Singapore. Contact Dermatitis 2005;52(3):130–132.

18. Handa S, Mahajan R, De D. Contact dermatitis to hair dye: an update. Indian J Dermatol Venereol Leprol 2012 Sep-Oct;78(5):583–90.

19. Hillen U, Grabbe S, Uter W. Patch test results in patients with scalp dermatitis: Analysis of data of the Information Network of Departments of Dermatology. Contact Dermatitis 2007;56:87–93.

20. Jacob SE, Castanedo-Tardan MP. A diagnostic pearl in allergic contact dermatitis to fragrances: The atomizer sign. Cutis 2008;82(5):317–318.

21. James WD, Berger TG, Elston D, eds. Andrews' Diseases of the Skin: Clinical Dermatology, 11th edition. Philadelphia: WB Sanders, 2010.

22. Jensen P, Johansen UB, Johansen JD, Thyssen JP. Nickel may be released fromiPhone(®) 5. Contact Dermatitis 2013 Apr;68(4):255–6.

23. Kind F, Sherer K, Bircher A. Allergic contact stomatitis to cinnamon in chewing gum mistaken as facial angioedema. Allergy 2010;65(2):274–280.

24. Koh D, Lee BL, Ong HY, Ong CN, Wong WK, Ng SK, Goh CL. Colophony in bindi adhesive. Contact Dermatitis 1995 Mar;32(3):186.

25. Kozuka I, Goh CL, Doi T, Yioshikawa K. Sudan I as a cause of pigmented contact dermatitis in "kumkum" (an Indian cosmetic). Ann Acad Med Singapore 1988 Oct;17(4):492–4.

26. Laxmisha C, Nath AK, Thappa DM. Bindi dermatitis due to thimerosal and gallate mix. J Eur Acad Dermatol Venereol 2006 Nov;20(10):1370–2.

27. Lazarov A. Sensitization to acrylates is a common adverse reaction to artificial fingernails. Journal of European Academy of Dermatology and Venereology 2007;21(2):169–174.

28. Lee PW, Elsaie ML, Jacob SE. Allergic contact dermatitis in children: Common allergens and treatment. A review. Curr Opin Pediatr 2009; 21(4):491–498.

29. Levin N. Rash on the upper arm. Geriatrics 2003; 58(8):16.

30. Litvinov IV, Sugathan P, Cohen BA. Recognizing and treating toilet-seat contact dermatitis in children. Pediatrics 2010;125(2):e419-422. doi: 10.1542/peds.2009-2430. Epub 2010 Jan 25.

31. Ma XM, Lu R, Miyakoshi T. Recent advances in research on lacquer allergy. AllergoInt 2012; 61(1):45–50.

32. Morris-Jones R, Robertson SJ, Ross JS, White IR, McFadden JP, Rycroft RJ. Dermatitis caused by physical irritants. Br J Dermatol 2002;147(2):270–275.

33. Mortz CG, Andersen KE. New aspects in allergic contact dermatitis. Current Opinion in Allergy and Clinical Immunology 2008;8(5):428–432.

34. Nath AK, Thappa DM. Kumkum-induced dermatitis: an analysis of 46 cases. Clin Exp Dermatol. 2007 Jul;32(4):385–7.

35. Nedorost S. Clinical patterns of hand and foot dermatitis: Emphasis on rubber and chromate allergens. Dermatologic Clinics 2009;27(3):281–287.

36. Onder M, Aksakal AB, Oztas MO, Gurer MA. Skin problems of a musician. International Journal of Dermatology 1999;38(3):192–195.

37. Orton DI, Salim A, Shaw S. Allergic contact cheilitis due to shellac. Contact Dermatitis 2001; 44(4):250.

38. Rietschel RL, Fowler JF, Fisher AA. Fisher's Contact Dermatitis, 5th edition. Philadelphia: Lippincott Williams & Wilkins, 2001.

39. Rietschel RL, Warshaw EM, Sasseville D, Fowler JF, DeLeo VA, Belsito DV, et al. Common contact allergens associated with eyelid dermatitis: Data from the North American Contact Dermatitis Group 2003-2004 Study Period. Dermatitis 2007; 18(2):78–81.

40. Ringborg E, Lidén C, Julander A. Nickel on the market: a baseline survey of articles in 'prolonged contact' with skin. Contact Dermatitis. 2016 Aug; 75(2):77–81.

41. Rodríguez-Martin M, Sáez-Rodríguez M, Carnerero-Rodríguez A, Cabrera de Paz R, Sidro-Sarto M, Pérez-Robayna N, et al. Pustular allergic contact dermatitis from topical minoxidil 5%. Journal of the European Academy of Dermatology & Venereology 2007;21(5):701–702.

42. Roul S, Ducombs G, Léauté-Labrèze C, Taïeb A. 'Lucky Luke' contact dermatitis due to rubber components of diapers. Contact Dermatitis 1998;38(6):363–364.

43. Schad K, Nobbe S, French LE, Ballmer-Weber B. Sofa dermatitis. Journal der Deutschen Dermatologischen Gesellschaft 2010;8(11):897-899. doi: 10.1111/j.1610-0387.2010.07386.x.

44. Schlosser BJ. Lichen planus and lichenoid reactions of the oral mucosa. Dermatol Ther 2010; 23(3): 251–267.

45. Sheard C. Electronic Textbook of Dermatology, Contact Dermatitis. Internet Dermatology Society, 1997 Available at: http://telemedicine.org/contact.htm. Accessed July 2, 2011.

46. Spring S, Pratt M, Chaplin A. Contact dermatitis to topical medicaments: A retrospective chart review from the Ottawa Hospital Patch Test Clinic. Dermatitis 2012;23(5):210–213.

47. Tewary M, Ahmed I. Bindi dermatitis to 'chandan' bindi. Contact Dermatitis 2006 Dec;55(6):372–4.

48. Torchia D, Giorgini S, Gola M, Francalanci S. Allergic contact dermatitis from 2-ethylhexyl acrylate contained in a wig-fixing adhesive tape and its 'incidental' therapeutic effect on alopecia areata. Contact Dermatitis 2008;58(3): 170–171.

49. Torres F, Maria das Graças M, Melo M, Tosti A. Management of contact dermatitis due to nickel allergy: An update. Clinical, Cosmetic and Investigational Dermatology 2009;2:39–48.

50. Tremblay S, Avon SL. Contact allergy to cinnamon: A case report. J Can Dent Assoc 2008l;74(5):445–461.

51. Valsecchi R, Imberti D, Martino D, et al. Eyelid dermatitis: An evaluation of 150 patients. Contact Dermatitis 1992;27:143–147.

52. Warshaw EM, Furda LM, Maibach HI, et al. Anogenital dermatitis in patients referred for patch testing: Retrospective analysis of cross-sectional data from the North American Contact Dermatitis Group, 1994-2004. Arch Dermatol 2008;144(6): 749–755.

53. Warshaw EM, Schram SE, Belsito DV, DeLeo VA, Fowler JF, Maibach HI, et al. Shoe allergens: Retrospective analysis of cross-sectional data from the North American Contact Dermatitis Group, 2001-2004. Dermatitis 2009;18(4):191–202.

54. Wentworth AB, Richardson DM, Davis MD. Patch testing with textile allergens: The Mayo Clinic experience. Dermatitis 2012;23(6):269–274.

55. Wentworth AB, Yiannias JA, Keeling JH, et al. Trends in patch-test results and allergen changes in the standard series: A Mayo Clinic 5-year retrospective review (January 1, 2006, to December 31, 2010). J Am AcadDermatol 2014;70(2): 269–275.

56. Wetter DA, Yiannias JA, Prakash AV, Davis MD, Farmer SA, el-Azhary RA. Results of patch testing to personal care product allergens in a standard series and a supplemental cosmetic series: An analysis of 945 patients from the Mayo Clinic Contact Dermatitis Group, 2000-2007. Journal of the American Academy of Dermatology 2010; 63(5):789–798.

57. Wetter DA, Yiannias JA, Prakash AV, et al. Results of patch testing to personal care product allergens in a standard series and a supplemental cosmetic series: An analysis of 945 patients from the Mayo Clinic Contact Dermatitis Group, 2000-2007. J Am Acad Dermatol 2010;63(5):789–798.

58. Yokota M, Fox LP, Maibach HI. Bilateral palmar dermatitis possible caused by computer wrist rest. Contact Dermatitis 2007;57(3):192–193.

59. Zirwas MJ, Moennich J. Antiperspirant and deodorant allergy: Diagnosis and management. J Clin Aesthet Dermatol 2008;1(3):38–43.

60. Zoli V, Tosti A, Silvani S, Vincenzi C. Moist toilet papers as possible sensitizers: Review of the literature and evaluation of commercial products in Italy. Contact Dermatitis 2006;55(4):252–254.

B. ALLERGIC CONTACT DERMATITIS

Taru Garg, Seema Rani, Soumya Agarwal

The term 'allergie' was first coined by the scientist von Pirquet in 1906 (Adams RM, 1983). The word was derived from the Greek *allos* and *ergon*, meaning other or different work (Ayto J, 1990). Contact dermatitis accounts for 4–7% of all dermatological consultations. Of all contact dermatitis cases, around 20% are caused by allergic contact dermatitis (ACD). It represents the classic cutaneous presentation of delayed type hypersensitivity response to exogenous antigens.

Definition

ACD can be defined as a delayed type IV allergic reaction of the skin presenting with varying degrees of erythema, edema, and vesiculation resulting from cutaneous contact with a specific allergen.

Epidemiology

ACD affects approximately 7% of the general population (Heine G *et al*, 2004). An Indian study reported positive patch test reactions in 50% of the patients (Sharma VK *et al*, 2010). Nickel sulfate was the most common sensitizer (43.7%), followed by fragrance mix (18.6%), paraben mix, potassium dichromate, cobalt, and formaldehyde. Westernization of lifestyle in India has resulted in an increased exposure to cosmetics, hair and other dyes, and packaged food.

Pathogenesis

Allergic contact dermatitis involves two main processes of sensitization (afferent or induction phase), and elicitation (efferent or challenge phase) (Flowchart 3.1). Most contact allergens/antigens are haptens (simple chemicals) with a molecular weight of 500–1000 daltons, so that they can penetrate the skin easily and combine with a carrier protein to produce contact hypersensitivity. The induction of sensitivity is the primary event which is initiated by binding of allergens to skin components, and association of these products

Flowchart 3.1: Pathogenesis of allergic contact dermatitis

Allergen + skin components → Recognition by T lymphocytes → Proliferation of specific CD8+ and CD4+ lymphocytes [Sensitization phase] → Re-exposure to specific allgergen → Local reaction [Elicitation phase]

with major histocompatibility complex (MHC) class II molecules (Lepoittevin J-P, 2006). These complete or conjugated antigens are recognized by lymphocytes in the presence of other co-stimulatory molecules such as IL-1α, TNF-β, and GM-CSF. This is followed by the proliferation of antigen-specific cytotoxic CD8+ and also CD4+ (Th1) lymphocytes (Kimber I *et al*, 2002). These T lymphocytes disseminate via the efferent lymphatics throughout the body and interact with Langerhans' cells and residual antigen in the skin. When a sensitised person is re-exposed to the specific allergen, reaction between the allergen residues and the sensitised T lymphocytes leads to elicitation of local reaction, termed as 'late' reaction.

Predisposing Factors (Flowchart 3.2)

Flowchart 3.2: Predisposing factors of allergic contact dermatitis

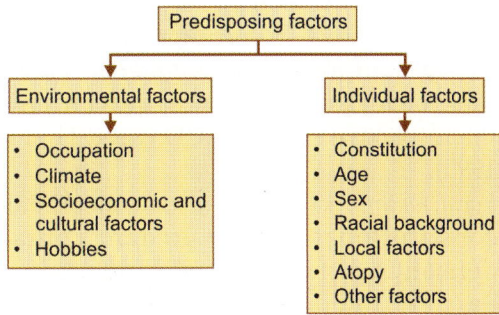

Individual Factors

1. *Constitution*: The capacity for sensitization varies individually, but some persons are more prone to develop sensitivity to a particular substance. Susceptibility to contact allergens may be a genetically determined trait (Menné T *et al*, 1986). On the contrary, studies on twins with hand eczema and nickel allergy indicate that environmental rather than genetic factors are important (Bryld LE *et al*, 2004).

2. *Age*: It has a little influence on capacity for sensitization (Kwangsukstith C *et al*, 1995). The inflammatory response decreases with increasing age. But the number of positive patch-test reactions tends to increase with age (Berit CC *et al*, 2007), due to the accumulation of allergies. Young adults are more likely to have occupational or cosmetic allergies, whereas elderly people are more liable to medicament (Green CM *et al*, 2007) and 'historic' sensitivities.

3. *Sex*: Gender differences in the development of ACD are largely unknown. Female preponderance in clinical patch-test studies can be explained by exposure (Modjtahedi BS *et al*, 2004); for example, the large number of metal sensitive females, is a result of ear piercing (Peltonen L *et al*, 1989), and the greater exposure to fragrances, cosmetics and hair dyes.

4. *Racial background*: Some differences in prevalence of sensitization to individual allergens among racial groups have been observed, but this could be a reflection of exposure rather than predisposition (Deleo VA *et al*, 2002). Some reports implicate darker skin to have a heightened barrier function for a few substances thus lowering the respective risk for ACD (Reed JT *et al*, 1995).

5. *Local factors*: Pre-existing or concomitant constitutional and/or irritant contact dermatitis damages the skin, affecting its barrier function and increasing per-cutaneous absorption of allergens and secondary sensitization. Hand eczema predisposes to nickel sensitivity and vice versa (Menné T *et al*, 1982), and the prevalence of chromate, cobalt and balsam sensitivity is increased in men with hand eczema (Wilkinson DS *et al*, 1970). Occlusion greatly promotes percutaneous absorption and contributes to the high incidence of medicament dermatitis in stasis eczema, otitis externa and perianal dermatitis, and is also a factor in dermatitis from shoes and rubber gloves.

   Many drugs may cause contact dermatitis with eczema after topical administration, presumably through type IV hyper-sensitivity mechanism. Medications that may cause eczema through systemic administration include penicillin, bleomycin and gold (Bruce T. Ryhal).

6. *Atopy*: The relationship of atopy, particularly atopic eczema, predisposition to allergic contact dermatitis is not clear. Atopics exhibit down-regulation of Th1 cells, which should result in a decreased tendency to develop ACD. However, clinical studies are conflicting, some showing an increase in prevalence of contact allergy, especially to medicaments (Brandmann HJ *et al*, 1972), others the same (Cronin E *et al*, 1970) or a decrease (Hanifin JH, 1982).

7. *Other factors*: Hormones may have some effect on ACD. Contact dermatitis may flare premenstrually, with patch-test reactivity to nickel being less intense during the ovulatory than the progestagenic phase (Bonamonte D *et al*, 2005). Drugs may also have an influence on ACD. Antihistamines have a little effect, whereas prednisolone (dose >15 mg/day), potent topical steroids (Moed H *et al*, 2004), immunosuppressants like azathioprine, cyclosporine, and UVB or psoralen UVA (PUVA) therapy suppress allergic patch-test reactions. Patients with acute or debilitating diseases like cancer, Hodgkin's disease and mycosis fungoides, have impaired capacity for contact sensitiza-tion (Grossman J *et al*, 1975).

Environmental Factors

1. *Occupation*: Occupational ACD is a common occurrence, and frequently complicates occupational irritant contact dermatitis. Individuals involved in carpet and footwear industry are exposed to various allergens like leather, formaldehyde, rubber (Fig. 3.28a), and dyeing agents.

2. *Climate*: Several factors like varying UV exposure, heat and relative humidity influence the seasonal liability to contact dermatitis. UVB exposure diminishes the skin's immune response to contact allergens. Seasonal variation of the lesions may point towards a plant allergen or photoaggravation or photoallergy (Fig. 3.28b).

3. *Socioeconomic and cultural factors*: Exposure to cheap (nickel releasing) metals used as jewellery is relatively higher in those with less disposable income. Similarly, the pattern of perfume and cosmetic exposure might vary according to social class. Cultural factors are also important, for example, hair dyes are used much more commonly by men in the Indian subcontinent, including use on the beard, Indian women may become sensitized to dyes and adhesives used in kumkum and bindi applied to the forehead (Dwyer CM *et al*, 1994) (Fig. 3.28c). The frequency of tattooing and body piercing has increased amongst young adults, thereby increasing their risk of contact with potential allergens including nickel and p-phenylenediamine (Fig. 3.29).

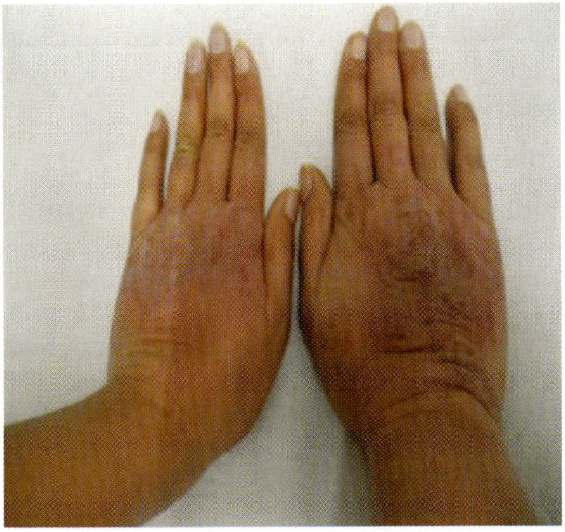

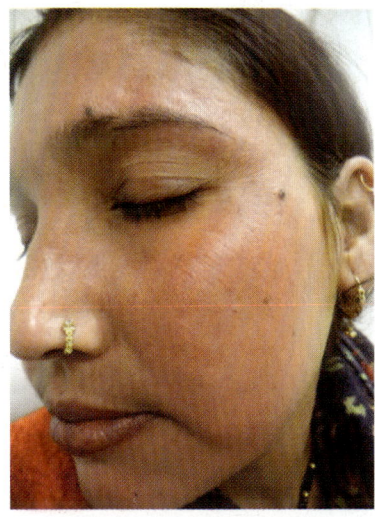

Fig. 3.28b: Allergic contact dermatitis with photo-aggravation

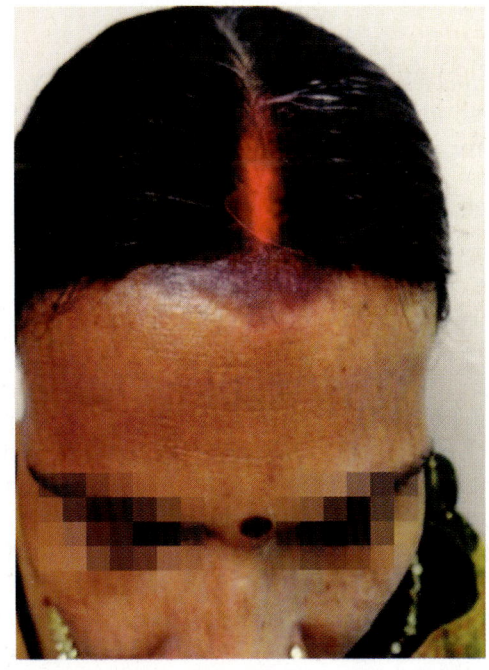

Fig. 3.28c: ACD on forehead to sindoor (kumkum)

Fig. 3.28a: Allergic contact dermatitis over bilateral hands in a staff nurse. The cause was latex gloves

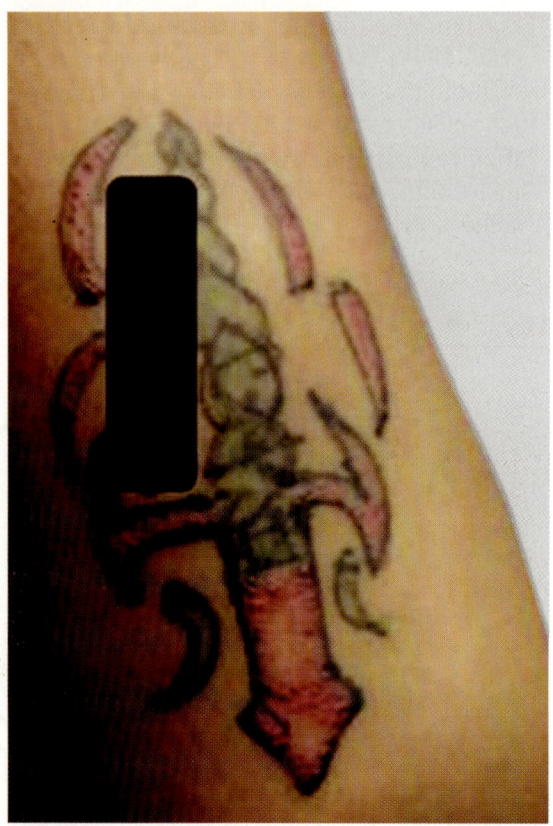

Fig. 3.29: Pruritic papules at the sites of red-colored tattoo

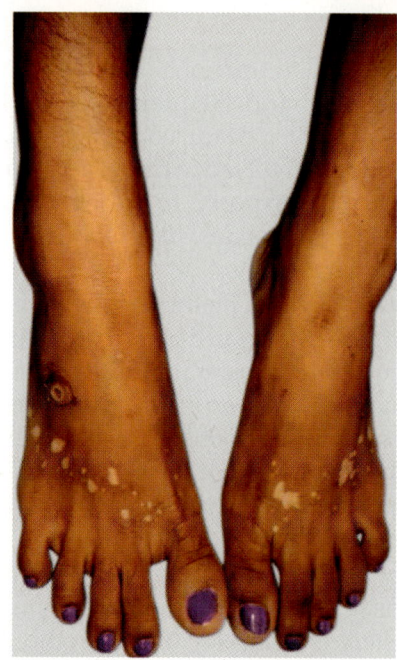

Fig. 3.30a: Contact leukoderma due to footwear

4. *Hobbies*: Interests in gardening, cookery, painting, photography, etc. are considered important factors in causing ACD.

Clinical Features

The dominant symptom of ACD is itching. The classical clinical presentation of ACD is pruritic eczematous dermatitis. In early stages, it presents as erythema, swelling, papules and papulovesicles. Continued or repeated exposure to allergen might lead to dryness, thickening, and scaling of skin along with lichenification and fissuring in more chronic cases. ACD might occasionally present as non-eczematous reactions such as contact urticaria, erythema multiforme-like, purpuric, lichenoid, lymphomatoid, pigmented, leukoderma (Fig. 3.30a), granulomatous, onycholysis and systematized contact dermatitis.

History

The important points in history are summarised in Table 3.11.

Examination

The location can be important for identification of the causal allergen, since contact dermatitis is generally restricted to the contact site (Table 3.12). A detailed discussion has been detailed in Chapter 3A, but a brief overview is given below:

Hand Dermatitis

About two-thirds of all cases of contact dermatitis involve the hands. The etiology is usually multifactorial, and includes both exogenous factors (exposure to irritants and allergens), and endogenous factors (atopy and defective skin barrier). Housewives' dermatitis, occupational dermatitis, and allergy to gloves are mostly confined to hands. Streaky dermatitis on the fingers, dorsa of the hands and forearms are typically caused by plants. Allergy to nickel, chromate and p-tertiary-butylphenol formaldehyde resin

Table 3.11: History taking in allergic contact dermatitis	
Primary site	*Important clue for diagnosis*
Duration and behavior	Did the condition spread and if so where? Has the problem been persistent or intermittent? Are there any obvious exacerbating factors? Repeated sudden exacerbations may point to an ACD
Previous history	Skin reactions to cheap metal, perfume and adhesive plasters, atopic diathesis (history of infantile or childhood flexural eczema, asthma, hay fever or conjunctivitis)
Sources of allergy	i. Occupation, past and present: Improvement of dermatitis during weekends or holidays favors an occupational origin ii. Hobbies (cement, glues, paint, wood and wood preservatives): Relapse at weekends suggests a hobby or non-occupational allergen. iii. Personal objects (textiles, footwear, protective clothing and gloves, jewellery, spectacles, hearing aids, medical appliances, cosmetics, toiletries, fragrances) iv. Home environment v. Current and previous topically applied medicaments: Dermatitis around a wound, especially leg ulcers, suggests sensitization to medicaments
Medical history	Drug allergies, concomitant diseases, medications, surgeries

Table 3.12: Common sources of ACD according to various sites			
S. No.	*Site*	*Common sources*	*Allergens*
1.	Hands	Gloves, plants, cement	Latex, rubber, plant allergens, chromate
2.	Wrists	Watch, watchstraps	Nickel, chromate, colophony
3.	Forearms	Bracelets, bangles, dust, textiles, cement	Nickel, chromate, colophony, 4-phenylenediamine
4.	Face	Cosmetics, hair dyes, spectacle frames, preservatives, nail varnish, leather airband	Fragrances, balsam of Peru, paraben, formaldehyde, 4-phenylenediamine, colophony, nickel plastics, chromate
5.	Eyelids	Eye make-up, eye make-up removers and applicators, nail varnish, eye drops and ointments, contact lens solutions, plants	Fragrances, parabens, epoxy resins, colophony, balsam of Peru, nickel, rubber, neomycin, gentamicin, preservatives plant allergens
6.	Lips and perioral area	Lipsticks, lip salves, medicaments, flavorings, garlic, cosmetics, toothpaste, chewing-gum, dentures	Eosin, nickel, neomycin, gentamicin, paraben, preservatives, food additives, cinnamic aldehyde, spearmint oil, peppermint oil, colophony

(Contd.)

Table 3.12: Common sources of ACD according to various sites (*Contd.*)

S. No.	Site	Common sources	Allergens
7.	Ears	Earrings and clips, medicaments, hairpins, matches, hearing-aids, headsets, spectacle frame, nail varnish	Nickel, chromate, neomycin, plastics, epoxy resins, colophony, phosphorus sesquisulphide, urea, rubber
8.	Neck	Necklaces, zip-fasteners, nail varnish, textiles, perfumes	Nickel, chromate, epoxy resins, 4-phenylenediamine, fragrances
9.	Axilla	Deodorants, perfumes	Fragrances, balsam of Peru
10.	Trunk	Clothes, buttons, zip-fasteners, elastic, leather belts, plants	Nickel, rubber, chromate, plant allergens
11.	Anogenital area	Medicaments, tights, toilet tissues and wipes, condoms	Neomycin, gentamicin, preservatives, local anesthetics, rubber
12.	Thighs	Textiles, coins	Nickel
13.	Lower legs	Medicaments, compression bandage, elastic hosiery	Topical antibiotics, rubber, colophony, nylon dye
14.	Feet	Shoes, stockings, topical medicaments, antiperspirants	Rubber, colophony, nickel, preservatives
15.	Scalp	Hair dyes, hair styling products, medicated shampoos, minoxidil	4-phenylenediamine, preservatives, tar, zinc pyrithione

may develop at the wrists from sensitivity to the metal, leather (Fig. 3.30b) and glue, in watch straps.

The forearms may be affected by the sensitizers that splash above protective gloves, particularly at work. Loose bracelets and bangles can also primarily involve forearms (Fig. 3.31a). Furthermore, repeated contact with sweat and saliva may accelerate the release of nickel ions from these metal devices (Linh K *et al*).

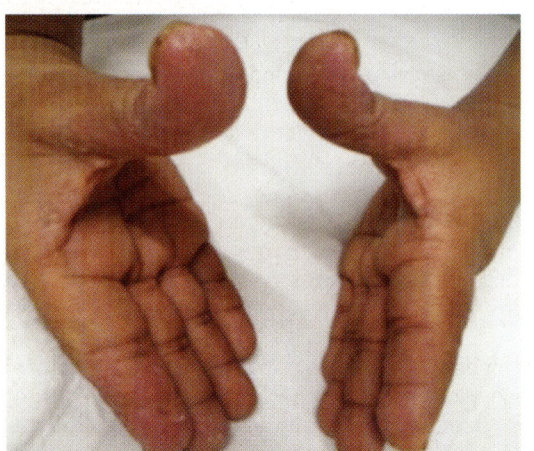

Fig. 3.30b: Allergic contact dermatitis over both hands in a patient employed in manufacture of leather purses

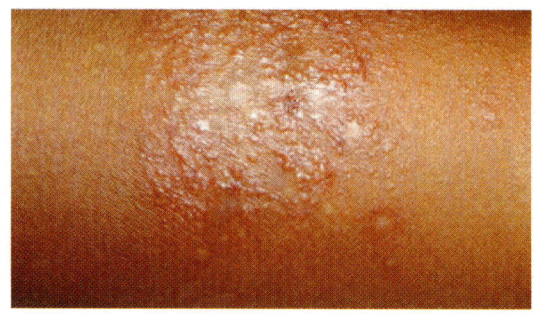

Fig. 3.31a: ACD on forearms due to metal (Ni induced) bangles

Face Dermatitis

Facial allergic contact dermatitis from fragrances, hair dyes, preservatives, emulsifiers and other constituents of skincare products and cosmetics, including nail varnish, is common. Nail varnish allergy often affects face in well-demarcated patches, and may be associated with eyelid dermatitis (Lidén C *et al*, 1993). A similar distribution may be seen from allergy to acrylic nails and rubber sponge applicators (Tucker SC *et al*, 1999). The forehead is affected by allergy to anything applied to the hair. Spectacle frames containing nickel or plastics may cause dermatitis on areas of contact with the cheeks, nose, eyelids and ears. Other causes include acne medications (e.g. benzoyl peroxide) (Fig. 3.31b) and aftershave lotions (Fig. 3.31c).

Eyelid dermatitis: The skin of the eyelids is thin, sensitive and may be sensitized by the fingers (e.g. nail varnish), airborne droplets

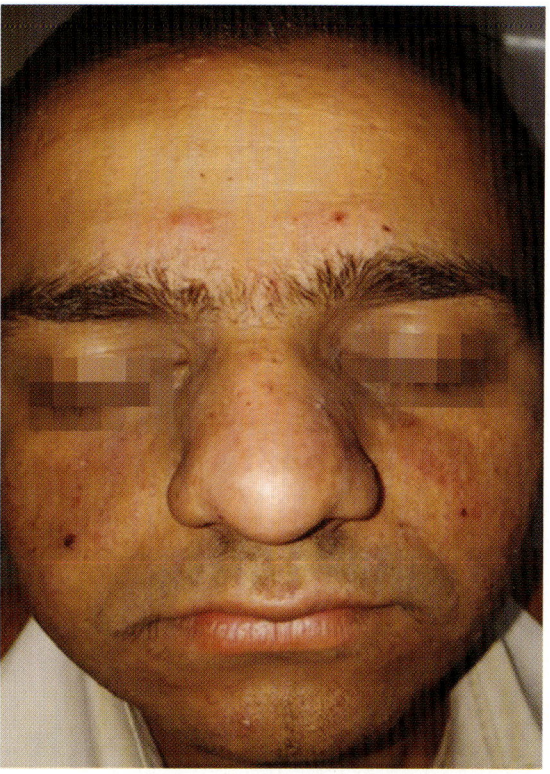

Fig. 3.31c: Allergic contact dermatitis over face, mimicking seborrheic dermatitis, due to aftershave lotion

(e.g. fragrance sprays) or volatile substances (e.g. epoxy resin). The common sources are eye creams, eye shadows, mascara, eye make-up removers, eyelash curlers and make-up applicators (nickel and/or rubber), eye drops and ointments, and contact lens solutions (preservatives).

Perioral dermatitis: ACD may occur from lipsticks and lip salves, nickel, medicaments, flavorings, garlic, and cosmetic excipients. Allergy to toothpaste (flavors), chewing gums (colophony), food additives (sodium metabisulphite), preservatives, colors, antioxidants, and badly fitting dentures are the potential causes of cheilitis and perioral eczema (Fig. 3.31d and e).

Earlobe dermatitis: The ear, particularly the helix, may be sensitized by hair sprays, shampoos, and hair dyes. Earlobe dermatitis

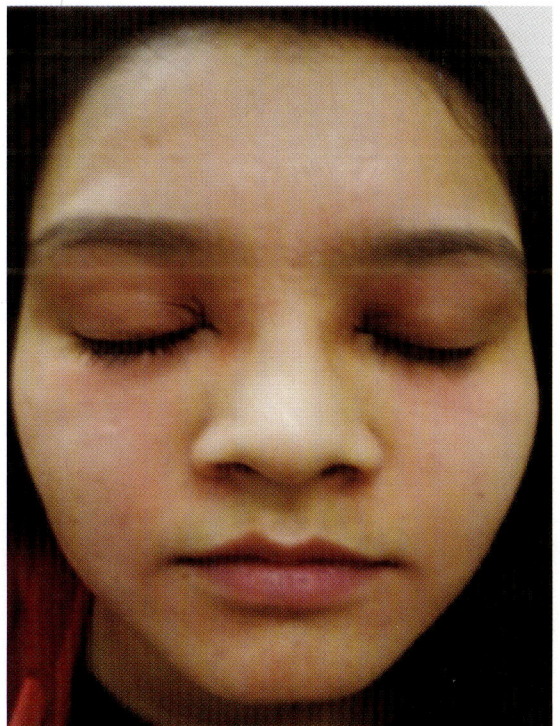

Fig. 3.31b: Contact dermatitis over face due to BPO gel for acne

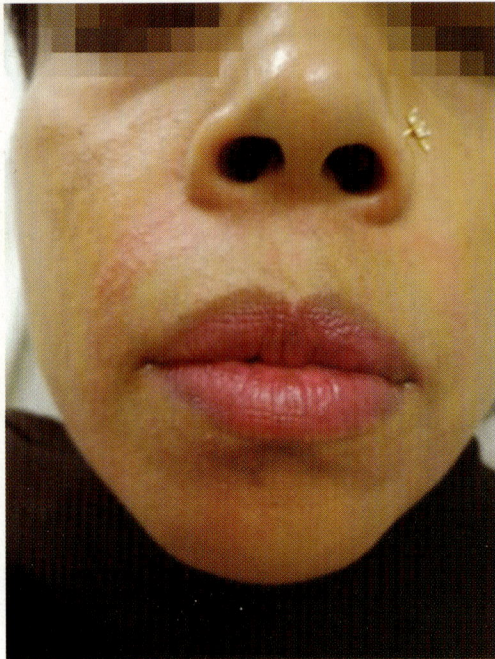

Fig. 3.31d: Perioral dermatitis

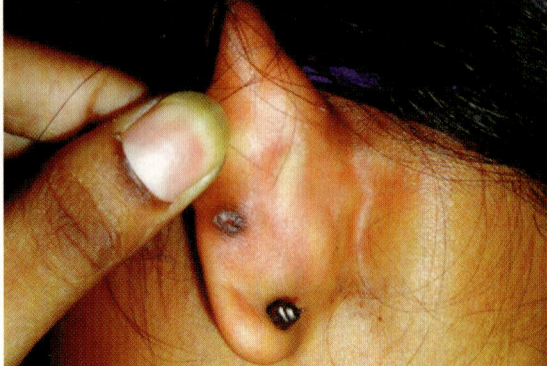

Fig. 3.32: ACD at the site of ear-piercing (nickel sensitivity)

Habitual scratching with hairpins, pens or pencils (nickel), matches (phosphorus sesqui-sulphide and chromate) (Tucker SC *et al*, 1999) or fingertips (nail varnish), sensitizing medications (neomycin) (Fig. 3.33), clips (nickel), plastic helmets or bathing caps, spectacle frames (nickel and palladium), hearing aids, headsets, earphones, or earplugs are other causes.

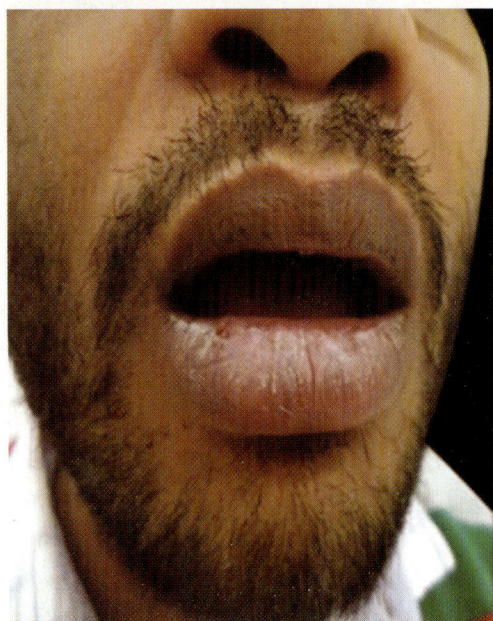

Fig. 3.31e: Contact cheilitis (after use of herbal toothpaste)

is a cardinal sign of nickel sensitivity in persons wearing artificial jewellery (Fig. 3.32). Ear-piercing is often a precipitating factor in nickel and gold sensitivity.

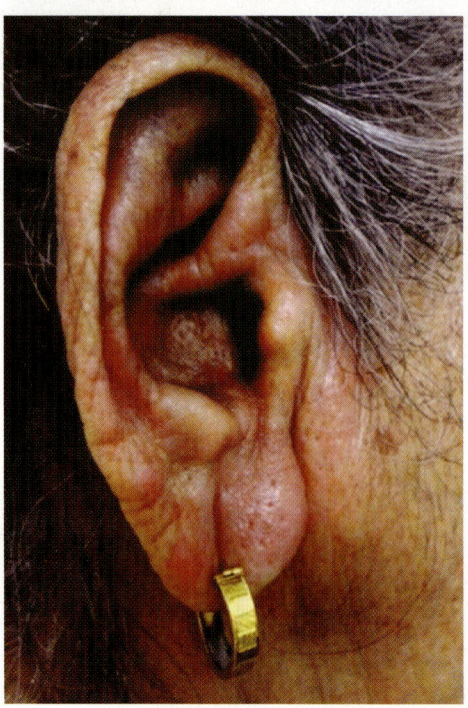

Fig. 3.33: Swelling and erythema as an allergic response to neomycin

Contact Eczema 61

Neck

ACD of neck can be caused by nickel in the clasps of necklaces or zip fasteners, nail varnish or primer from fingertips, perfume (sides of the neck), textiles (finishes in collars, dyes) and necklaces (nickel, exotic wood) which cause collar-like dermatitis, or eruptions on the sides of the neck. Dermatitis from airborne allergens and photosensitizers is sharply limited by the collar to the 'V' of the neck if blouses or open-necked shirts are worn.

Axilla

Allergic sensitivity may occur to fragrances in deodorants, and perfumes. The dermatitis produced by textiles tends to be periaxillary.

Trunk

Nickel buttons and zip fasteners may cause dermatitis localized to where they are worn, but a more widespread secondary spread eruption is often associated. Chromate sensitivity from leather, and rubber allergy from elastic may present as truncal eczema (Fig. 3.34). Dermatitis from dresses, blouses and sweaters (textile dyes and finishes) usually predominantly affects the neck and folds of the axilla, and spares areas of skin covered by undergarments (Beck MH *et al*, 2010). Fragrances, preservatives in moisturizing lotions, topical medication, sunscreens, poison

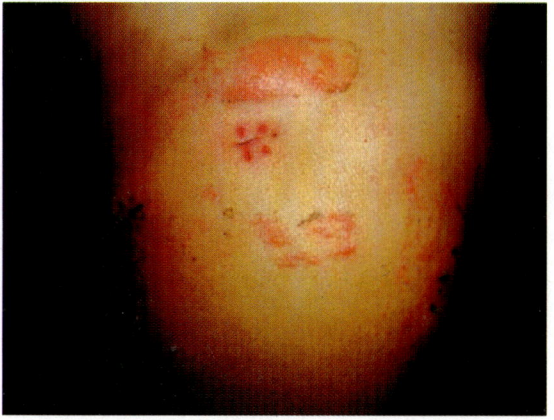

Fig. 3.34: ACD due to adhesive tape

ivy, plants (phototoxic reactions) can also cause truncal eczema. Laundry detergents rarely cause allergic contact dermatitis.

Anogenital

The anogenital region is a common site for sensitization by medicaments for pruritus, skin eruptions and hemorrhoids (perfume, local anesthetics), neomycin, hydroxy-quinolines, ethylenediamine, corticosteroids, topical antifungals, moist toilet tissues and wipes (preservative), feminine hygiene sprays, condoms (rubber accelerators), nail varnish and tights (nylon dyes) (Beck MH *et al*, 2010). Poison ivy (transferred by hand) can also cause allergic dermatitis in the genital area.

Thighs

Textile dermatitis starts at the edge of the underwear, and is more pronounced in the popliteal spaces or gluteal folds. Finishes in the material of the pockets or objects kept in the pockets (e.g. nickel coins or boxes of matches) may produce a patch of dermatitis on the underlying skin as allergens may penetrate working clothes.

Lower Legs

ACD from medicaments and dressings predominates, especially in those with varicose eczema and ulcers. The common medicament allergens are topical antibiotics and components of creams and paste bandages such as lanolin, cetearyl alcohol and preservatives (Wilson CL *et al*, 1991). ACD can also be caused by compression bandaging (rubber, colophony) and elastic hosiery (rubber, nylon dye), rubber boots.

Foot

Dermatitis may result from shoe materials including leather, rubber, glues and nickel (Fig. 3.35a to c), stockings, topical medicaments, antiseptics and antiperspirants. It presents as pruritic papular and oozy rash on dorsae of toes and feet, sparing the toe webs.

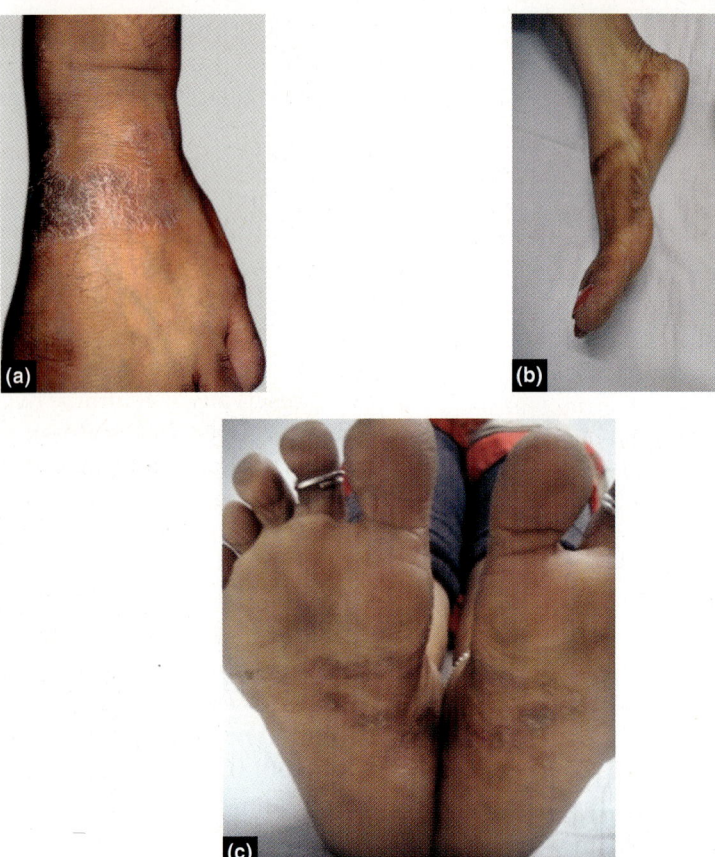

Fig. 3.35a to c: Contact dermatitis due to footwear

Scalp

It tends to be relatively spared from involvement by ACD. Dermatitis may still be caused by permanent hair dye, p-phenylene-diamine, and related semi-permanent dyes (Fig. 3.36), hair-styling products such as mousses, gels, waxes and holding sprays, medicated shampoos (tar extract, zinc pyrithione, preservatives), and topical minoxidil (Friedman ES *et al*, 2002).

Generalized

Generalized erythroderma may be the result of a chronic contact dermatitis maintained by continued exposure to multiple allergens, including components of topical medicaments (Beck MH *et al*, 2010).

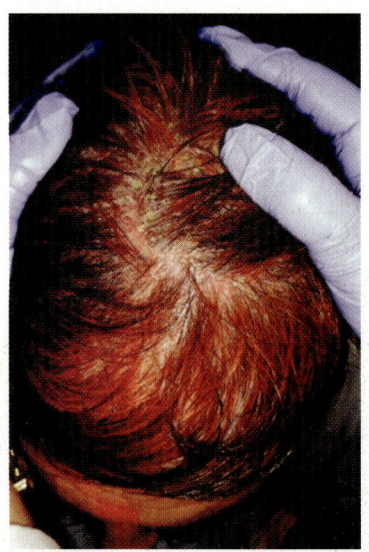

Fig. 3.36: Erythema and crusting on scalp (ACD to henna/mehendi)

Systemically Reactivated Contact Dermatitis

Ingestion or other systemic exposure to a contact allergen in an already sensitized person may result in a number of different patterns of skin eruption. Reactions may occur after systemic exposure to the primary allergen as well as closely related allergens. The most frequent types of reaction are focal flares of previous patch tests and sites of previous dermatitis, vesicular hand eczema, or more widespread eczema and erythema, sometimes with additional urticarial features. The agents include cinnamic aldehyde, balsam (cosmetics, topical medications, suppositories, dental liquids, and flavorings), paraben (food preservatives) and contaminants in foodstuffs such as nickel.

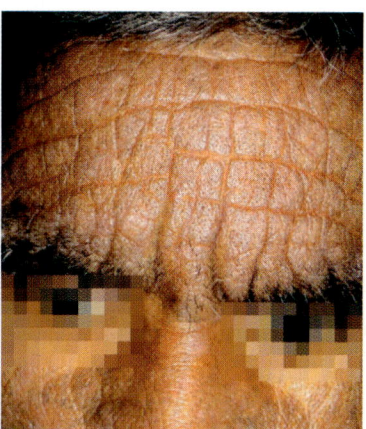

Fig. 3.37a: Involvement of face in photoallergic contact dermatitis

Mucosal

Most patients allergic to allergens applied intra-orally have cheilitis but not stomatitis; individual who react to nickel, mercury, palladium, or gold in dental amalgams present with a systemic contact dermatitis with or without a localized stomatitis (Thomas P. Habif).

Photoallergic Contact Dermatitis

Certain substances are transformed into irritants or sensitizers (photosensitizers) after irradiation with UV or short-wave visible radiation (280–600 nm). Photoallergic dermatitis is usually localized to exposed areas of the skin (Fig. 3.37a to c), with well-demarcated margins where the skin is covered by clothing, for example, at the collar and 'V' of the neck, below the end of the sleeves and trouser leggings. The area below the chin and **'Wilkinson's triangle'** behind the earlobe is usually spared (Wilkinson DS, 1962). The common photoallergens are UV filters, including *p*-aminobenzoic acid and its derivatives, cinnamates, benzophenones, perfumes (musk ambrette), halogenated salicylanilides used as antibacterials in soaps and detergents, topical non-steroidal anti-inflammatory agents like ketoprofen, pheno-

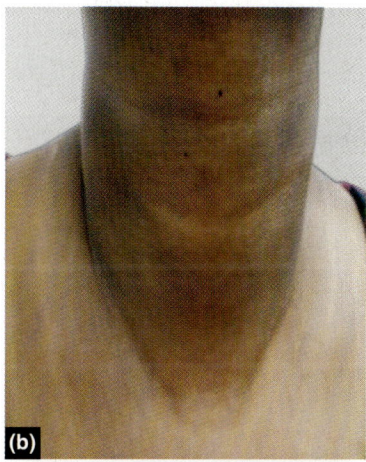

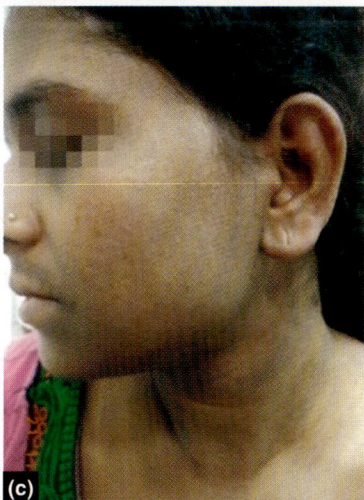

Fig. 3.37b and c: Photocontact dermatitis sparing the neck fold, due to prolonged used of mustard oil

thiazines, topical sulphonamides, eosin in lipsticks, thiourea (in design paper), and garlic.

DIAGNOSIS

Patch testing is the universally accepted method for the detection of causative contact allergens. A proper patch test uses a specific purified etiologic agent reproducing the clinical disease in a susceptible host and causing no disease outside the proper clinical settings (Fig. 3.38). To perform this test, specific allergens are applied on the upper back in Finn chambers (occlusive aluminum discs) under occlusion. Standard series include those allergens which most commonly cause reactions in the population, and to detect other less common ones which may not be considered by history or distribution of dermatitis

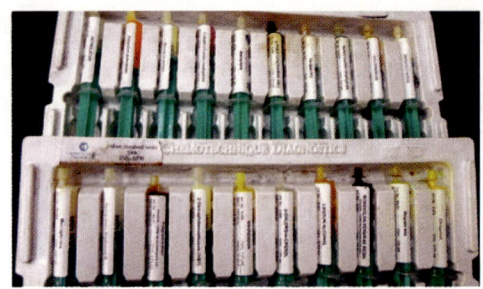

Fig. 3.38: Battery of allergens in Indian standard series patch test kit

being investigated. The allergens in Indian standard series are listed in Table 3.13.

Readings are made after 2 and 4 days, one hour after removal of patch tests. The patch test reactions are recorded as follows (International Contact Dermatitis Research Group) (Wilkinson DS *et al*, 1970):

S. No.	Compound	Conc. % (W/W)	Vehicle	Common sources
	Table 3.13: Allergens in Indian standard series and their common sources			
1.	Petrolatum white (pet)	100.0	Pet	Base/vehicle
2.	Potassium dichromate	0.5	Pet	Cement, antirust paints, dust liberated by drilling, cutting or sandpapering of painted metals
3.	Neomycin sulfate	20.0	Pet	Topical antibiotic, cross reaction with kanamycin, framycetin (soframycin), gentamicin, tobramycin
4.	Cobalt chloride hexahydrate	1.0	Pet	Hard metal used for metal cutting and drilling, magnets, jewellery, alloys, paints, glass, china pottery, ceramics
5.	Benzocaine	5.0	Pet	Local anesthetic
6.	4-phenylenediamine base	1.0	Pet	Hair dyes, tattoos, henna, textile azo dyes
7.	Paraben mix	15.0	Pet	Preservative in topical and parenteral medicaments, paste bandages, cosmetics, ultrasound gels and foods
8.	Nickel sulphate hexahydrate	5.0	Pet	Alloys, plated objects, jewellery and metal components of clothing, coins, keys, scissors, knitting needles, other metallic tools, utensils, diet
9.	Colophony	20.0	Pet	Pine trees and wood, adhesive dressings, glues, balms and salves, printing ink, herbal medicaments

(Contd.)

Table 3.13: Allergens in Indian standard series and their common sources (*Contd.*)

S. No.	Compound	Conc. % (W/W)	Vehicle	Common sources
10.	Gentamicin	20.0	Pet	Topical antibiotic
11.	Epoxy resins	1.0	Pet	Coatings including paints, varnishes and metals, construction industry, dental fillings, cardiac pacemakers
12.	Fragrance mix	8.0	Pet	Perfumes, cosmetics, moisturizers, deodorants, aftershaves, soaps, bath additives, aroma-therapy oils, toilet tissues and wipes
13.	2-mercaptobenzothiazole	2.0	Pet	Rubber industry, rubber gloves, shoes, gloves, clothing, condoms, electric cords, tubes, masks, rubber bands
14.	Nitrofurazone	1.0	Pet	Topical antibiotic
15.	Chlorocresol	1.0	Pet	Corticosteroid creams, topical medicaments
16.	Wool alcohols	30.0	Pet	Cosmetics (creams, lotions, ointments), topical drugs
17.	Balsam of Peru	25.0	Pet	Perfumes, cosmetics, medicaments, e.g. hemorrhoid preparations, balms for wounds, sprains, joint pains, flavor in tobacco, spices, drinks
18.	Thiuram mix	1.0	Pet	Rubber industry, rubber gloves, shoes, gloves, clothing, condoms, electric cords, tubes, masks, rubber bands
19.	Clioquinol	5.0	Pet	Topical medicaments
20.	Black rubber mix	0.6	Pet	Rubber industry, rubber gloves, shoes, gloves, clothing, condoms, electric cords, tubes, masks, rubber bands
21.	4-tert-phenol formal-butyl-aldehyde resin	1.0	Pet	Electrical appliances, glues, plywood, fiber glass, brake linings, telephones and steering wheels
22.	Formaldehyde	1.0	Aqueous (aq)	Cosmetics, clothing resins, shampoos, paints/lacquers, glues, printing ink, used for preservation of pathological specimens, orthopedic casts, renal dialysis
23.	Polyethylene glycol	100.0	Aqueous	Cosmetics (shampoos, hair dressings), topical medicaments, detergents
24.	Parthenolide	0.1	Pet	Herbal medicaments

– Negative

?+   Doubtful reaction; faint erythema only

+   Weak positive reaction; palpable erythema, infiltration, possibly papules

++   Strong positive reaction; erythema, infiltration, papules, vesicles

+++   Extreme positive reaction; intense erythema and infiltration and coalescing vesicles

IR   Irritant reaction of different types

NT   Not tested

Reading at day 4 is important to distinguish an allergic from a false-positive non-allergic irritant reaction. No infiltration, lack of itching, deep redness or a brown hue, and sharp delineation corresponding to the margins of the patch test point to an irritant reaction. It is important to rule out false positive and false negative reactions.

A positive reaction confirms the person has allergic contact sensitivity (Fig. 3.39), although this does not necessarily mean that the substance is the cause of the presenting clinical dermatitis, and it is important to establish relevance by carefully re-examining the patient's history, distribution of rash and materials with which there has been contact.

The adverse patch test reactions include active sensitization, folliculitis, irritant reactions, ectopic flare of dermatitis, Koebner's phenomenon, hyper- or hypopigmentation at test sites, scarring, and anaphylaxis (rare).

Other adjunctive tests for diagnosis of ACD include open test, TRUE test, repeat open application test, usage test, and intradermal test. Photoallergic contact dermatitis is diagnosed by photopatch testing.

DIFFERENTIAL DIAGNOSIS

Allergic contact dermatitis should be differentiated from irritant contact dermatitis, atopic dermatitis, asteatotic dermatitis, dyshidrotic

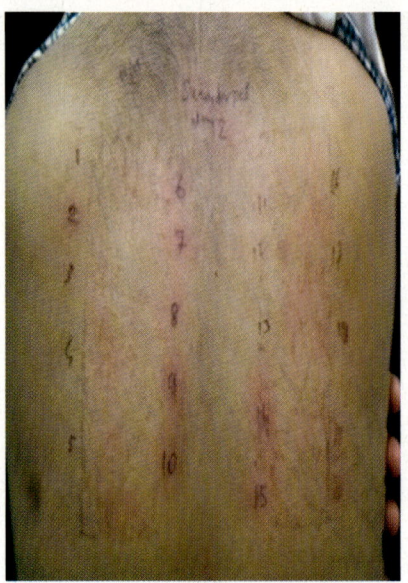

Fig. 3.39: A patch test done with Indian standard series showed positive reaction against multiple allergens

eczema, nummular dermatitis, autosensitization, insect bite reaction, fungal infection and systemic drug reaction, psoriasis and mycosis fungoides (patch or plaque) (Table 3.14).

PREVENTION

Principles of prevention can be divided into primary, secondary and tertiary. Primary prevention focuses on the induction of contact sensitization and control of exposure. Secondary prevention relates to elicitation, and tertiary to measures for established and continuing dermatitis. Avoidance is the mainstay of treatment for ACD. Educating patients about avoidance of the allergen and its potentially related substances, and providing suitable alternatives are crucial to a good outcome.

Containment, replacement and elimination of potential allergenic hazards can be helpful in both the domestic and working environments, for example, perfume-free cosmetics and medicaments, non-latex gloves, high molecular-weight epoxy resins (Thorgeirsson A et al, 1978), and white spirit instead of

Table 3.14: Differential diagnosis	
Diseases	*Important clue for diagnosis*
Irritant contact dermatitis (ICD)	Physical findings can be indistinguishable clinically; in general there is an absence of vesiculation (only very strong irritants produce vesicles) and burning exceeds itching. Does not spread beyond the area of contact with continued exposure
Atopic dermatitis	Distribution of skin findings can be helpful; atopic patients can and do develop contact allergies. Worsening disease can indicate new contact allergy development
Nummular dermatitis (ND)	Widespread ACD can assume this pattern in certain patients; nonetheless, the classical morphology of coin-shaped, well-demarcated plaques on the legs, dorsal hands, and extensor surfaces favors ND
Seborrheic dermatitis	Greasy and scaly papulosquamous plaques usually located in the hairbearing regions, glabella, and nasolabial folds
Asteatotic eczema	Parchment-like patches with no edema or vesiculation on the lower legs
Stasis dermatitis	Papulosquamous plaques with dyschromia located on the shins and medial surfaces of the lower legs, with presence of concomitant varicosities
Pompholyx and/or dyshidrotic eczema	Deep-seated vesicles on palms, soles, sides of the fingers, and volar edges
Psoriasis	When the lesions are a few and limited to the hands and/or feet differentiation can be more difficult. Classical location and predominance in areas of trauma (Koebnerization) can be helpful as well as the presence (if any) of concomitant arthritis
Mycosis fungoides (patch or plaque stage)	The well demarcated, atrophic, poikilodermatous, scaly patches and plaques of MF are usually found in nonsun-exposed areas of the skin, such as the trunk, breasts, hips, and buttocks (bathing suit distribution)
Insect bite reaction	Bites, particularly those from bedbugs, often cause a linear eruption that may occasionaly be confused with Rhus dermatitis (poison ivy)
Autoeczematization (Id reaction)	Widespread aute eczematous eruption that is presumably triggered by secondary bacterial infection of eczema, with resultant circulating immune complexes released from the site of eczema. It is hypothesized that patients become sensitized to their own tissue breakdown products
Fungal infection	When the lesion present over palm and sole, but well-demarcated plaques with positive KOH or fungal culture clinches the diagnosis
Systemic drug reaction	Especially lichenoid or morbilliform eruptions. Detailed history is important

turpentine. Housewives' dermatitis can be prevented by wearing cotton-lined gloves when the hands are in contact with irritants, including food, cleaning agents and polishes. Skin protection courses and education have been shown to reduce occupational dermatitis.

TREATMENT

The first principle of management is to give advice on avoidance of the possible sources of sensitizer and cross-reacting substances. Examples of specific avoidance measures include plastic instead of rubber gloves, cosmetics and medicaments free of an identified allergen, and clothing free of nickel-containing studs, zips, etc. It should be stressed that allergy does not disappear when the dermatitis clears but that the risk of relapse after further contact with the allergen persists throughout life.

Topical steroids are used in the acute stage and are gradually replaced by hydrating emollients as the skin lesions improve. It is important to choose the topical corticosteroid to which the patient is not allergic. Topical calcineurin inhibitors should be considered when steroid-sparing agents are required, and for certain areas like face, axilla, groins where chances of steroid-induced atrophy are high. In severe and widespread cases, systemic corticosteroids may be indicated for a short period of time. Secondary infection requires antibiotics, and a sedative antihistamine is indicated for pruritus, particularly at night. Recalcitrant, disabling cases may require treatment with immunosuppressive therapy such as azathioprine (Verma KK et al, 2000) and ciclosporin.

Hyposensitization

Many attempts have been made to down-regulate the immune response to allergens in an already sensitized individual. Some success has nevertheless been claimed in India for hyposensitization against Parthenium hysterophorus **(Mark Wilkinson).**

Prognosis

The prognosis of ACD depends on its cause and the feasibility of avoiding repeated or continued exposure to the causative allergen. Associated irritant dermatitis and constitutional factors are also important. Prognosis of ACD is worse than irritant contact dermatitis. It is clear from a number of studies that poor compliance and understanding results in a higher rate of ongoing exposure to the causative allergen, and is associated with a worse prognosis (Agner T et al, 1999). Once relevant allergens are identified by patch test and successfully avoided, improvement of dermatitis is the rule.

Sensitivity to ubiquitous allergens, such as nickel and chromate (Thormann J et al, 1979), and to strong allergens, such as primin and PPD (Fisher AA et al, 1958), is reported to persist, whereas sensitivity to other weaker and avoidable allergens may disappear.

Bibliography

1. Adams RM. Diagnostic patch testing. In: Occupational Skin Disease. New York: Grune and Stratton 1983: 136.

2. Agner T, Flyvholm MA, Menné T. Formaldehyde allergy: a follow-up study. Am J Contact Dermatitis 1999; 10: 12–7.

3. Ayto J. Dictionary of Word Origins. London: Bloomsbury 1990: 18.

4. Bandmann H-J, Breit R, Leutgeb C. Kontakallergie und Dermatitis atopica. Arch DermatolForsch 1972; 244: 332–4.

5. Beck M. H, Wilkinson B.M. Allergic contact dermatitis. In: burns T, Breathnach SM, Cox N, Griffiths C, editors. Rook's Textbook of Dermatology. 8th Ed. Oxford. Blackwell; 2010: 26.1–106.

6. Berit CC, Menné T, Johansen JD. 20 years of standard patch testing in an eczema population with focus on patients with multiple contact allergies. Contact Dermatitis 2007; 57: 76–83.

7. Bonamonte D, Foti C, Antelmi AR, Biscozzi AM et al. Nickel contact allergy and menstrual cycle. Contact Dermatitis 2005; 52. 309–13.

8. Bruce T. Ryhal, M.D. Drug hypersensitivity and allergy. In: M.Eric Gershwin, M.D. Stanley M. Naguwa, MD editors. Allergy & Immunology Secrets. 2nd edition. Philadelphia: Elsevier publishers; 2006. p. 233.

9. Bryld LE, Hindsberger C, Kyvik KO et al. Genetic factors in nickel allergy evaluated in a population-based female twin sample. J Invest Dermatol 2004; 123:1025–9.

10. Cronin E, Bandmann H-J, Calnan CD et al. Contact dermatitis in the atopic. Acta DermVenereol (Stockh) 1970; 50:183–7.

11. Deleo VA, Taylor SC, Belsito DV et al. The effect of race and ethnicity on patch test results. J Am Acad Dermatol 2002; 46:S107–12.

12. Dwyer CM, Forsyth A. Allergic contact dermatitis from bindi. Contact Dermatitis 1994; 30: 174.

13. Fisher AA, Prelzig A, Kanof NB. The persistence of allergic eczematous sensitivity and the cross-sensitivity pattern to paraphenylenediamine. J Invest Dermatol 1958; 30:9–12.

14. Friedman ES, Friedman PM, Cohen DE et al. Allergic contact dermatitis to topical minoxidil solution: etiology and treatment. J Am Acad Dermatol 2002; 46:309–12.

15. Green CM, Holden CR, Gawkrodger DJ. Contact allergy to topical medicaments becomes more common with advancing age: an age-stratified study. Contact Dermatitis 2007; 56:229–31.

16. Grossman J, Baum J, Gluckman J et al. The effect of aging and acute illness on delayed hypersensitivity. J Allergy Clin Immunol 1975; 55:262–75.

17. Hanifin JH. Atopic dermatitis. J Am AcadDermatol 1982; 6:1–13.

18. Heine G, Schnuch A, Uter W, Worm M. Frequency of contact allergy in German children and adolescents patch tested between 1995 and 2002: results from the Information Network of Departments of Dermatology and the German Contact Dermatitis Research Group. Contact Dermatitis 2004; 51:111–7.

19. Kimber I, Dearman RJ. Allergic contact dermatitis: the cellular effects. Contact Dermatitis 2002; 46: 1–5.

20. Kwangsukstith C, Maibach HI. Effects of age and sex on the induction and elicitation of allergic contact dermatitis. Contact Dermatitis 1995; 33: 289–98.

21. Lepoittevin J-P. Molecular aspects of allergic contact dermatitis. In: Frosch PJ, Menné T, Lepoittevin J-P, eds. Contact Dermatitis, 4th edn. Berlin: Springer, 2006: 45–68.

22. Lidén C, Berg M, Farm G et al. Nail varnish allergy with far-reaching consequences. Br J Dermatol 1993; 128:57–62.

23. Linh K. Erin M. Warshaw, and Cory A. Dunnick. In, Prevention of nickel allergy: The case for Regulation? Robert P. Dellavalle Editor. Dermatologic Clinics: Dermatologic Epidemiology and Public Health. Elsevier publication, 2009; vol 27:Issue 2: P 157.

24. Mark Wilkinson. David Orlon.In Allergy contact dermatitis.Christopher E. Jonathan Barker. Tanya Bleiker. Robert Chalmers. Daniel Creamer. Editors. Rooks Textbook of Dermatology. 9th edition. Wiley Blackwell publisher. Chapter 128; Vol 2:p-128.75.

25. Menné T, Borgan O, Green A. Nickel allergy and hand dermatitis in a stratified sample of the Danish female population. Acta DermVenereol (Stockh) 1982; 62:35–41.

26. Menné T, Holm V. Genetic susceptibility in human allergic sensitization. SeminDermatol 1986; 5: 301–6.

27. Modjtahedi BS, Modjtahedi SP, Maibach HI. The sex of the individual as a factor in allergic contact dermatitis. Contact Dermatitis 2004; 50:53–9.

28. Moed H, Stoof TJ, Boorsma DM, et al. Identification of anti-inflammatory drugs according to their capacity to suppress type-1 and type-2 T cell profiles. ClinExp Allergy 2004; 34:1868–75.

29. Peltonen L, Terho P. Nickel sensitivity in schoolchildren in Finland. In: Frosch P, Dooms-Goossens A, LaChapelle J-M, et al., eds. Current Topics in Contact Dermatitis. Heidelberg: Springer, 1989: 184–7.

30. Reed JT, Ghadially R, Elias PM. Skin type, but neither race nor gender, influence epidermal permeability barrier function. Arch Dermatol 1995; 33:289–98.

31. Sharma VK, Asati DP. Pediatric contact dermatitis. Indian J DermatolVenereolLeprol 2010; 76: 514–20.

32. Thomas P. Habif. In Contact Dermatitis and patch testing. Clinical Dermatology. Elsevier publication. 5ed; p:133.

33. Thorgeirsson A, Fregert S, Fammas O. Sensitization capacity of epoxy resin oligomers in the guinea pig. Acta DermVenereol (Stockh) 1978; 58:17–21.

34. Thormann J, Jesperson NB, Joensen HD. Persistence of contact allergy to chromium. Contact Dermatitis 1979; 5:261–5.

35. Tucker SC, Beck MH. A 15-year study of patch testing to (meth) acrylates. Contact Dermatitis 1999; 40:278–9.

36. Tucker SC, Lyon CC, Beck MH. Persistent otitis externa due to allergic contact dermatitis to phosphorus sesquisulphide in 'strike-anywhere' matches (Minerva). BMJ 1999; 318:1566.

37. Verma KK, Manchanda Y, Pasricha JS. Azathioprine as a corticosteroid sparing agent for the treatment of dermatitis caused by the weed Parthenium. Acta DermVenereol (Stockh) 2000; 80:31–2.

38. Wilkinson DS, Bandmann H-J, Calnan CD, et al. The role of contact allergy in hand eczema. Trans St John's Hosp DermatolSoc 1970; 56:15–9.

39. Wilkinson DS, Fregert S, Magnusson B, et al. Terminology of contact dermatitis. Acta Derm Venereol (Stockh) 1970; 50:287–92.

40. Wilkinson DS. Patch test reactions to certain halogenated salicylanilides. Br J Dermatol 1962; 74:302–6.

41. Wilson CL, Cameron J, Powell SM et al. High incidence of contact dermatitis in leg-ulcer patients: implications for management. Clin Exp Dermatol 1991; 16:25–03.

4

Non-eczematous Contact Dermatitis

Seema Rani, Abir Saraswat

Besides the classic eczematous form of contact dermatitis (CD) detailed in Chapter 3, a number of non-eczematous clinical variants has also been described, which are often misdiagnosed, a few of which are being detailed below.

1. Erythema Multiforme-like Contact Dermatitis

Of all the types, this is believed to be the most common type in the West and is commonly due to exotic woods, primula medicaments, and ethylenediamine. PPD in hair dye and temporary tattoos, rubber chemicals and clothing dyes are also recognized causes of this reaction pattern.

Clinical Features

Early lesions are eczematous and localized at the allergen contact site. After 1 to 15 days delay, the erythema multiforme-like eruption follows, involving the area around the original lesions or extending to the whole cutaneous surface. The generalized spread is due to systemic exposition to drugs which the patient had previously been sensitized to topically.

Target-like, erythematovesicular, or urticarial lesions are characteristic. Resolution is slow-paced; these manifestations persist usually much longer than the original eczematous lesions (or sometimes appearing after regression of the latter).

2. Purpuric Contact Dermatitis (PCD)

This particular form of noneczematous contact dermatitis is frequently misdiagnosed. Pigmented purpuric reactions are uncommon and eruption evolves in several weeks after the withdrawal of the offending agent and resolves with more or less persistent pigmentation. Purpuric reaction can present as pigmented purpuric reaction to textile azo dyes, resins and allergic contact purpura due to rubber chemical-IPPD (isopropyl-p-phenylenediamine) less commonly observed with PPD, diphenylthiourea in heat retainer and secondary spread eruption from balsam of Peru (Mark Wilkinson). Hence purpuric contact dermatitis is more frequently to allergic mechanism rather than irritant.

Causes

a. *Rubber:* This has been associated with the use of rubber boots, rubber diving suits, elasticized shorts, and rubberized support leg bandage. It has also been seen due to the use of orthopedic elastic bandages.

b. *Textile:* This was initially associated with optical whiteners, but has been described due to various dyes added to clothing. A petechial and itchy dermatitis is seen in those areas which are typically subject to tighter contact with clothes (armpits, arms, upper limbs folds, neck and thighs, Fig. 4.1a and b).

Clinical Features

Purpuric contact dermatitis can be either toxic or allergic in nature. Palpable purpuric lesions are seen followed by persistent pigmentation.

At times, clinical extension represents a useful feature in differentiating the 2 forms, the irritant being strictly limited to contact sites.

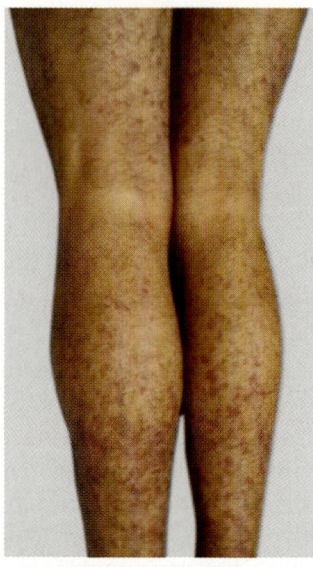

Fig. 4.1a: Contact purpura over back of lower extremity with textile (jean cloth)

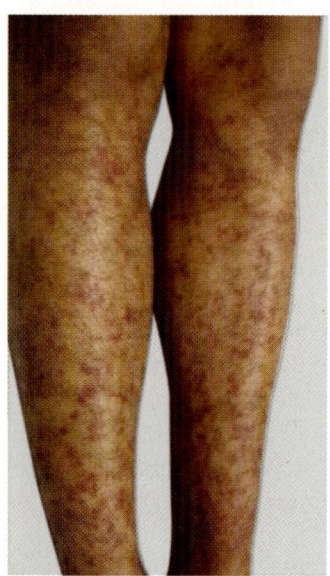

Fig. 4.1b: Contact purpura with textile over front of lower extremity

3. Lichenoid Contact Dermatitis

A particularly uncommon form of non-eczematous contact dermatitis which presents with clinical features resembling those of lichen planus. It affects both skin and mucosal membranes.

Causes

Color developers, substances derived from paraphenylenediamine, are the most common cause of allergic contact lichenoid eruption. As a general rule, the eruption from color developers spares the oral mucosa. Cases from paraphenylenediamine in hair dyes, P. obconica, nickel, epoxy resins, aminoglycoside antibiotics and methacrylic acid esters for industrial use have been reported. Oral mucosae can be involved due to copper, zinc, and mercury contained in dental restorations. Lichen planus-like reactions of the buccal mucosa may represent allergy to metals, other materials used in dental treatment, cinnamal and spearmint.

Clinical Features

Eczematous lesions evolve into lichenoid papular lesions. Though the eruption mostly involves contact sites, it can spread widely but usually spares the mucosa. The course is prolonged and leaves variably intense pigmentary changes lasting up to some months.

4. Pigmented Contact Dermatitis/Riehl's Melanosis/Pigmented Cosmetic Dermatitis

One of the reasons that this is being covered here is that this condition is often misdiagnosed as lichen planus pigmentosus or ashy dermatoses and the patient is put on various topical and systemic agents which rarely help, complicating the condition as the irritation caused by the topical agents aggravates the condition. As this is caused commonly by cosmetics, which is a largely unregulated industry, it is author's belief that a large number of such cases are missed in clinical practice!

Pigmented contact dermatitis was first reported by Osmundsen in Denmark in 1969. In 8 months, he had 120 patients, seven of whom showed a pronounced and bizarre hyperpigmentation. In four of these seven cases, contact dermatitis preceded the hyperpigmentation, while the other three did not notice any signs of dermatitis, such as itching or erythema, before the pigmentation appeared.

Hyperpigmentation, with or without dermatitis, was located mostly in covered areas, such as the chest, back, waist, arms, neck, and thighs. The hyperpigmentation was brown, slate-colored, grayish-brown, reddish-brown, bluish-brown, etc. according to the case, and often had a reticulate pattern.

The cause was linked to the use of washing powders that contained a new optical whitener, Tinopal or CH3566. This was one of numerous optical whiteners that became available at that time to make textiles "whiter than white." Another cause was azo dyes and affected workers in a textile factory.

Pigmented cosmetic dermatitis is seen mainly in Asian women. Slight dermatitis may precede or coexist with the hyperpigmentation, which occurs mainly on the cheeks. The allergens associated with this have been found to be fragrances and pigments, cosmetics and soaps. Pigmented cheilitis has occurred from allergy to ricinoleic acid in castor oil used in lipsticks. Components of kumkum, applied as a cosmetic to the forehead, commonly cause a pigmented dermatitis. The signs of pigmented cosmetic dermatitis are diffuse or reticular, black or dark brown hyperpigmentation of the face, which cannot be cured by the use of corticosteroid ointments or the continuous ingestion of vitamin C.

Another common but under-recognized cause in Indian patients is perfumed hair oil. These oils contain various fragrances and cooling agents like menthol and camphor. They are used not only for hair cosmesis but are also very popular as headache-relieving

medicine. Ylang-ylang oil positivity has been seen in many of these patients (unpublished observation).

Japanese dermatologists gradually became aware of the role of cosmetics in this hyperpigmentation. First, it occurred only in those women, and very exceptionally men, who used cosmetics, and secondly, even though the bizarre brown hyperpigmentation was so conspicuous, the presence of slight, recurrent, or preceding dermatitis was observed in most cases clinically or on taking a history.

The border of pigmented cosmetic dermatitis is not sharp, as in lichen planus or melasma (Fig. 4.2a to c). In some cases, the dark brown or black hyperpigmentation is also seen on skin other than on the face (Fig. 4.3). The neck (Figs 4.3 and 4.4), chest, and back can be involved and, in a few exceptional cases, hyperpigmentation may extend to the whole body.

In these cases, the allergens cinnamic alcohol and its derivatives sensitize the patients first to cosmetics and then provoke allergic reactions to soaps, domestic fabric softeners, and food, all of which sometimes contain cinnamic derivatives. Pigmented contact dermatitis over face might be misdiagnosed as LPP (lichen planus

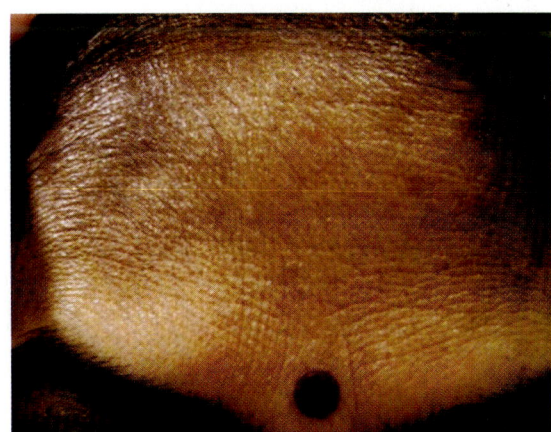

Fig. 4.2a: A case of PCD (pigmented cosmetic dermatitis) on the forehead in a patient who was allergic to PPD and had been using hair dyes for more than 7 years

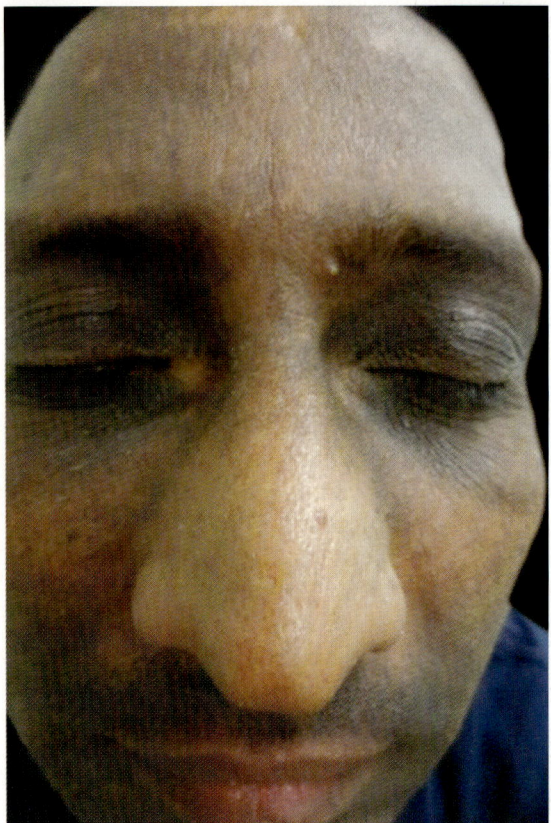

Fig. 4.2b: Pigmented contact dermatitis after use of hair dye

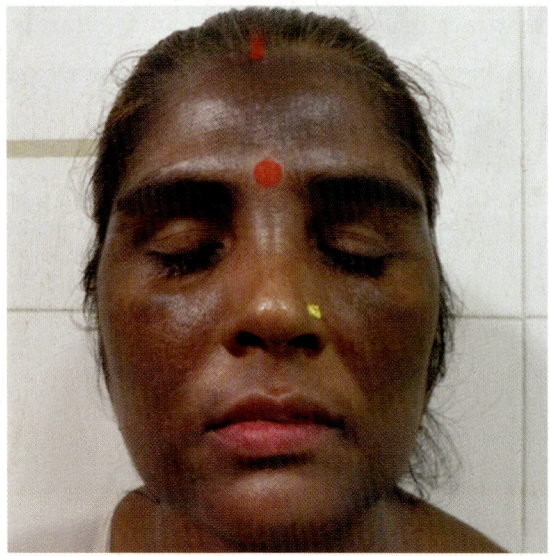

Fig. 4.2c: Pigmented cosmetic dermatitis due to use of various cosmetic products for longtime

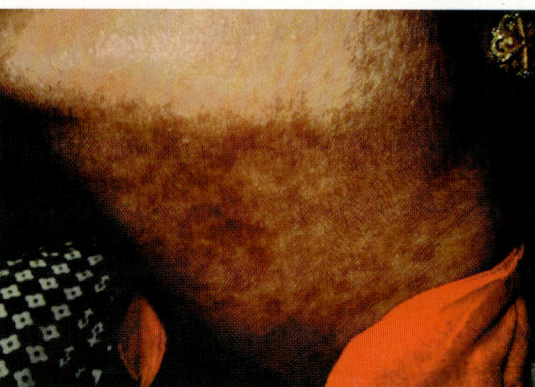

Fig. 4.3: A female with PCD extending to the neck, diagnosed as a case of lichen planus pigmentosus

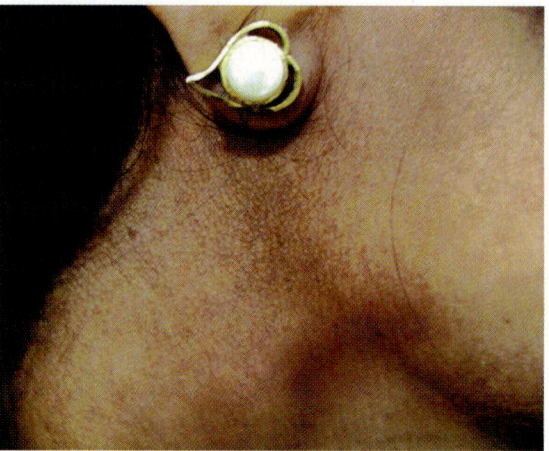

Fig. 4.4: An early case of PCD in a female using a fragrance on the jawline "pulse point"

pigmentosus). Tienthavorn found some similarities and differences between ashy dermatosis (AD), lichen planus pigmentosus (LPP) and pigmented contact dermatitis (PCD). Also a recent study (Sharma VK) found that a relevant patch test was seen in 17 (34%) patients: Paraphenylenediamine (n = 5), nickel (n = 3), colophony, perfume mix and fragrance mix (n = 2 each), thiuram mix and 3, 3, 4, 5-tetrachlorosalicylanilide (n = 1 each), and patients' own products (n = 9), in case of LPP on the face.

Causative agents: Jasmine absolute, ylang-ylang oil, cananga oil, benzyl salicylate, hydroxycitronellal, sandalwood oil, artificial sandalwood, geraniol, geranium oil, D and C Red 31, Yellow No. 11 and PPD (Fig. 4.2). Other rare causations of pigmented cosmetic dermatitis include fragrances (Fig. 4.4), musk ambrette, musk moskene, pigment orange F2G, and diisostearyl malate in the lipsticks.

Prevention and Treatment

The problem in preventing lies in a knowledge of the countless chemicals that are used even now in the textile industry. The purity of dyes is, in general, very low and some of the many impurities are allergenic. The experiences accumulated in the past show that when entirely new textile finishes are introduced to the textile industry, the minimum safety evaluation tests such as LD50, Ames test, and skin irritation test should be performed, and their sensitization potential should be investigated by a research team including dermatologists.

1. Stopping all kinds of facial creams, specially fairness creams and avoiding facials, perfumes, foundations and sunscreens is a tough protocol to follow, but we have seen patients with near complete improvement with such a protocol. This is as most of the causative allergens are difficult to find and thus it is best to stop whatever is possible. It is usually required 1–2 years for a patient to regain normal non-hyperpigmented facial skin.

2. The dermatologist may choose to administer a topical product with a long history of safety, but using a triple combination creams or a skin lightening cream is of a little use.

3. In early lesions, topical tacrolimus can hasten the clearance and low fluence Q-switched Nd: YAG laser has been reported to be effective in late stage disease.

4. In most cases, contamination with ordinary soaps and cosmetics is a decisive factor inhibiting therapeutic results, because such ordinary daily necessities contain the allergens that cause the condition. Thus, it

is a good advice to ask the patient to visit the dermatologist once a month to be checked for improvement where the patient is persuaded every time to avoid products used in beauty parlors.

Though not a definitive list, Table 4.1 elucidates the common allergens that can cause this dermatosis.

Table 4.1: A list of agents that can cause pigmented contact and cosmetic dermatitis*

Optical whiteners	Tinopal CH3566
Dyes	• Naphthol AS • Sudan I • Brilliant lake red • Vacanceine • Red solvent orange 8
Cosmetics	Pigments: • Pigment orange 3 • Pigment red 3 • Pigment red 49 • Pigment red 53 • Pigment red 64 Azoic solvents: • Solvent orange 2 • Solvent orange 8
Fragrances	• Cananga • Geraniol
Fragrances	• Hydroxycitronellal • Jasmine • Patchouli • Sandalwood oil • Ylang-ylang oil
Miscellaneous agents	• Formaldehyde • Nickel • Rubber • Primula obconica • Musk ambrette • Cinnamic alcohol • Benzyl salicylate
Lightening creams	Kojic acid
Hair dye	PPD

*Hideo Nakayama. Pigmented Contact Dermatitis and Chemical Depigmentation. JD Johansen et al. (eds.): Contact Dermatitis, DOI: 10.1007/978-3-642-03827-3_19, © Springer-Verlag Berlin Heidelberg 2011.

5. Lymphomatoid Contact Dermatitis

This uncommon dermatitis manifests with the clinical features of plaque parapsoriasis or an early stage mycosis fungoides. These have been seen at the site of ear piercing in those sensitized to gold. Other reported causes include matches, nickel, dental amalgam, medicament components, PPD, isopropyl-diphenylenediamine and PTBPFR (para-tertiary butylphenol formaldehyde resin). Lymphomatoid contact dermatitis and mycosis fungoides alike present with infiltrative patches; the former, however, demonstrates a bright erythematous color and undefined margins.

6. Pustular Contact Dermatitis

Pustules are usually associated with irritant reactions. Nevertheless, allergic pustular reactions are known from nitrofurazone, black rubber and minoxidil.

7. Depigmentation

Irritant and allergic contact dermatitis can induce hypopigmentation as a post-inflammatory effect or by koebnerization of vitiligo. It has been difficult to ascertain whether the cause was post-inflammatory or melanocytotoxic. In particular, it is reported from hair dyes (Fig. 4.5) and is commonly seen from tempo-

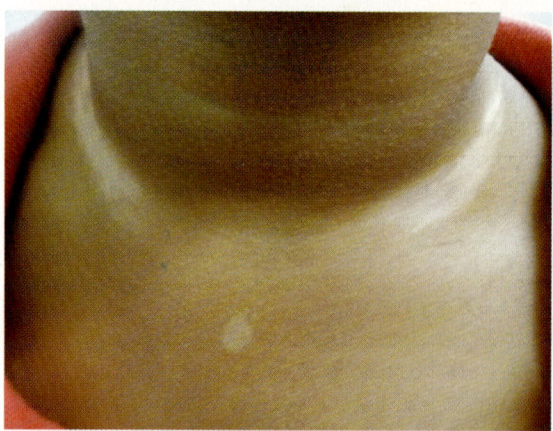

Fig. 4.6: Contact (chemical) leucoderma around the neck as the child used to hang water bottle over the neck

rary tattoos. Other causes are epoxy resin components, rubber (Fig. 4.6), methacrylates, perfumes, alstroemeria, chloroxylenol and primula allergy.

8. Granulomatous Reactions

Some topically applied metal salts, like zirconium in deodorants, immunization with aluminium-adsorbed vaccines, produce non-allergic granulomatous skin reactions. Gold and palladium in earrings and pigments in tattoos may cause allergic granulomatous and lichenoid reactions. Orofacial granulomatosis has been associated with allergy to gold crowns and mercury fillings.

9. Baboon Syndrome

First described in 1983 from Japan. The term 'baboon syndrome' was introduced by Andersen *et al* in 1984, used as the specific skin eruption resembled the red gluteal area of baboons. Clinically, the lesions were characterized by pruritic and confluent maculo-papular light red eruption over the buttocks, upper and inner surface of the thigh and axilla without any systemic symptoms and signs. Pustules are sometimes present on the red plaques. The most common cause is mercury, others are nickel, different antibiotics, heparin, aminophyllin, pseudoephedrine, terbinafine

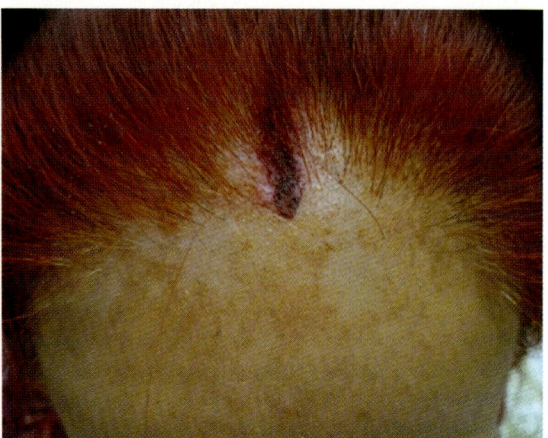

Fig. 4.5: Contact leucoderma noticed after used of heena and kumkum

and immunoglobulins. Epstein-Barr virus and cytomegalovirus can cause baboon like syndrome in children. After initial sensitization, subsequent topical or systemic exposure produces the typical morphology of the rash within a few hours to days. Baboon syndrome caused by systemic medications without a known history of previous cutaneous sensitization in the patient is termed drug-related baboon syndrome (DRBS) or symmetric drug-related intertriginous and flexural exanthema (SDRIFE). The following diagnostic criteria are proposed:

1. Exposure to a systemically administered drug either at the first or repeated dose (excluding contact allergens).
2. Sharply demarcated erythema of the gluteal/perianal area and/or V-shaped erythema of the inguinal/perigenital area;
3. Involvement of at least one other intertriginous/flexural localization.
4. Symmetry of affected areas.
5. Absence of systemic symptoms and signs.

Bibliography

1. Andersen K, Hjorth N, Menne T. The baboon syndrome: systemically-induced allergic contact dermatitis. Contact Dermatitis 1984;10:97–100.

2. Hideo Nakayama. Pigmented Contact Dermatitis and Chemical Depigmentation. Johansen JD et al. (eds.), Contact Dermatitis, DOI: 10.1007/978-3-642-03827-3_19, © Springer-Verlag Berlin Heidelberg 2011.

3. Mark Wilkinson. David Orton. Allergic contact dermatitis. In: Christopher E.M. Griffiths. Jonathan Barker. Tanya Bleiker. Robert Chalmer. Daniel Creamer, Editors. Rooks Text Book of Dermatology. Ninth edition Wiley Blackwell publishers, UK, 2016. p 3552.

4. Rietschel RL, Fowler JF, "Noneczematous contact dermatitis". Hamilton, Rietschel RL, Fowler JF, (Eds), In Fisher's Contact Dermatitis 6. pp. 88-109, BC Decker, 2008.

5. Sharma VK, Gupta V, Pahadiya P, Vedi KK, Arava S, Ramam M. Dermoscopy and patch testing in patients with lichen planus pigmentosus on face: A cross-sectional observational study in fifty Indian patients. Indian J Dermatol Venereol Leprol 2017 Nov-Dec; 83(6):656–62.

6. Textbook of Contact Dermatitis. Goh CL. "Non-eczematous contact reactions." in, Rycroft, RJG, Menn T, Frosh PJ, Lepoittevin JP, (Eds), pp. 413–31, Springer, Berlin, Germany, 3rd edition, 2001.

7. Tienthavorn T, Tresukosol P, Sudtikoonaseth P. Patch testing and histopathology in Thai patients with hyperpigmentation due to erythema dyschromicum perstans, lichen planus pigmentosus, and pigmented contact dermatitis. Asian Pac J Allergy Immunol 2014 Jun;32(2):185–92.

5

Photosensitive Eczema

Seema Rani, Shivani Bansal, Kabir Sardana

A. PHOTOALLERGIC AND PHOTOTOXIC DERMATITIS

Photoallergy is an immune reaction to a UVA-modified chemicals, commonly topical sunscreen agents, antimicrobials and topical nonsteroidal anti-inflammatory agents. Photoallergic reactions are usually triggered by sunlight and can persist in a chronic state as seen in chronic actinic dermatitis. The rash is seen on the areas exposed to the sun, its exact location is dictated by the clothes worn by the patient (Fig. 5.1). Generally speaking, it will be confined to the face, exposed area of the neck, nape of the neck, dorsum of the hands and the forearms (Fig. 5.2). However, the dermatitis may subsequently involve covered sites due to the presence of circulating activated T lymphocytes.

In cases of contact photosensitization, the rash is confined to the areas to which the photoallergen has been applied. Thus, a photoallergic reaction to a daily care cream will occur only on the face (Fig. 5.3), a reaction to a topical anti-inflammatory agent will cause a rash on the treated joint; with phyto-photodermatosis, only the areas directly in contact with the plant will present the typical vesicular-bullous lesions.

In the event of systemic photosensitization, the photoallergen spreads evenly throughout the skin in such a way that all sun-exposed areas are affected simultaneously with only slight variations in intensity due to the impact of the sun's rays.

TYPES OF RASH

The appearance of the rash varies depending on the patho-physiological mechanisms underlying the photosensitivity reaction.

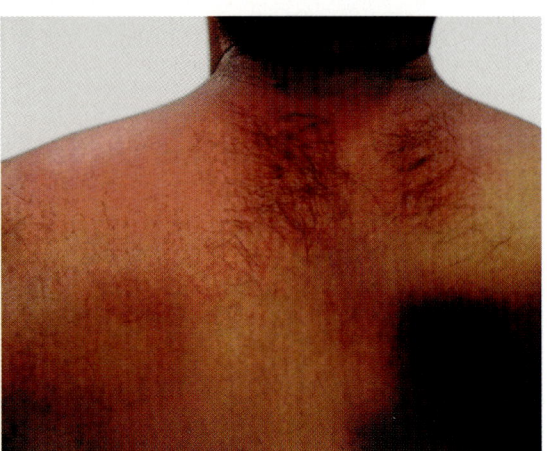

Fig. 5.1: A patient with an acute phototoxic reaction involving the upper back following exposure to sunlight while on a beach holiday

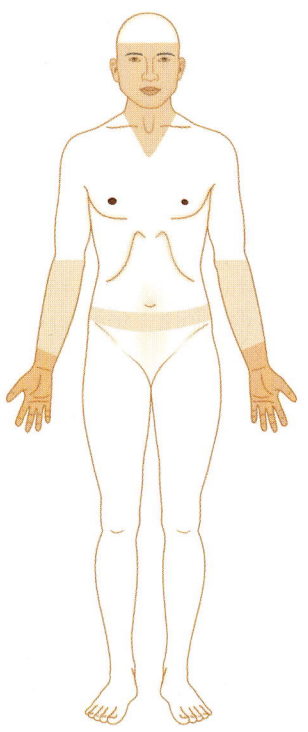

Fig. 5.2: A depiction of the distribution of a photoinduced reaction, which involves the exposed sites but spares the submental, supraorbital and periorbital area. Note the involvement of midriff in Indian patients

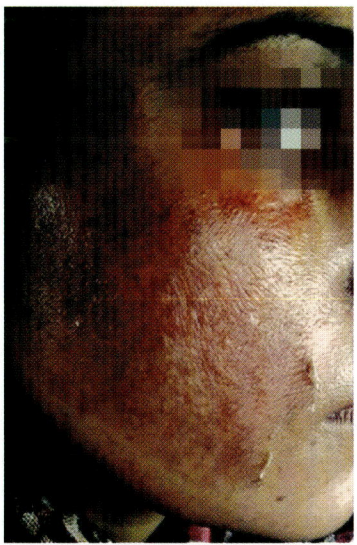

Fig. 5.3: An intense photoallergic reaction in a patient who used a herbal face pack. The peeling noticed is due to the use of topical corticosteroids that abates the intense erythema

PHOTOTOXICITY

Acute phototoxicity occurs within hours of exposure to the phototoxic agent and UV radiation with burning and stinging sensation on exposed areas, such as forehead, nose, V area of the neck, and dorsa of the hands with sparing of nasolabial folds, postauricular and submental areas, and areas covered by clothing. A phototoxic reaction causes intense erythema (Fig. 5.1) sometimes with blistering and peeling resembling a sunburn. Once the rash heals, a marked post-inflammatory pigmentation is seen.

Histopathology

Acute phototoxicity is characterized by individual necrotic keratinocytes and, in severe cases, epidermal necrosis.

There may be epidermal spongiosis, dermal edema, and a mild infiltrate consisting of neutrophils, lymphocytes, and macrophages.

PHOTOALLERGY

Photoallergy is a photoimmunologic reaction which, like contact dermatitis, involves the patient's immune system. It presents as

Table 5.1: Clinical patterns of drug associated photosensitivity	
Predominant in phototoxicity	*Predominant in photoallergy*
Exaggerated "sunburn"	Urticaria in sun-exposed area
Pseudoporphyria eczema	Acute or subacute
Photoonycholysis	Cheilitis
Hyperpigmentation	Erythema multiforme-like
Hypopigmentation (vitiligo-like lesions)	
Telangiectasia	Subacute or chronic lupus
Purpura	erythematosus
Pellagra-like reactions	
Actinic keratosis and squamous cell carcinoma	

eczema-like, lichenoid, or urticaria-like lesions. In sensitized individuals, exposure to the photoallergen and sunlight results in the development of a pruritic, eczematous eruption within 24 to 48 hours after exposure. To begin with, the lesions are confined to sun-exposed areas usually with well-demarcated margins where the skin is covered by clothing, for example at the collar and 'V' of the neck, below the end of sleeves on the backs of the hands, but may spread to protected zones if the patient does not avoid the sun completely. The area below the chin is usually spared as in the Wilkinson's triangle, i.e. area behind the earlobe (Fig. 5.4).

Histopathology

There is epidermal spongiosis associated with infiltrate of mononuclear cells in the dermis.

ETIOLOGY

In cases of contact photosensitization, the culpable substance is identified by carefully interviewing the patient to establish a list of all the topical agents, cosmetics (Fig. 5.3) and plants with which he or she has come into contact. Though a photopatch is frequently used, it must be borne in mind that any phototoxic substance will induce a positive photopatch-test result if sufficiently UV-irradiated. This means that an allergen cannot be identified on the basis of a positive photopatch-test result alone.

It is much more difficult to identify the responsible substance in cases of systemic photosensitization. All the medications taken by the patient, together with the doses taken and the dates started, must be noted down. Usually days started 3 to 14 days before the rash is the usual culprit (Table 5.2).

Drugs

The clinical patterns of systemic drug photosensitivity vary from urticaria through eczema or subacute LE up to vitiligo-like lesions or NMSC.

They can be very typical as in acute exaggerated sunburn, but sometimes, the diagnosis or even the suspicion of drug photosensitivity is not so obvious (Table 5.1).

With drugs as a cause, skin reactions can occur immediately after sun exposure in vemurafenib-induced photosensitivity, but skin lesions may be delayed 1 or 2 days in most phototoxic or photoallergic contact dermatitis or systemic photoallergy, several days or weeks in pseudoporphyria or subacute LE or even years in skin cancers associated with a long exposure to the sun and the photoactive drugs.

In systemic drug photosensitivity, the reaction usually involves, in a symmetric distribution, the face and forehead, the V-shaped area of the neck and upper chest, dorsum of the hands and forearms. Shaded areas in the face (upper eyelids, upper lip, deep wrinkles) are usually spared (Fig. 5.4) as well as retroauricular areas, submandibular areas and areas covered by the beard or scalp hair. In more extensive sun exposure, large body folds, like the axillae, groins, finger webs and areas covered by clothing or other accessories (watch strip, shoes) are also usually spared. Involvement of the shaded areas suggests an airborne dermatitis, which may occur in occupational exposure to photo-active drugs, in nurses and caregivers who crush tablets or during drug manufacture.

A different pattern in the distribution of skin lesions can occur when sun exposure is asymmetric, as in car drivers who only expose the left arm. Sometimes, in systemic photo-sensitivity, the lower lip is mainly or almost exclusively involved, because of its higher exposure and, very probably, because the corneal layer is thinner and, therefore, more prone to photosensitivity.

In photoallergic or phototoxic contact dermatitis from topical drugs, lesions are coincident with the area of drug application and concomitant sun exposure, but distant lesions can occur in areas of accidental contact, as in a contralateral limb (kissing faces of the legs), or in areas of inadvertent spread by the

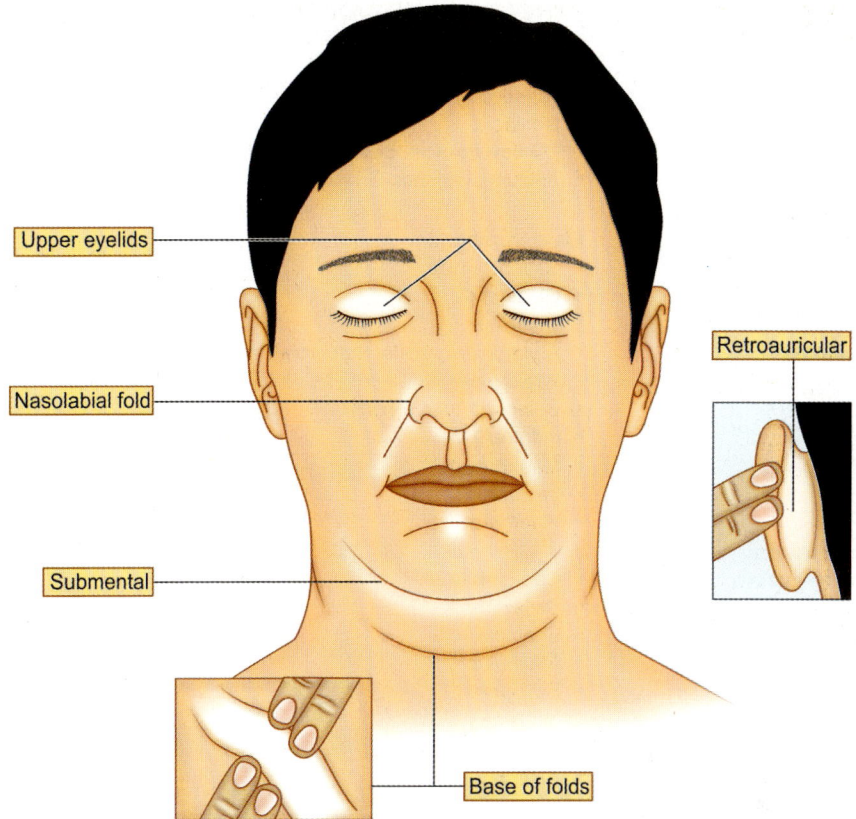

Fig. 5.4: Sites of sparing in photodistributed dermatoses of the head and neck (e.g. chronic actinic dermatitis and photoallergic dermatitis). Relatively sun-protected sites include the upper eyelids, nasolabial folds, retroauricular areas, submental region, and deepest portion of skin furrows. In airborne contact dermatitis, these areas may be involved

hands or contaminated objects. Cases of connubial dermatitis have been described, mainly ketoprofen and benzydamine. When used in the mouth these NSAIDs induce mostly lip and chin dermatitis. Some topical drugs can be considerably absorbed through the skin, and lesional distribution can be similar to systemic photosensitivity.

INVESTIGATION

Currently, the most effective and widely used method for investigating in a patient is to perform photopatch testing (Fig. 5.5). In this process, agents under investigation are prepared in a vehicle (often petrolatum) and a small volume is placed within plastic or metal chambers, which have low chemical

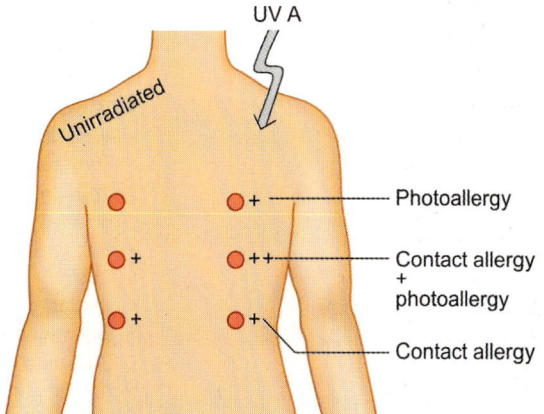

Fig. 5.5: Exogenous chemical-induced photosensitivity: Interpretation of photopatch tests. This schematic demonstrates the interpretation of photopatch tests. The UV A dose is usually the lower of 5 J/cm², or 50% of the MED to UV A

Table 5.2: The list of medicines with known photosensitizing potential

Antibacterials	• Azithromycin • Tetracycline (doxycycline, lymecycline, minocycline)[a] • Isoniazid • FQ (levofloxacin, ciprofloxacin, norfloxacin, ofloxacin)[a] • Antifungal agents: Griseofulvin[b], itraconazole, voriconazole[b]
Antimalarial agents	
Antiviral agents	Efavirenz ribavirin
Antidiabetic agents	• Glibenclamide • Glimepiride • Glipizide
Anti-inflammatories	• Arylpropionic acids: Ketoprofen[c, d], naproxen, ibuprofen • Piroxicam[c, d] • Celecoxib, diclofenac[d] • Indomethacin
Antineoplastic agents	• Methotrexate • Imatinib • Fluorouracil
Proton pump inhibitors	
Antihypertensive agents, anti-arrhythmic agents	• Captopril • Diltiazem • Enalapril • Nifedipine • Ramipril
Diuretics	
Lipid-lowering agents	
Neuroleptics, antidepressants	• Amitriptyline • Carbamazepine • Chlorpromazine • Fluoxetine • Imipramine • Levomepromazine • Paroxetine
Topical drugs	• Diclofenac • Diphenhydramine • Fluorouracil • Benzole peroxide
Antiseptics	• Bithionol • Fentichlor • Triclosan
Cosmetics	• Para-aminobenzoic acid, cinnamates, octocrylene, benzophenones, dibenzoylmethane, benzylidene camphor (sun filters) • Peru balsam • Eosin • Bergamot essence • Oak moss, 6-methylcoumarine (fragrances), paraphenylenediamine (hair dyes)
Botanics	Furocoumarins (angelica, celery, lemon, Fig, parsnip, parsley) Sesquiterpinic lactones (artichoke, chrysanthemum, dahlia, frullania, lettuce, lichen, dandelion)

[a]Mainly phototoxic

[b]An increase of actinic keratosis, NMSC and, occasionally, melanoma have been related with these drugs

[c]Mainly photoallergic

[d]Often also from topical exposure or airborne exposure, mainly in occupational settings

reactivity and are mounted on hypoallergenic adhesive tape. After the chamber preparation, they are then applied in duplicate sets to the skin of the patients' back. Ideally, the tape and chambers should not be placed on the paravertebral area 5 cm on either side of the midline, but should be placed lateral to this area on the left and/or right side(s). After a variable period of time, the tape and chambers are removed and the skin at the site of one set is irradiated with a UV source. At variable times after irradiation, usually multiples of 24 hours, both test sites are then visually inspected and the strength of any reaction is recorded using a grading scale.

Though beyond the scope of this book a overview of the various common photo-dermatoses is given in the (Fig. 5.6). Should be considered int he differential of photosensitive eczema.

TREATMENT

For a photosensitive reaction to occur, both a photosensitizing substance and the requisite radiation must be present. The condition can be cured if one or other of these two triggers is removed from the equation. It is obviously much easier to eliminate the photosensitizer in question than to control the sun exposure.

General Measures

I. *Elimination of antigen:* Eliminating the topical agent or medicine responsible for the reaction should lead to a cure. With a systemic photosensitivity reaction, the suspected drug must be replaced with a medicine from another therapeutic class. For a photoallergic reaction, the medicinal product responsible must be identified and eliminated because not only will the rash spread to protected areas of skin, but it will also occur at low doses and after mild exposure. In patients presenting with a phototoxic reaction (dose-dependent, requiring intense UV exposure and a high concentration of the drug in the skin), the risk of phototoxicity can be attenuated by reducing the dose prescribed and changing the time of intake to the evening (to ensure

that the concentration in the skin is lower during the day). It should be noted that photosensitivity does not decrease immediately after the medication presumed responsible is withdrawn. Photoallergy to UV filters should be eliminated. Patients should be informed of the INCI name (name of the agents/UV absorber) to which they are sensitive.

II. *Photoprotection:* Reducing exposure to radiation is the only solution when it has not been possible to identify the photo-allergen or when the patient's life depends on the drug considered to be the source of the reaction. Such patients must avoid going out in the mid-day sun when UV irradiation is at its peak. Clothing providing sufficient protection against UV rays and a wide-brimmed hat must be worn. Protective clothing is much more effective than sun protection products, which must nonetheless also be used.

Filters are synthetic chemical substances which absorb either UVB rays or UVB and UVA rays. Since most photosensitivity reactions are triggered by UVA, patients must be advised to use "Very High Protection 50+" products with the highest possible UVA protection factor. However, chemical filters may also cause contact photoallergic reactions. Patients presenting with medicinal product-related photosensitization should therefore be advised to use sun protection products containing physical screens only, consisting of minute particles of titanium dioxide, zinc oxide or mica. Nonetheless, it is important to be aware of the limitations of sun protection products since, although they certainly reduce the level of irradiation absorbed by the skin, there are currently no products available on the market actually capable of preventing a photosensitivity reaction.

Specific Measures

Corticosteroids: Topical corticosteroids are used for treating localised forms. In severe ones, though, depending on the extent of the affected skin, systemic corticosteroids may additionally be required.

Prevention

A list of days liable to induce phototoxic and photoallergic reactions (Table 5.2) can be used as a guide to eliminate at risk days. Photoallergic reactions are difficult to prevent since they depend on the immune status of the patient. Nonetheless, potentially phototoxic substances must be used with extreme caution during sunny periods. Patients must be told to avoid using fragrances and deodorants before going out into the sun.

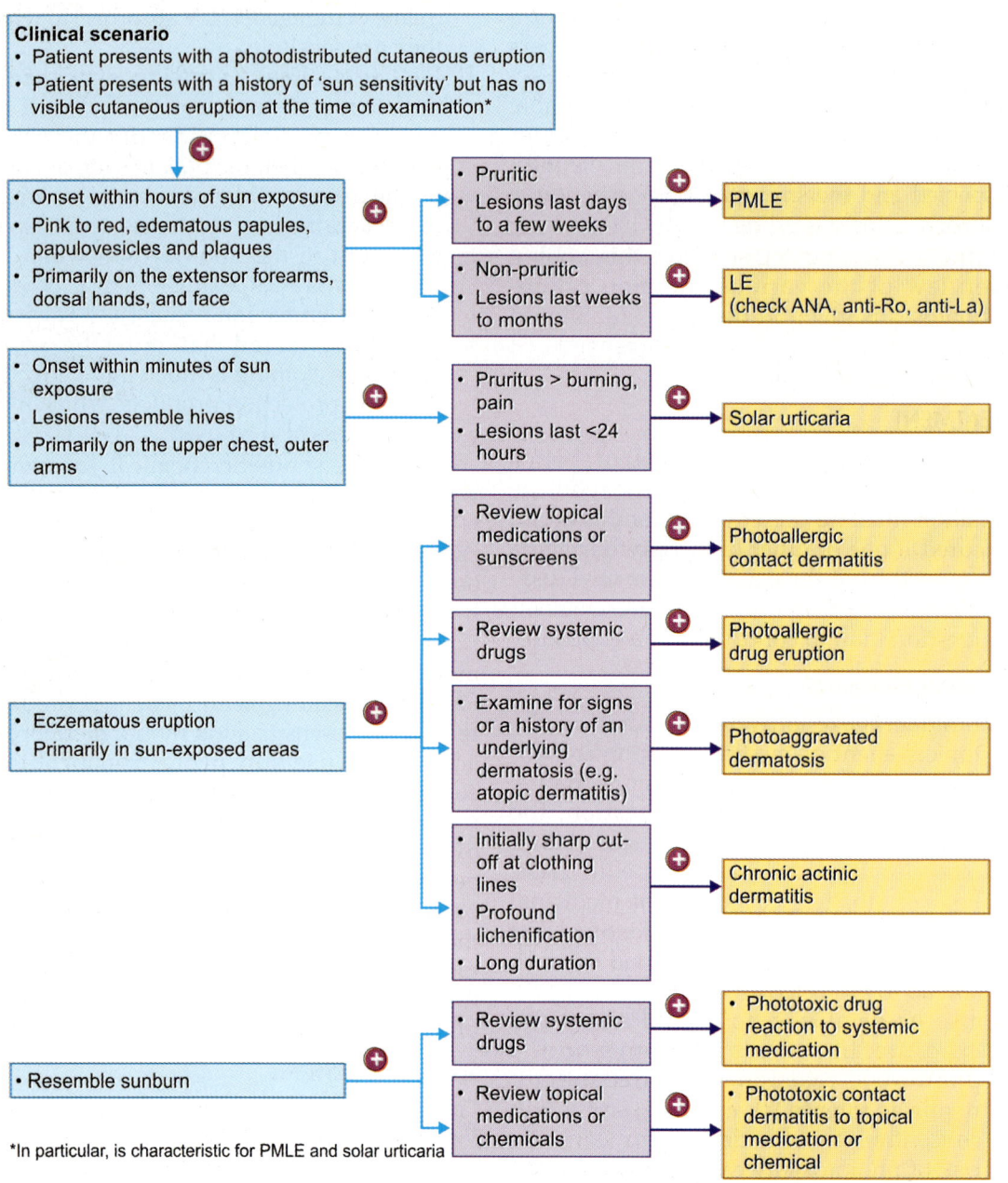

Fig. 5.6: Clues to the diagnosis of specific photodermatoses in adults. PMLE—polymorphic light eruption; LE—lupus erythematosus; ANA—antinuclear antibody

B. CHRONIC ACTINIC DERMATITIS (CAD)

The term 'CAD' was first proposed by Hawk and Magnus in 1979 and includes four previously reported diagnosis. These were actinic reticuloid, photosensitive eczema, photosensitivity dermatitis (PD)/actinic reticuloid (AR) and persistent light reactor **(Hawk JLM)**. Formerly known as persistent light reaction or actinic reticuloid syndrome, chronic actinic dermatitis is a rare photodermatitis generally affecting men aged over 50 who have worked outdoors. Persistent eczematous eruption of exposed skin, sometimes having pseudolymphomatous features.

The pathogenesis of CAD is not fully characterized, although evidence points to an underlying T cell mediated delayed cellular hypersensitivity to an undefined photo-induced antigen.

Clinical Features

The lesions of CAD are eczematous, patchy or confluent, and acute, subacute, or chronic. In severe cases, lichenification is common. Less commonly, scattered or widespread erythematous, shiny, infiltrated pseudo-lymphomatous papules or plaques are present on a background of erythematous, eczematous or normal skin, developing on photo-exposed areas where, owing to its chronic nature (Figs 5.7 and 5.8), it gives the skin an infiltrated lichenified appearance, gradually spreading into the covered zones. It can be a cause of erythroderma. It is estimated that resolution of the condition occurs in approximately 10% of those affected after 5 years (Dawe *et al.* 2000).

This is a highly debilitating condition causing a severe reaction even to minimal exposure. The patient is allergic to UVB, UVA and even visible wavelengths. The patient can also be allergic to plants of the Asteraceae family, sesquiterpenic lactones, colophane, fragrances and certain sun filters.

Pseudolymphomatoid features, such as lymphocyte exocytosis, may also be seen in severe cases which may lead to suspicion of cutaneous T cell lymphoma. Further characterisation of the T cell infiltrate, however, demonstrates predominantly CD8+ T cells, and T cell receptor gene rearrangement studies are negative.

Investigations

Assessment of the ANA and ENA is advisable in all patients to exclude the unlikely possibility of cutaneous LE. In severe or erythrodermic CAD, there may be a large numbers of circulating CD8+ Sézary cells without other suggestions of malignancy (Fitzpatricks).

As patients with chronic actinic dermatitis may also have contact allergy to airborne

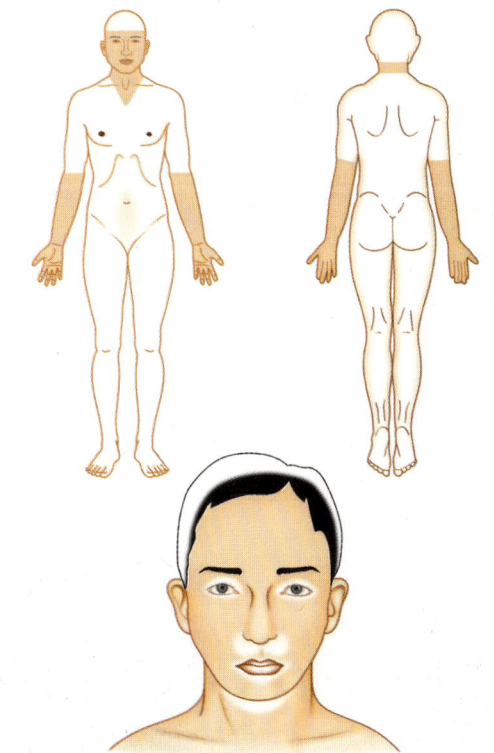

Fig. 5.7: Distribution of lesions in a classic case of CAD

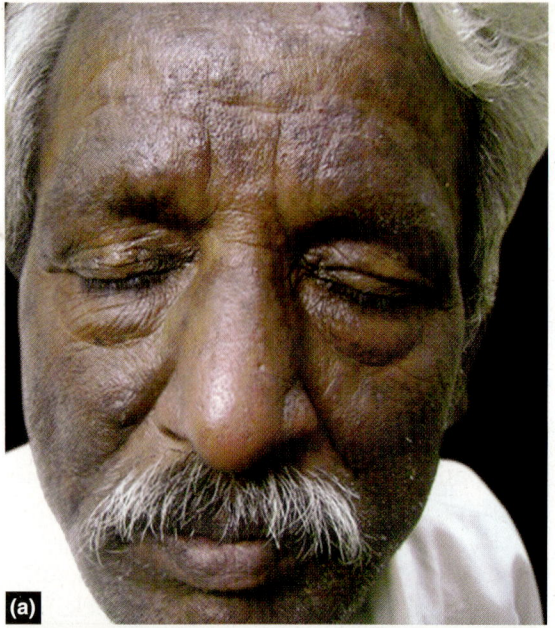

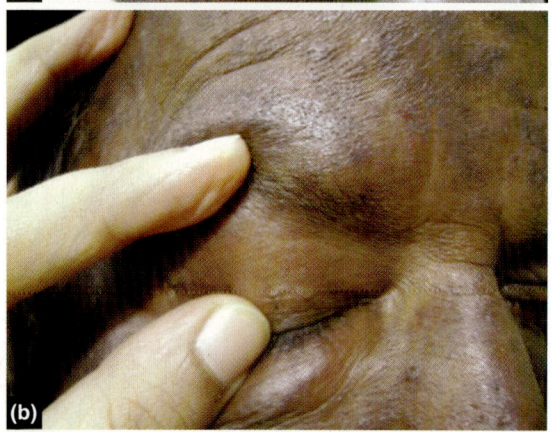

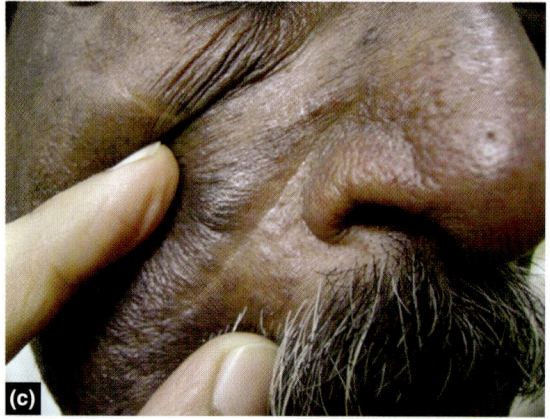

Fig. 5.8a to c: Lichenified appearance of CAD sparing the upper eyelid and the skin folds

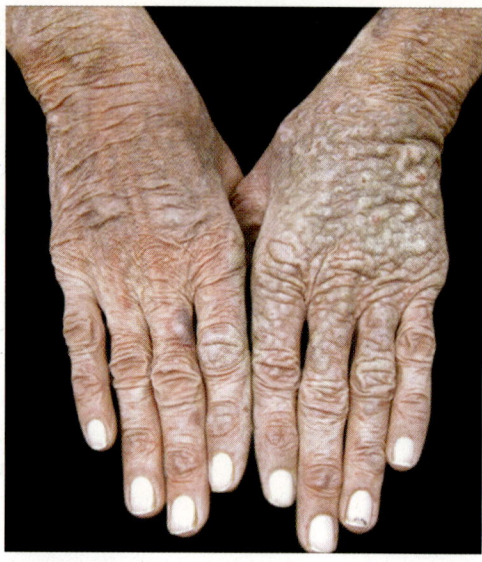

Fig. 5.8d: Lichenified pseudolymphomatous lesions on dorsum of hand

allergens, including plant antigens and fragrances, patch and photopatch testing (Fig. 5.9) is done to identify precipitating allergens and to differentiate chronic actinic dermatitis from other conditions.

Treatment

Management is broadly divided into *preventative, behavioral* and *environmental* avoidance methods to limit the clinical manifestations of photosensitivity and suppressive method to reduce the immune and inflammatory nature of disease (Table 5.3).

The results obtained with *topical treatments* are disappointing. The protection afforded by suncreams is insufficient, even when very high protection factor products are used, in preference those containing mineral screens only should be used since many patients can also be allergic to chemical filters. Protective clothing is effective but is not appropriate for certain parts of the body such as the face and hands.

a. *PUVA therapy* is the first line treatment for severe forms but is often poorly tolerated. Before treatment is started, the UVA MED must be established using the light tubes

Table 5.3: Line of treatment of CAD based on best available evidence			
	Topical	*Systemic*	*Others*
First line	**Dermocorticoids** (mometasone furoate cream; clobetasol propionate)	**Oral antihistamines**	**Photoprotection** **Allergen avoidance**
Second line	**Calcineurin inhibitors** 0.1% topical tacrolimus	**Azathioprine** (100 mg/d) **MMF:** 2 gm **Cyclosporine:** 2.5 mg/kg/day **HCQS:** 200 mg BD	**Phototherapy** PUVA, with starting UVA doses of 0.25 J/cm^2 and increases of 0.25–1 J/cm^2 up to a maximum 10 J/cm^2
Third line		**Danazol:** 600 mg/day for 3 weeks **Thalidomide** (100 mg/day reduced to 50 mg twice weekly) over 5 months	
Emergency measure		**Prednisolone** 40 mg × 5 d	

that will later be used for the treatment sessions. The initial UVA dose delivered must be less than the UVA MED (i.e. very low, about 0.25 to 0.50 J/cm^2), and should then be gradually increased (by about 0.25 J/cm^2 at each session) depending on tolerance. Generally, a patient will have three sessions per week for a total of 10 weeks. Treatment can be stopped when light tolerance has reached an acceptable level, but if photosensitivity persists, maintenance treatment should be offered (one PUVA therapy session a week during the summer and one session every two weeks in winter).

A combination with steroids known as *cortico-PUVA therapy* renders the first photo-therapy sessions more bearable. The patient is given systemic corticosteroids at a dose of 1 mg/kg/day starting 8 days before PUVA therapy and continued at the same dose for 4 weeks and then gradually withdrawn.

b. Narrow band UVB phototherapy (TL01 tubes) has been used in some cases, starting at a dose well below the MED (about 10 to 20 mJ/cm^2) and gradually increasing the dose delivered.

c. *Immunosuppressants* are the second-line treatment. These include cyclosporine 3.5–5 mg/kg/day, mycophenolate mofetil 2.5–4 mg/kg/day and azathioprine 1–2.5 mg/kg/day.

A questionnaire survey of 253 UK dermatologists demonstrated that 68% use azathioprine in CAD, 66% alone, and the others as a steroid-sparing agent. Most used 100 mg daily, only 13% prescribing it by body weight. CAD had the highest proportion of perceived efficacy (62%) of all disorders treated with azathioprine.

Hydroxyurea 500 mg once or twice daily was shown to induce remission of CAD in one patient (Gramvussakis S). Successful treatment with etretinate, attenuated androgen and danazol 600 mg/day and intramuscular injection of natural alpha-interferon (3 MU three times weekly) has also been reported (Alastair C Kerr and Sally H Ibbotson).

d. Immunomodulation, without the short- and long-term adverse events associated with a more general approach to immuno-suppression, would produce major advances in the treatment of this disease. The biological agents that are now being increasingly used for recalcitrant chronic skin diseases provide hope and may be the future developments in understanding of CAD. Availability of appropriate targeted immunomodulatory drugs may provide further answers for the management of this condition.

In summary, following photoprotection and topical steroids, most require azathioprine (50–200 mg/day). PUVA and oral steroids can be used. We usually initiate the patient on hydroxychloroquine (200 mg once or twice daily) and use cyclosporine as an emergency intervention.

REFERENCES

1. Alastair C Kerr and Sally H Ibbotson. In Chronic actinic dermatitis. Expert review of dermatology 2010. Aramuc India Ltd. Mumbai. Chapter 227; p 272–282.

2. Eczema, in. Sardana k, Mahajan S, Garg VK. Diagnosis and Management of Skin Disorders: An Evidence-Based Approach, 1/e.: Lippincott Williams and Wilkins, 2012 (reprint 2015).

3. Fast Facts: Eczema and Contact Dermatitis By John Berth-Jones, Eunice Tan and Howard I Malbach Published 2004.

4. Gramvussakis S, George SA. Chronic actinic dermatitis(photosensitivity dermatitis/actinic reticuloid syndrome): beneficial effect from hydroxyurea. Br. J. Dermatol. 143, 1340(2000).

5. Hawk JLM, Magnus IA. Chronic actinic dermatitis-an idiopathic photosensitivity syndrome including actinic reticuloid and photosensitive eczema. Br. J. Dermatol. 101(Suppl.17), 24(1979).

6. Norris PG, Hawk JLM. Chronic actinic dermatitis-a unifying concept. Arch. Dermatol. 126, 376–378(1990).

7. Thieme Clinical Companions Dermatology. Sterry, Dermatology© 2006 Thieme.

Seema Rani, Sanjay Ghosh, Saurav Kundu

6

Airborne Contact Dermatitis

INTRODUCTION

Airborne contact dermatitis (ABCD) denotes a unique subtype of contact dermatitis that originates from *plants*, especially compositae, *natural resins, woods, plastic, rubber, glues, metals, pharmaceutical chemicals, insecticides and pesticides* **(Huygens)**. Other causes include, dust, spray, pollens or volatile chemicals by airborne particles that settle on the exposed skin as well as body folds (Handa *et al*). This form of dermatitis commonly involves face, neck, V-area of chest, eyelids as well as non-exposed skin such as axilla and waist lines. Sometimes this form of dermatitis can be generalized (Gordon, Bajaj).

ABCD often causes diagnostic problems in terms of identifying the causative agent and the treatment is equally challenging. ABCD is clinically identified on the basis of history, morphology and distribution of lesions and proved by allergic patch test.

In this chapter, the various epidemiological aspects of ABCD, newly identified occupational and nonoccupational airborne contactants, clinical manifestations and treatment modalities available in ABCD will be discussed.

EPIDEMIOLOGY

Epidemiologically, ABCD can be classified into occupational and nonoccupational ABCD.

It can affect any individual, at any age and both men and women are affected by this condition. This is no racial, ethnic, or geographical predominance.

It is believed that airborne *irritant* dermatitis is much common than the *allergic* type.

Incidence of airborne dermatoses has increased considerably during recent years (Huygens and Goossens). There is great diversity in the nature of airborne reactions, which may be irritant, allergic, phototoxic, photoallergic or contact urticarial. Some agents may cause more than one type of reaction. Lists of airborne allergens have been published and updated by Huygens and Goossens. Plants, natural resins and woods are among the commoner causes of this distribution of contact allergy. In the USA, the oleoresins of ragweed commonly cause allergic contact dermatitis. A similar pattern in the UK during the summer months is caused by other compositae (asteraceae) weeds which, when they occur in other parts of the world, also produce an 'airborne' pattern of dermatitis. In India Parthenium has been associated with widespread epidemics of severe dermatitis and even deaths [Mark Wilkinson]. Colophony can also give an exposure pattern of dermatitis from its presence in solder fluxes, paper dust, polish and linoleum flooring [Mark Wilkinson]. Resin systems, particularly epoxy resins, including the more volatile amine hardeners, may induce an airborne pattern of allergy, especially in the occupational setting. Other causes of this pattern include perfumes, metals, many industrial and pharmaceutical chemicals, pesticides, fungicides, animal feed additives, textile dyes and matches [Handa S]. Equivalent patterns of airborne dermatitis may be seen with type I allergens, such as housedust mite antigens in atopics (Hostetler SG). Photocontact allergy causes a similar distribution, and is discussed in a separate section in this chapter.

Cabanillas *et al* reported a 3% prevalence of allergic ABCD to plant antigens among patients attending contact dermatitis unit. Sharma *et al* reported that in India, parthenium dermatitis caused by *Parthenium hysterophorus*, is an important cause of ABCD. In a study by Agarwal *et al* from South India, 50 patients of Parthenium dermatitis were studied. Among them, 90% were farmers by occupation and lesions were aggravated in summer. The most common type of dermatitis was the classic ABCD pattern (46%), followed by mixed pattern (30%), erythroderma (14%) and chronic actinic dermatitis (10%).

As per the previous reports by Nandakishor *et al* and Pasricha *et al*, ABCD in Indian patients has been attributed exclusively by pollens of plants like *Parthenium hysterophorus, Xanthium strumarium, Chrysanthemum coronarium, Helianthus annus and Dahlia pimrata*. The recent reports by Ghosh and Johnson *et al* have shown that the scenario has been changing rapidly in **urban and semiurban perspective in** developing countries where *cement, perfumes, deodorants, volatile paints*, etc. have become the commonest allergens contributing to ABCD.

In another study by Singhal *et al*, 75 patients with clinically suspected contact dermatitis were patch tested with the Indian Standard Series and indigenous antigens. Parthenium was the most common contact sensitizer (20%) followed by potassium dichromate (16%), xanthium (13.3%), nickel sulphate (12%), chrysanthemum (8%) and mercaptobenzothiazole (6.7%).

PATHOGENESIS

In ABCD, on initial exposure to the antigen, there is no response which is referred to as refractory phase. This is followed by an induction phase where the hapten penetrates the skin, conjugates with an epidermal protein and comes in contact with antigen presenting cells, migrates to the draining lymph nodes followed by stimulation of naïve T cells. This leads to proliferation of activated T cells to produce effector and memory cells which then enter the circulation. Reexposure to the specific hapten leads to the release of mediators producing skin inflammation (Lakshmi and Srinivas).

A personal history of atopy is also associated with increased risk for both ACD and ICD (Cashman *et al*).

ALLERGENS

Antigens which cause ABCD (modified from Santos *et al* and Huygens *et al*) have been listed in Table 6.1, 6.2.

CLINICAL FEATURES

Dooms-Goossens and Deleu classified airborne dermatitis into 5 types:

1. Airborne irritant contact dermatitis
2. Airborne allergic contact dermatitis
3. Airborne phototoxic reactions
4. Airborne photoallergic reactions
5. Airborne contact urticaria

Table 6.1: Antigens contributing to airborne contact dermatitis (allergic ABCD)

Plants and natural resins	Plastics, rubber and glues	Metals	Industrial chemicals and drugs	Miscellaneous
• Parthenium hysterophorus	• Epoxy resins	Chromate Cobalt Gold	• Organophosphorus Pesticides	• Agricultural Dust
• Eucalyptus pulverulenta	• Formaldehyde and formaldehyde resins	Mercury Nickel Silver	Animal feed	• Disperse dyes • Cigarettes
• Cedar pollen • Citrus fruits • Compositae • Cinnamon			• Antibiotics • Paraphenylenediamine	
• Chrysanthemum • Sunflower • Garlic	• Rubber additives • Fragrance mix		• Potassium metabisulphite • Quaternerium-15 • Potassium Dichromate	
• Essential oils • Tropical and domestic woods • Latex • Psyllium • Soybean	• Colophony		• Metaproterenol • Rhodium solution	

Table 6.2: Specific antigens contributing to ICD, photoallergic and contact urticaria (Santos R et al and Huygen S)

ICD	Photoallergic reaction	Contact urticaria
Phosphates	Carprofen	Amoxycillin
Synthetic fibers	Chlorpromazine	Epoxy resins
Mustard gas, Ethylene oxide	Olaquindox	Hyacinth
Metal dust	Pesticides	Pine processes
Carbon dust		Weeping fig

The occurrence of airborne irritant dermatitis, i.e. irritant contact dermatitis due to agents carried by or through the air, has been underestimated offending agents are present in the air under various physical forms: fibers, dust particles, sprays, vapors, and gases.

Some agents, such as *P. hysterophorus*, can produce both allergic CD and phototoxic reactions. Mixed pattern is also seen in **formaldehyde** and **phosphorus sesquisulfide** where allergic CD can coexist with contact urticaria (Dooms-Goossens and Deleu).

In **classical ABCD**, there is involvement of the exposed areas of face (Figs 6.1 and 6.2),

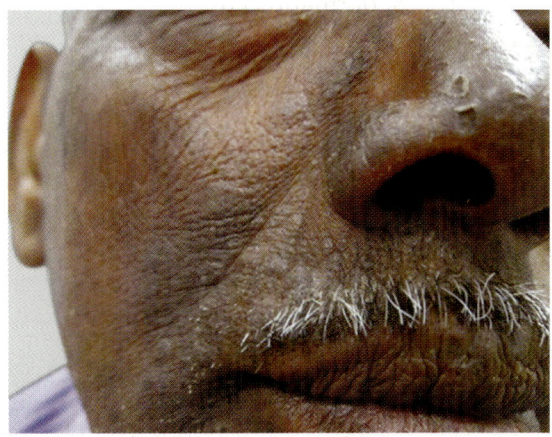

Fig. 6.1: Face affected by airborne contact dermatitis, note the involvement of the folds of the skin

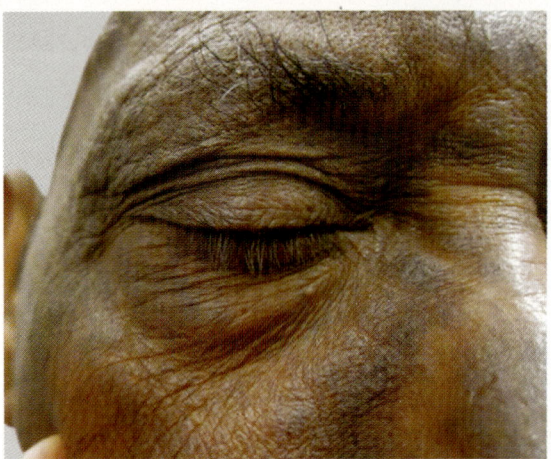

Fig. 6.2: Marked involvement of the eyelids

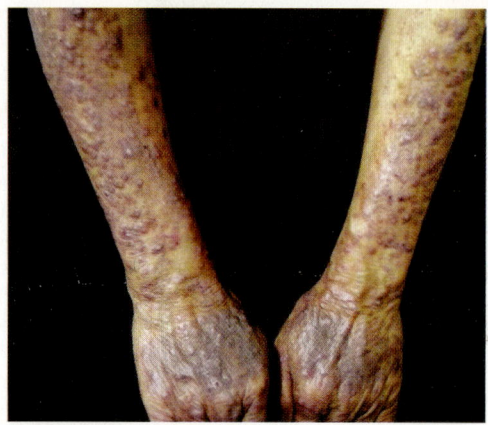

Fig. 6.4: Forearm affected by airborne contact dermatitis (lichenoid morphology)

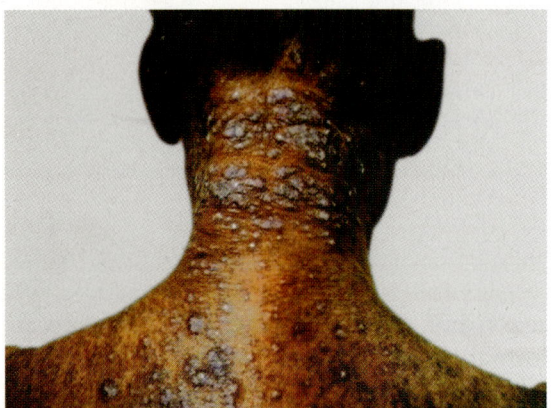

Fig. 6.3: Nape of the neck and upper back affected by airborne contact dermatitis (lichenoid morphology)

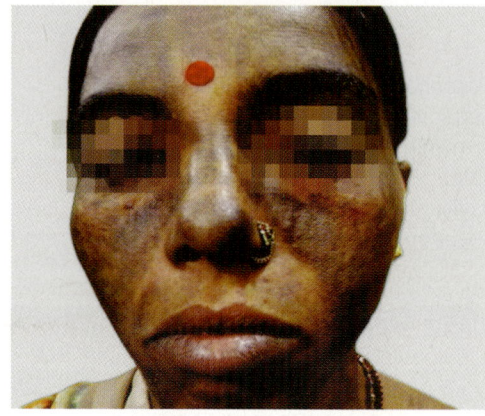

Fig. 6.5: A female patient affected by airborne contact dermatitis

V-area of neck, hand and forearms, 'Wilkinson's triangle', eyelids, nasolabial folds and under the chin. Other than these, areas of skin where the dust and fibers can be trapped such as neck (under shirt collar) (Fig. 6.3), forearms (under cuffs) (Fig. 6.4), lower legs (inside trouser leg) can also be affected. Contact dermatitis from prolonged and repeated exposure to small quantities of airborne allergens such as pollens and dust may produce diffuse, dry and lichenified eruptions.

ABCD and photoallergic dermatitis have similar presentation, as both photoexposed and covered areas are involved in ABCD (Sharma and Sethuraman). However, in

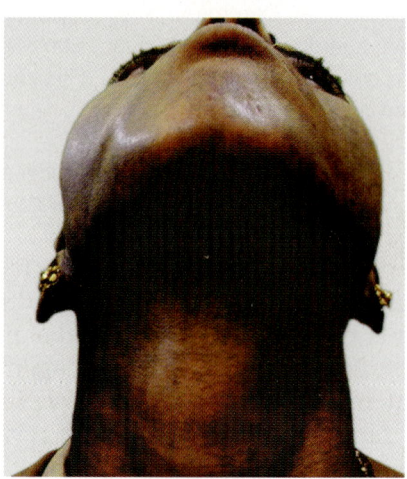

Fig. 6.6: Submental area affected by airborne contact dermatitis (contrasting from photoallergic dermatitis)

photoallergic dermatitis, submental and post-auricular area is *spared* (Ghosh) (Figs 6.5 and 6.6). Sawdust from teak and mahogany contains sensitizers that produce a dry dermatitis of face, penis and scrotum of carpenters (Sharma and Sethuraman).

Contact dermatitis from prolonged, repeated exposure to relatively small quantities of airborne allergens, such as pollens, dusts and vapors, produces diffuse, dry and lichenified eruptions with vesiculations. The exposed portions of the body as well as wrinkles and folds are most markedly involved (Fig. 6.7a and b).

1. The most commonly seen **parthenium dermatitis** classically presents as ABCD but may occasionally present with photo-sensitive lichenoid eruptions or erythroderma (more than 90% body surface area involvement) may develop. The flowers, leaves, stems, and pollens of these plants are coated with sesquiterpene lactones, which are the primary substances respon-sible for producing an allergic reaction upon exposure. Airborne exposure can occur via direct contact with sesquiterpene lactones coating the pollen or through the release of these chemicals into the air through incineration (Habif TP).

2. Dermatitis from **wood dust** is common in carpenters and cabinet makers. It normally starts on the eyelids or the lower half of the face, and is often preceded by a period of itching. Swelling and redness spread to the neck, hands and forearms. By the time the patient attends for treatment, a diffuse dermatitis may have developed, distinctly limited at the margins of the sleeves and collar. Because of the accumulation of dust and sweat, the elbow flexures and the skin under a tight collar are often lichenified.

3. **Cabinet makers** frequently develop a genital dermatitis from the accumulation of sawdust on the clothes during sawing and planing, and by hand contact. Swelling and redness of the eyelids may be the only signs of recurrence. Exotic woods are more likely to sensitize than fir or spruce, although the latter may cause dermatitis in patients sensitive to colophony and turpentine.

4. Dermatitis **in woodworkers** may additionally be caused by liverworts and lichens on the bark of trees.

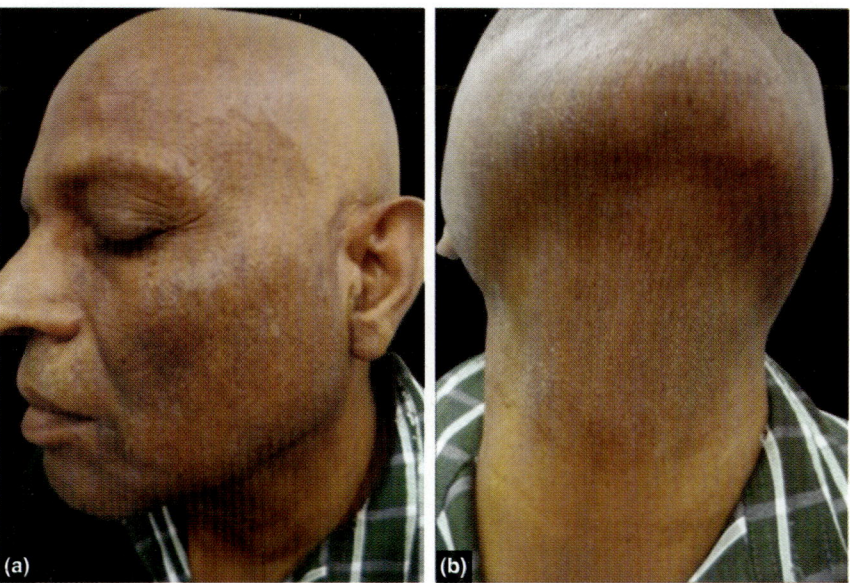

Fig. 6.7a and b: Airborne photocontact dermatitis involving face and submental area

5. **Cement dust** usually presents as a dry, lichenified dermatitis due to the presence of chromates.

6. **Household** sprays, insecticides and occupational volatile chemicals can produce eyelid dermatitis (Rietschel and Fowler).

7. **Airborne** chloromethyl and methylisothiazolinone dermatitis may appear on face of sensitized individuals who stay in newly painted rooms (Bohn, Niederer, Brehm *et al*).

8. Airborne **contact urticaria** can be associated with rhinitis, conjunctivitis and asthma in patients with hypersensitivity to latex proteins in rubber gloves (Christophe, Le, Ducombs). Airborne transmission of latex allergens is enhanced by their adsorption onto the cornstarch. Airborne contact urticaria is also reported in person exposed to cinchona dust (Dooms-Goossens).

DIFFERENTIAL DIAGNOSIS

The differential diagnoses of airborne contact dermatitis must include contact allergic reactions caused by directly applied agents, by occasional contacts with allergens, by transfer of the allergens ("ectopic") dermatitis, connubial or consort dermatitis, an id-like spread of a dermatitis elsewhere on the body, systemic eczematous contact dermatitis-type reactions, and photo-induced dermatosis. Other eczematous skin conditions, particularly atopic dermatitis and also seborrheic dermatitis, must be considered.

Diagnosis

The diagnosis of airborne dermatitis is usually made on the basis of history of the patient, the distribution and morphology of the lesions and patch test, prick test or radioallegro-sorbent test.

After clinically suspecting a case as ABCD, it needs to be confirmed with patch test or prick test. The patch test is used to find the causative allergens. In case of volatile allergens, high dilution should be used during patch test as there is a chance of developing irritant reaction. For testing wood dust, it should not be moistened as it increases irritancy. Photopatch test can be used for excluding light as a precipitating factor.

In a study by Green and Ferguson, sesquiterpene lactone (SL) mix detected only 35% of compositae allergy and hence is not a very useful screening test. These patients could be diagnosed by additional compositae mix testing which is more useful.

TREATMENT

Treatment of ABCD can be broadly divided into:
- Preventive management
- Treatment of existing dermatitis.

Preventive Management

In cases of ABCD due to Parthenium, one should avoid going outdoors on days when pollen are present in high concentration specially in summers and in the month of September to November. Air conditioning also decreases indoor pollen load. Simple routine like taking a bath after coming indoors, wearing fresh clothes and eliminating grasses and weeds in the house garden can be of great benefit. Other preventive measures include photoprotection, change of job and residence, if possible (Nicholson, Llewellyn, English). In some countries, addition of ferrous sulphate to cement converts the hexavalent chromates into trivalent ones, thereby reducing the sensitizing potential.

Treatment of Existing Dermatitis

Topical

- Topical steroids are the mainstay of therapy.
- Emollients can be co-prescribed in lichenified lesions, whereas in oozing lesions drying agents such as aluminum sulfate and calcium acetate can be given.

Systemic

- Systemic steroids are indicated when more than 25% of body surface area is involved
- Psoralens and UVA
- UVB
- In a therapeutic study of patients with parthenium dermatitis azathioprine was given as weekly pulse doses (Verma KK et al)
- Parthenium dermatitis, unresponsive to topical treatment has been treated with oral methotrexate in a dose of 15 mg/week (Sharma et al)
- Handa et al evaluated the effect of oral hyposensitization as an alternative therapeutic modality and observed a gradual improvement in the clinical status of 70% of those patients who completed the study.

CONCLUSION

Evidence indicates that up to 50% of patients with ABCD experience adverse effects on quality of life, daily function and personal relationship and take time off work on sick leave because of their skin disease. It is emphasized that avoidance of further exposure can lead to recovery from dermatitis in many cases. With respect to ABCD secondary to parthenium dermatitis, there are continuing attempts to control the spread of weed through biological measures like introduction of exotic arthropods, use of antagonistic plants and bioherbicides as well as selective chemical herbicides.

Airborne irritants are certainly more common than allergic reactions, although they are more difficult to demonstrate. Recognizing the characteristic nature of the reactions can greatly facilitate the diagnosis. Such reactions could be strongly suspected when symmetric lesions occur on the exposed body parts (sometimes even on occluded areas!), and especially the eyes and the face in general, when the patient denies having applied any topical agents and when the symptoms clear when the patient changes environment.

Bibliography

1. Agarwal KK, Souza MD. Airborne contact dermatitis induced by parthenium: A study of 50 cases in South India. Clin Exp Dermatol 2009; 34:e4–6.

2. Bajaj AK. Contact dermatitis. In IADVL Textbook and Atlas of Dermatology. In: Valia RG, Editor, 2nd Ed, Vol 1. Mumbai: Bhalani; 2001, p.453–97.

3. Bohn S, Niederer M, Brehm K, et al. Airborne contact dermatitis from methylchloroisothia-zolinone in wall paint. Abolition of symptoms by chemical allergen inactivation. Contact Dermatitis 2003; 31:275–6.

4. Cabanillas M, Fernandez-Redondo V, Toribio J. Allergic contact dermatitis to plants in a Spanish dermatology department: A 7-year review. Contact Dermatitis 2006; 55:84–91.

5. Cashman MW, Reutemann PA, Ehrlich A. Contact dermatitis in the United States:epidemiology, economic impact and workplace prevention. DermatolClin 2012; 30: 87–98.

6. Christophe J, Le Coz, Ducombs G. Plants and plant product contact dermatitis. In: Frosch PJ, Menne T, Lepoittevin JP, Editors, 4th ed. Heidelberg: Springer; 2006. p.751–800.

7. Dooms-Goossens A, Deveylder H, Duron C, et al. Airborne contact urticaria due to cinchona. Contact Dermatitis 1986; 15:258.

8. Ghosh S. Airborne contact dermatitis of non-plant origin: An overview. Ind J Dermatol 2011; 56:(6)711–4.

9. Ghosh S. Airborne contact dermatitis: An urban perspective. Perils of urban pollution: Proceedings National Seminar on Pollution in Urban Industrial Environment. In:Mitra AK, Editor. Kolkata: St Xavier's College; 2006 p. 9–12.

10. Ghosh S. Atlas and Synopsis of Contact and Occupational Dermatology. Jaypee Brothers, New Delhi 2008:20–4.

11. Gordon LA. Compositae dermatitis. Australas J Dermatol 1999; 40:123–30.

12. Green C, Ferguson J. Sesquiterpene lactone mix is not an adequate screen for Compositae allergy. Contact Dermatitis 1994; 31:151–3.

13. Habif TP. Contact dermatitis and patch testing. In: Habif TP, ed. Clinical Dermatology: A Color Guide to Diagnosis and Therapy, 5th edn. St Louis, MO: Mosby (Elsevier), 2009: 130–153.

14. Handa F, Handa S, Handa R. Environmental factors and the skin. In: Valia RG, Editor. IADVL Textbook and Atlas of Dermatology. 2nd ed, Vol.1. Mumbai: Bhalani; 2001; p. 81–91.

15. Handa S, De D, Mahajan R. Airborne contact dermatitis current perspectives in etiopathogenesis and management. Indian J Dermatol 2011; 56: 700–706.

16. Hostetler SG, Kaffenberger B, Hostetler T, et al. The role of airborne proteins in atopic dermatitis. J Clin Aesthet Dermatol 2010; 3: 22–31.

17. Huygen S, Goossen A. An update on airborne contact dermatitis. Contact Dermatitis 2001; 44:1–6.

18. Lakshmi C, Srinivas CR. Parthenium dermatitis caused by immediate and delayed hypersensitivity. Contact Dermatitis 2007; 57:64–5.

19. Mark Wilkinson. David Orton. Allergic contact dermatitis. In: Christopher E.M. Griffiths. Jonathan Barker. Tanya Bleiker. Robert Chalmer. Daniel Creamer, Editors. Rooks Text Book of Dermatology. Ninth edition Wiley Blackwell publishers, UK, 2016, p. 3544–47.

20. Nandakishore TH, Pasricha JS. Pattern of cross-sensitivity between four Compositae plants Parthenium hysterophorus, Xanthiumstrumarium, Chrysanthemum coronarium, Helianthus annusin Indianpatients. Contact Dermatitis 1994;30:162–7.

21. Nicholson PJ, Llewellyn D, English JS. On behalf of the Guidelines Development Group. Evidence-based guidelines for the prevention, identification and management of occupational contact dermatitis and urticaria. Contac Dermatitis 2010;63:177–86.

22. Pasricha JS, Verma KK, D'souza P. Airborne contact dermatitis caused exclusively by Xanthium strumarium. IndianJDermatolVenerolLeprol1995; 61:354–5.

23. Rietschel RL, Fowler JF. Fisher's Contact Dermatitis. Hamilton: BC Decker Inc; 2008, p. 69–101.

24. Santos R, Goossens AR. An update on airborne contact dermatitis: 2001-2006. Contact Dermatitis 2007;57:353–60.

25. Sharma VK, Bhat R, Sethuraman G, et al. Treatment of parthenium dermatitis with methotrexate. Contact Dermatitis 2007; 57:118–9.

26. Sharma VK, Sethuraman G, Bhat R. Evaluation of clinical patterns of Parthenium dermatitis: A study of 74 cases. Contact Dermatitis 2005;44: 49–50.

27. Sharma VK, Sethuraman G, Tejasvi T. Comparison of patch test contact sensitivity to acetone and aqueous extracts of Partheniumhysterophorusin patients with airborne contact dermatitis. Contact Dermatitis 2004;50:230–2.

28. Sharma VK, Sethuraman G. Parthenium dermatitis. Dermatitis 2007;18:183–90.

29. Singhal V, Reddy BS. Common contact sensitizers in Delhi. J Dermatol 2000;27:440–5.

30. Verma KK, Bansal A, Sethuraman G. Parthenium dermatitis treated with azathioprine weekly pulse doses. Indian Dermatol Venereol Leprol 2006; 72:24–7.

7

Parthenium Dermatitis

Ananta Khurana

Allergic contact dermatitis (ACD) to *Parthenium hysterophorus* is the most common cause of plant dermatitis in India. Parthenium dermatitis (PD) is caused by airborne dry and friable plant particles, especially trichomes.

In India, *Parthenium hysterophorus* is commonly known as "Congress grass" or "Congress weed," probably referring to the US congress which allocated the contaminated wheat shipment, containing the herb, for Pune in 1956 (Figs 7.1 and 7.2). The plant is a native of tropical America but now has a worldwide presence. *P. hysterophorus is* thought to be a natural hybrid of *Parthenium confertum* and *Parthenium bipinnatifidum* and belongs to the family Asteraceae (Compositae). It is an annual plant, growing all round the year except in extreme winters. Further, it can grow in all soils except the saline soil near

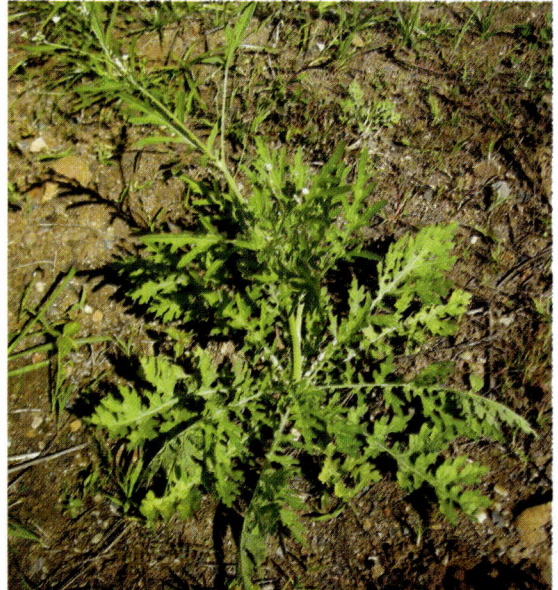

Fig. 7.1: Juvenile plant: Grows like a rosette. Lower leaves are spread on the ground; are relatively large and deeply divided (bi-pinnatifid or bi-pinnatisect). Leaves on the upper branches decrease in size and are also less divided

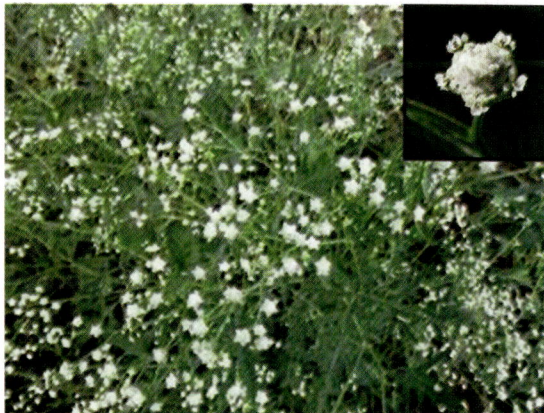

Fig. 7.2: Mature plant with flowering. Each flower-head (capitulum) in borne on a stalk (pedicel) and has five tiny 'petals' (ray florets). They also have numerous tiny white flowers (tubular florets) in the centre and are surrounded by two rows of small green bracts (involucre)

sea shores. It is a rapid colonizer showing allelopathic effects, meaning that it competes out any vegetation in its vicinity and thus can destroy natural ecosystems. It also has detrimental effects on the livestock consuming it, with reduction in the quality of milk and meat, liver and kidney damage and skin and hair disorders. It not only produces dermatitis but is widely implicated in causing respiratory allergies. Thus, it is aptly called the "Scourge of India".

ALLERGENS IN *PARTHENIUM HYSTEROPHORUS*

The most important allergens responsible are sesquiterpene lactones(SQLs). These are present in the leaf, stem, flower and pollen, but the highest concentrations are present in the small glandular hairs (trichomes) present on the under surface of the leaves and stem. SQLs are biologically active plant chemicals identified in many plant families, with Compositae having the greatest numbers (more than 3000 different SQLs). They are classified on the basis of their carbocyclic skeletons into germacranolides, guaianolides, eudesmanolides, pseudoguaianolides and xanthonolides. Parthenin is the major SQL in *P. hysterophorus* seen in India (Box 7.1). As SQLs are found in other Compositae and non-Compositae plants as well, there may be cross-reaction to other plants in patients with PD. Other members of the compositae family in North India include *Xanthium strumarium, Chrysanthemum morifolium* (chrysanthemum), *Dahlia pinnata* (dahlia) and *Tagetes indica* (marigold). *P. hysterophorus* and

X. strumarium have shown a high rate of cross-sensitivity in Indian patients whereas the prevalence of cross-reaction with *Chrysanthemum* is generally low.

PATHOGENESIS

Parthenium dermatitis is mainly caused by dried leaves and trichomes. Pollen mainly play a role in respiratory allergy. These may not pass beyond the nasal mucosa and hence more often cause allergic rhinitis than bronchial asthma. Skin sensitization by parthenium antigen propagates as a cell-mediated hypersensitivity immune response with early sensitization phase and a subsequent elicitation phase, if antigen exposure persists. Antigen presentation to T lymphocytes in the regional lymph nodes is followed by T cell proliferation and production of effector and memory T cells. There is subsequent infiltration of these T cells into re-exposed skin sites leading to cutaneous inflammation. Elevated levels of TNF-α, IL-6, IL-8 and IL-17 and reduced levels of anti-inflammatory cytokines IL-4 and IL-10 have been demonstrated in patients with PD. A further report demonstrates that the concentration of Th1 cytokines (IL-2 and IFN-γ) and Th-17 cytokine (IL-17) are increased significantly in PD as compared to controls, while levels of Th2 cytokine (IL-10) and T-regulatory cytokine (TGF-β) are low. This suggests that the lower circulating level of IL-10 (an anti-inflammatory and immunosuppressive cytokine) might be insufficient to counter-regulate the proinflammatory signals and lead to a hypersensitivity immune response. Khatri et al demonstrated that a low serum level of IL-10 in patients is associated with a high prevalence of low IL-10-producing genotypes due to IL-10 (-) 1082 G>A and(-) 819 C>T polymorphisms. The concerned IL-10 genotypes at these loci may impose a strong genetic predisposition to PD and function as a risk factor.

In addition to this well-accepted model of type IV delayed type hypersensitivity, some

---

Box 7.1: Allergens in Parthenium hysterophorus

- Parthenin (major allergen in India; belongs to pseudoguinolide class of SQLs)
- Coronopilin
- Tetraneurin A
- Hymenin
- Hysterin
- Ambrosin
- Dihidroisoparthenin

authors have postulated that type I hypersensitivity may also be playing a role, especially in those with an atopic diathesis. This may be demonstrated by a positive skin prick test.

SQLs are not photosensitizers, they have neither phototoxic nor photoallergic properties. The absorption spectrum of SQL of parthenium has not been characterized. There are a few reports of phototoxicity due to *Chrysanthemum* extract but it is not from contact sensitizing SQL component. There is only one suspected case of photocontact dermatitis to *Parthenium*. Recently, photo-reactivity of α-methylene-γ-butyrolactone ring (an SQL model) has been reported toward thymidine and it has been postulated that this may contribute to the development of photosensitivity in PD. Reduced MED to UVB, and reduced MPD to UVA have also been well-described with PD and may contribute to the CAD pattern described.

CLINICAL FEATURES

Males are more commonly affected than females (with male: female ratio being reported between 5.5:1 and 20:1). The difference is related to outdoor exposure and nature of clothing but cannot be completely explained by these alone, as women also work in fields. On the other hand, PD has been reported in housewives and indoor workers without direct handling, in areas of widespread growth of parthenium, suggesting incidental exposure may also sensitize. Parthenium dermatitis is rare in the teenagers and children.

PD may present with a variety of morphologies (Box 7.2). In sensitized individuals, the clinical manifestations usually start within 24 hours of exposure, but it may be delayed for up to 2–3 days or even longer in milder cases. The severity varies from brief periods of erythema and itching to persistent erythema, swelling, papules or papulovesicles with itching and burning in moderate cases and extensive vesiculation and exudation

> **Box 7.2:** Clinical patterns of parthenium dermatitis
> - Airborne pattern contact dermatitis (ABCD)
> - Chronic actinic dermatitis (CAD)
> - Mixed pattern dermatitis (combination of ABCD and CAD)
> - Pseudophotodermatitis
> - Exfoliative dermatitis
> - Hand and feet dermatitis
> - Photosensitive lichenoid eruption
> - Prurigo nodularis-like
> - Perianal dermatitis
> - Vesicular hand eczema
> - Seborrheic pattern
> - Dermatitis simulating lichen nitidus
> - Atopic pattern
> - Polymorphic light eruption like

associated with edema in severe ones. Contact sensitivity to parthenium is everlasting and hence the disease runs a chronic course with exacerbation during summers initially and some reduction in winters. In southern parts of India, there are often flares in September, October and November which may be owing to increased growth of the plant following monsoons. The seasonal pattern seen initially gradually evolves into a persistent eruption with pruritic lichenified dermatitis over years.

The classical pattern, also known as airborne contact dermatitis (ABCD) pattern, affects the face, especially eyelids and/or neck, V of chest, cubital and popliteal fossae (Fig. 7.3). The eruption is termed pseudophotodermatitis as the skin of the upper eyelids, the retroauricular and submental areas, which are spared in photodermatitis, are involved in PD (Fig. 7.4). Phytophotodermatitis is not to be confused with plant dermatitis as it is a cutaneous phototoxic inflammatory eruption, resulting from contact with light-sensitizing botanical substances and long wave ultraviolet (UV-A 320–380 nm) radiation. Phytophotodermatitis typically manifests as a burning erythema in a bizarre pattern that may subsequently blister. It is not caused by parthenium. CAD pattern presents with lichenified papules, plaques, or

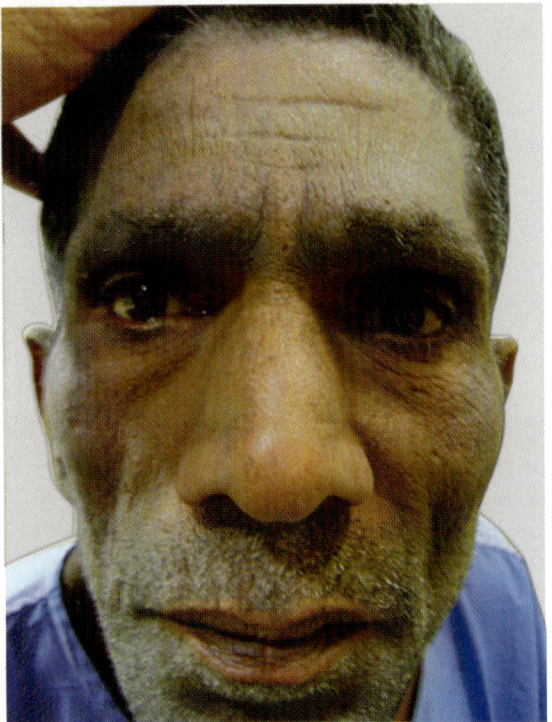

Fig. 7.3: Parthenium dermatitis involving the folds of the forehead

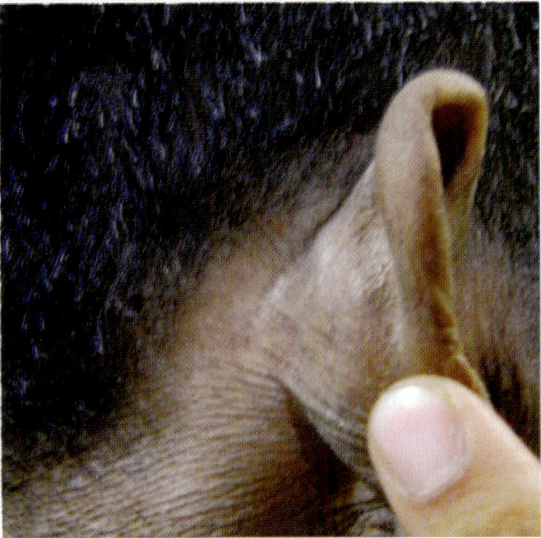

Fig. 7.4: Involvement of the retroauricular folds

forehead, ears, cheek, upper chest and back, extensor aspect of forearms and dorsae of hands. Exfoliative dermatitis with widespread erythema and scaling can develop in severely affected patients (Fig. 7.5). Recurrent erythroderma may also develop in some.

The photoaggravation of PD has been reported, but interestingly improvement is observed in patients after avoiding further exposure to plant, even if they move to a sunny area. The pattern of involvement with PD also changes over time. In a study conducted by Sharma et al, out of 60 patients with an initial ABCD pattern, 27 changed to CAD pattern and 11 to mixed pattern after an average period of 4.2 years, which suggests the clinical pattern of PD undergoes a significant change after the onset, i.e.

nodules over the exposed areas. The photosensitive lichenoid eruption pattern presents with pruritic, discrete, flat, violaceous papules and plaques over sun-exposed parts such as

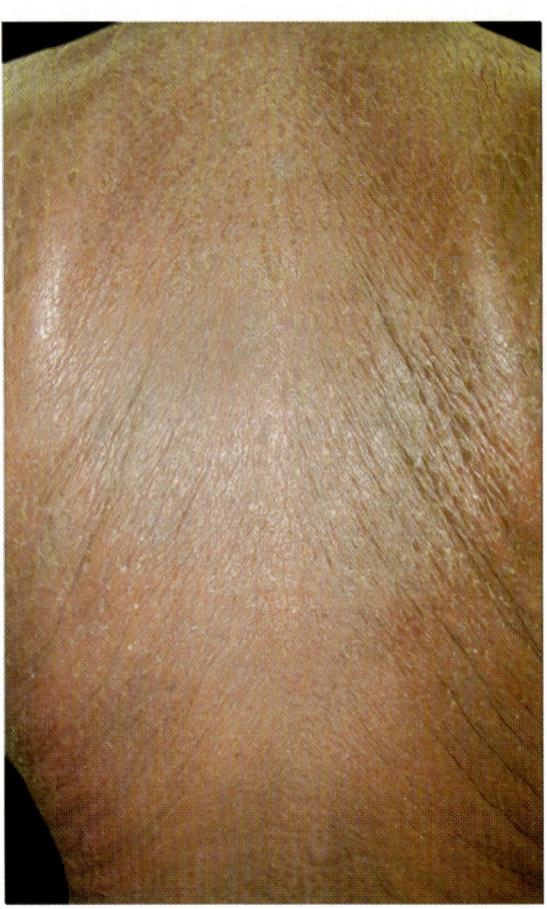

Fig. 7.5: Diffuse involvement in a severe case

progresses from ABCD to mixed or CAD pattern. Vitiliginous skin is thought to be spared in PD due to the vacuolization of Langerhans cells of the area.

DIAGNOSIS

1. **Patch testing:** Patch test detects the delayed type (IV) hypersensitivity to tested antigens. It is carried out with the plant material "as is". In addition, parthenium antigen from the Indian Standard Series (ISS) may also be applied. ISS by chemotechnique diagnostics contains 0.1% parthenolide which may not always pick-up sensitivity to parthenium. Further, neither any single SQL nor the commonly used "SQL mix" of three common SQLs (alantolactone, dehydrocostus lactone and costunolide) serves as a reliable screen for SQL allergy. This mix which has been widely tested detects only 30% cases of sensitization. Thus using plant extracts is essential. Acetone extract of dried plant material is more sensitive than water extract. Ethanol extracts of dried plant are more stable but with evaporation of the solvent, concentration increases with time. Ether extracts are prepared from fresh plant extracts.

2. **Photopatch testing:** Perfomed in PD confined to exposed parts, but is uncommonly positive.

3. **Prick test:** Detects the immediate (type I) hypersensitivity, which is also proposed to play a role. It is performed with the parthenium leaf solution and antigen extract containing 500 PNU, with glycerinated saline as negative control and histamine as positive control. Plant materials can be crushed and diluted with saline (1:9 parts) in order to obtain a parthenium leaf solution that can be easily pricked. Both the immediate reaction at 15 min and the late phase reaction (LPR) at 24–48 h should be recorded.

4. **Optional tests:** RAST (radioallegrosorbent test); serum IgE levels, histopathology (to differentiate from other dermatoses, if required).

TREATMENT (Table 7.1)

1. **Eradication of the antigen:** As the plant is ubiquitous, this is not a practical option but removal of the weed from the patient's immediate environment may be worth while where feasible.

2. **Protection from exposure:** Patient must be instructed to cover as much skin as possible with clothing. Barrier creams should be repeatedly applied, with washing off of the area before each application. The clothes must be dried indoors to reduce antigen load as pieces of cloth dried outside are reported to elicit a positive patch test in a sensitive patient. The need to take a bath after coming indoors and wearing fresh clothes must be impressed upon. No documented studies are available for sunscreen use in parthenium dermatitis. However, if patients have photosensitivity, sunscreens can be used. Gloves may not offer protection since SQL permeates vinyl, polyethylene, and latex gloves.

3. **Drugs:**
   a. *Topical steroids:* For limited involvement
   b. *Topical tacrolimus ointment* has been effectively used in management of chronic actinic dermatitis.
   c. *Systemic steroids:* These form the mainstay of treatment in the acute stage with extensive involvement. Starting doses of 0.5–1 mg/kg/day of prednisolone or 2–3 mg/day of betamethasone are commonly employed and are generally adequate. Complete remission usually occurs within 3 months. Long- term use must be avoided and early effort should be made to taper the steroids and add adjuvants, if required.
   d. *Azathioprine (Aza):* Aza has been used in daily regimens in the dose of 1–2 mg/kg/day, with or without monthly 300 mg boluses. It has also been successfully used in a 300 mg weekly regimen, with advantages of greater compliance and reduced cost of therapy. The drug takes

Table 7.1: Treatment of parthenium dermatitis		
GENERAL MEASURES		
• Removal of the plant from immediate vicinity (If possible) • Protection with appropriate clothing • Repeated application of barrier creams after washing the exposed parts • Drying clothes indoors • Sun protection, if photoexaggeration • Bathing and changing into fresh clothes following outdoor exposure		
TOPICAL DRUGS: Steroids, tacrolimus, pimecrolimus		
SYSTEMIC DRUGS		
Oral Steroids	Prednisolone: 0.5–1 mg/kg/day Betamethasone: 2–3 mg/day	Mainstay for acute flares
Azathioprine	1–2 mg/kg/day Daily regimen: Daily Aza ± monthly 300 mg boluses Weekly regimen: 300 mg once a week	Mainstay of long-term maintenance
Cyclosporine	2.5 mg/kg/day	Very quick remission reported in 2 atopics with PD. Unpublished observations support the role in rapid clearance of flares
Methotrexate	15 mg/week	Mtx + tapering steroids showed faster clearance than Aza+tapering steroids

4–6 weeks to act and thus concomitant use of steroids is helpful in the initial phase. It must be continued for 6–12 months beyond remission of the disease. Verma et al. found azathioprine 100 mg daily to be as effective as betamethasone 2 mg daily for 6 months, and with a better adverse effect profile and lesser relapses.

e. *Cyclosporine:* Successful use with rapid response (within 10 days) reported in 2 atopic PD patients at a dose of 2.5 mg/kg/day. The authors also mention unpublished observation of using cyclosporine for control of flares while on Aza treatment, avoiding the need of systemic steroids.

f. *Methotrexate:* Has been used in a dose of 15 mg/week with and without concomitant oral steroids. De et al compared combination of Mtx vs Aza with oral steroids (in tapering doses in the initial phase) and demonstrated >75% reduction in clinical severity score (CSS) within 5.6 weeks with the Mtx combination and in mean time period of 9.5 weeks for Aza combination. The cost of therapy was also much lower with the Mtx combination.

g. Combination/sequential therapies have been suggested, which consists of giving cyclosporine +Aza for 4–6 weeks followed by daily Aza for 6 weeks and then weekly Aza as maintenance for 2–5 years.

h. *Oral desensitization:* Has not produced consistent results in PD and is associated with uncomfortable adverse effects and hence not widely used.

i. *Others:* Chloroquine, PUVA with steroids, ethinyl estradiol. Unsuccesful use of dexamethasone-cyclophosphamide pulse (DCP) therapy is also reported.

Bibliography

1. Akhtar N, Verma KK, Sharma A. Study of pro- and anti-inflammatory cytokine profile in the patients with parthenium dermatitis. Contact Dermatitis 2010;63:203–8.

2. Akhtar N1, Satyam A, Anand V, Verma KK, Khatri R, Sharma A. Dysregulation of T(H) type cytokines in the patients of Parthenium induced contact dermatitis. Clin Chim Acta 2010 Dec 14;411(23-24):2024–8.

3. Bhutani JK, Rao DS. Photocontactdermatitiscaused by Parthenium hysterophorus. Dermatologica 1978, 157, 206–209.

4. De D, Sarangal R, Handa S. The comparative efficacy and safety of azathioprine vs methotrexate as steroid-sparing agent in the treatment of airborne-contact dermatitis due to Parthenium. Indian J Dermatol Venereol Leprol 2013 Mar-Apr;79(2):240–1.

5. Dogra S, Parsad D, Handa S. Narrow band ultraviolet B in air borne contact dermatitis: a ray of hope! Br J Dermatol 2004; 150: 367–399.

6. Fuchs S, Berl V, Lepoittevin JP. Chronic actinic dermatitis to sesquiterpene lactones: (2 + 2) photo reaction toward thymidine of (+) and (?) alpha-methylene-hexahydrobenzofuranone with cis ring junction. Photochem Photobiol 2010, 86, 545–552.

7. Khatri R1, Mukhopadhyay K, Verma KK, Sethuraman G, Sharma A. Genetic predisposition to parthenium dermatitis in an Indian cohort due to lower-producinggenotypes of interleukin-10 (-) 1082 G>A and (-) 819 C>T loci but no association with interferon-? (+) 874 A>T locus. Br J Dermatol 2011 Jul;165(1):115–22.

8. Lakshmi C, Srinivas CR, Jayaraman A. Ciclosporin in parthenium dermatitis—a report of 2 cases. Contact Dermatitis 2008;59: 245–248.

9. Lakshmi C, Srinivas CR. Parthenium the terminator: An update. Indian Dermatol Online J 2012 May-Aug; 3(2): 89–100.

10. Nousari HC, Anhalt GJ, Morison WL. Mycophenolate in psoralen-UV-A desensitization therapy for chronic actinic dermatitis Arch Dermatol 1999; 135: 1128–1129.

11. Pasricha JS. Story of pulse therapy in pemphigus and other dermatoses. In: Shankar PS, Biradar PM, editors. Advances in Dermato-Venereo-Leprology. Gulbarga: South Zone conference of IADVL; 1992. pp. 53–60.

12. Sharma VK, Bhat R, Sethuraman , Manchanda Y. Treatment of parthenium dermatitis with methotrexate Contact Dermatitis 2007; 57: 118–119.

13. Sharma VK, Verma P, Maharaja K. Parthenium dermatitis. Photochem Photobiol Sci 2013;12: 85–94.

14. Sharma VK, Verma P. Parthenium dermatitis in India: Past, present and future. Ind J Dermatol Venereol Leprol 2012;78(5): 560–8.

15. Verma KK, Mahesh R, Srivastava P, Ramam M, Mukhopadhyaya AK. Azathioprine versus betamethasone for the treatment of parthenium dermatitis: a randomized controlled study. Indian J Dermatol Venereol Leprol 2008, 74, 453–457.

16. Verma KK1, Bansal A, Sethuraman G. Parthenium dermatitis treated with azathioprine weekly pulse doses. Indian J Dermatol Venereol Leprol 2006 Jan-Feb;72(1):24–7.

17. Verma KK1, Manchanda Y, Pasricha JS. Azathioprine as a corticosteroid sparing agent for the treatment of dermatitis caused by the weed Parthenium. Acta Derm Venereol 2000 Jan-Feb;80(1):31–2.

8

Diaper Dermatitis

Deepshikha Khanna, Ananta Khurana

INTRODUCTION

Diaper dermatitis also known as napkin dermatitis, nappy rash or diaper rash is one of the most common skin conditions affecting neonates and infants. Classically, the term is used to describe irritant contact dermatitis of the diaper area and needs to be differentiated from other dermatoses that can affect that area.

PATHOGENESIS (Tables 8.1 and 8.2)

Prolonged contact with a mixture of urine and feces is central to the pathogenesis of diaper dermatitis (Scheinfeld et al). Presence of urine produces excessive hydration and subsequent maceration of the skin of the anogenital region predisposing this area to effects of friction by the diaper. Overhydration also impairs the

Table 8.1: Main pathogenetic factors for irritant contact diaper dermatitis	
Maceration	Maceration of the stratum corneum is likely to be the most critical predisposing factor. The stratum corneum is almost exclusively responsible for the barrier function of the epidermis. Excessive wetness has a deleterious effect on the stratum corneum, making the outer layer of the skin more liable to frictional damage, and interfering with barrier function, allowing increased permeation of irritant substances.
Friction	Friction between the skin and the fabric of the nappy appears to be an important factor in most cases. This role is strongly suggested by the increased susceptibility to the rash of the convex skin surfaces in the napkin area rather than the folds.
Urine	Newborn babies pass urine more than 20 times in 24 h. This frequency reduces through infancy to an average of seven times in 24 h at 12 months. It has been shown that the higher the pH of the urine, the greater the risk of development of irritant diaper dermatitis (IDD).
Feces	Babies' feces contain variable amounts of residual proteolytic and lipolytic digestive enzymes, which are highly irritating to the skin. Fecal contamination causes breaks down of urea to ammonia, ↓ Increase in skin pH ↓ ↑ Activity of fecal enzymes ↓ Further increases skin permeability ↓ Irritation with bile salts and acids in feces

Table 8.2: Factors that may decrease threshold to develop IDD or worsen an existing one

- Gastrointestinal factors: Diarrhea or developmental abnormalities
- Use of antibiotics: Disrupt the balance of gut microflora
- Inadequate skin care or use of certain topical therapies, such as liquid soap or talcum powder
- Allergic sensitization to certain chemicals, such as fragrances and preservatives
- Presence of microorganisms on the epidermis
- Formula feed

Table 8.3: Factors responsible for reduction in incidence of IDD especially in developed world

Improved design and greater use of modern superabsorbent nappies (compared with the traditional cotton napkins, modern disposable napkins reduce the contact time of the skin with urine)	• Surface emollient layer (transfers emollient to skin during use) • Topsheet to absorb urine and feces • Acquisition layer beneath the top layer that spreads urine laterally • Storage layer with AGM • Breathable backsheet, reducing occlusive effect • Stretchiness for comfortable fit • Wetness indicators to guide diaper change
Improved design of wipes	• Now made with non-woven soft absorbent fabric • With an acidic pH to counteract alkaline urine • Without preservatives and fragrances
Improved use of barrier emollients	• Standard practice for most educated caretakers
Improved general skin care of infants	• With avoidance of harsh soaps and talc • Appropriate emollient use

barrier function of the skin increasing its permeability for various irritants. Fecal contamination leads to breakdown of urea present in urine to ammonia that increases the pH of skin. This promotes the activity of various fecal enzymes such as proteases, ureases and lipases, that subsequently increases the permeability of skin and render it susceptible to irritant action of bile salts and acids. Exposure to such irritants under occlusion for a prolonged period of time leads to epidermal barrier disruption and erythema of skin (Scheinfeld et al).

The incidence of diaper dermatitis is related inversely to frequency of diaper change and directly to frequency of bowel movements and presence of diarrhea (Jordan et al, Adalat et al). Exclusively breastfeeding infants have a lower incidence of moderate to severe diaper dermatitis as compared to formula fed infants possibly due to lower stool pH and enzyme activity in former (Berg et al, Jordan et al, Pratt et al). No difference has been found in the flora of skin of diaper area of infants wearing disposable diapers with cellulose pulp core with or without absorbent gel material and cloth diapers (Keswick et al). However, candidal superinfection is a common cause of persistence of inflammation in the diaper area and should be excluded in every diaper dermatitis that lasts beyond 48–72 hours (Murat-Susiæ et al, Shin et al). Irritant diaper dermatitis usually resolves when the child becomes toilet trained. The incidence of IDD has probably decreased over the years (especially so in the developed world) and the factors enlisted in Table 8.3 may have contributed to this trend.

CLINICAL FEATURES

The most common presentation is irritant contact diaper dermatitis (IDD) typically affecting convex areas of buttocks and perianal areas, mons pubis, upper thighs, lower abdomen, scrotum and outer surface of labia majora (Fig. 8.1). The sites with maximum contact with the diaper have the greatest severity of lesions. Inguinal folds are spared in classical IDD due to disposable diapers as they are protected from contents of the diaper. IDD initially presents as localized sharply demarcated mildly scaly erythema that may progress to painful confluent erythema, erosions and frank ulceration. Regression of lesions leaves wrinkled skin resembling cigarette paper.

In a Chinese study, where cloth diapers are being used, found IDD to be rare on buttocks or genitalia but common in perianal and intertriginous areas, possibly due to accumulation or residual collection of mixture of urine and feces trickling into the inguinal folds as cloth diapers have minimum absorptive and holding capacity (Liu et al). The typically erosive form, with crater-like punched out erosions and ulcerations with heaped up borders affecting the perianal areas, glans penis or urinary meatus, known as Jacquet dermatitis (Fig. 8.2a) occurs due to infrequent diaper changes compounded by frequent liquid stools (Bluestein et al). Pseudo-verrucous papules and nodules present with shiny, smooth, flat topped moist or ulcerated papules (Fig. 8.2b). This is a rare condition which was first described in patients with urostomies. It was attributed to chronic irritation from leakage of urine. This eruption has more recently been reported to also occur in the perianal area of children in association with chronic faecal soiling. In the reported cases, stool leakage was due to severe constipation with secondary encopresis or followed surgical colonic reanastomosis in patients with Hirschsprung disease. Granuloma gluteale infantum presents with large

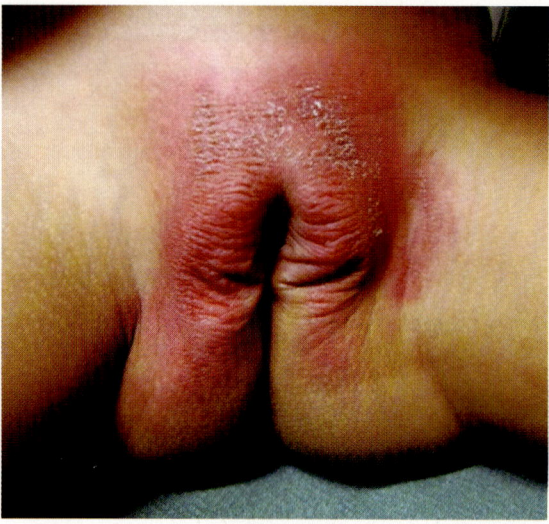

Fig. 8.1: Irritant diaper dermatitis affecting the convex surfaces of labia majora and mons pubis while sparing the vulva and inguinal folds

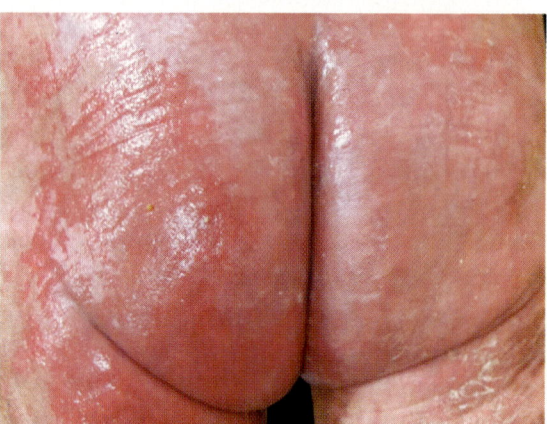

Fig. 8.2a: Jacquet dermatitis

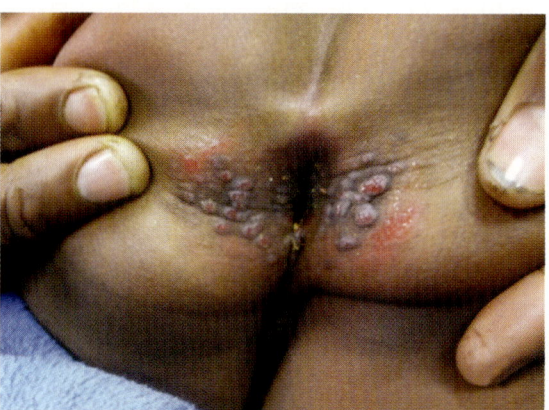

Fig. 8.2b: Pseudoverrucous papules

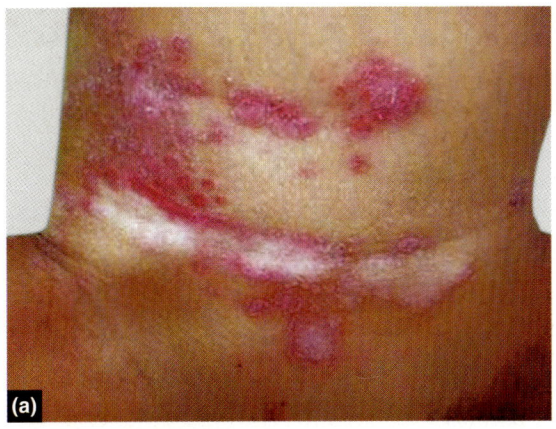
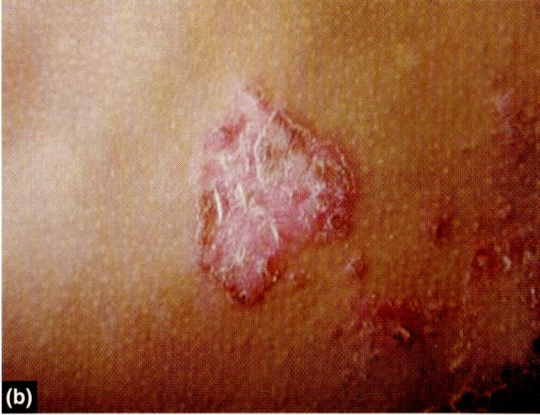

Fig. 8.3a and b: (a) Psoriasiform ID secondary to diaper dermatitis; (b) Close up view

violaceous papules and nodules with erosions over the buttocks, lower abdomen, groin, penis and even axillae and neck. The name granuloma gluteale infantum is a misnomer as no granulomas are found histopathologically and the condition is basically an IDD aggravated due to repeated and prolonged application of topical steroids and *Candida* superinfection (Murat-Susiæ et al, Scheinfeld et al, Humphrey et al). It is usually self-limiting, resolving in a few weeks to months often with residual scarring (Shin et al, Bluestein et al). Diaper dermatitis may also lead to ID eruption occurring beyond the diaper area (Rattet et al) (Fig. 8.3).

DIFFERENTIAL DIAGNOSIS

IDD needs to be differentiated from other conditions that affect the diaper area (Table 8.4). *Candida albicans* is a frequent secondary offender and leads to worsening of the pre-existing diaper dermatitis (Fig. 8.4). Severe chronic candidal diaper dermatitis and napkin dermatitis may sometimes indicate underlying immunodeficiency including HIV (Thiboutot et al). An unusual erosive napkin dermatitis with deep gluteal cleft ulceration has been reported as a presenting sign of HIV infection. In addition, ulcerative eruptions in the anogenital area of HIV-infected infants can be due to, or complicated by, infection with

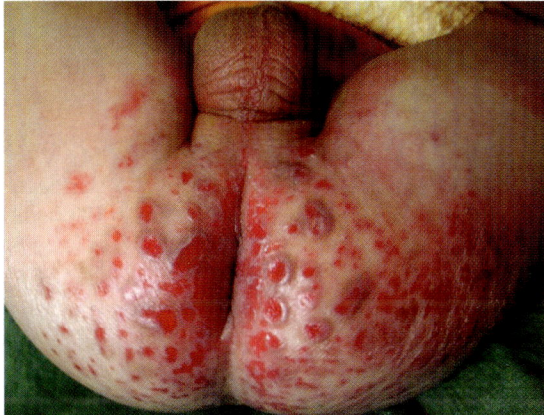

Fig. 8.4: Irritant diaper dermatitis around a urostomy in an infant, secondarily complicated by candidiasis

herpes simplex, cytomegalovirus and other opportunistic agents. Therefore, HIV infection should be considered in infants with unusually severe or erosive napkin dermatitis. Allergic contact dermatitis is rare in children less than 2 years due to the incompletely developed immune response.

Uncommon systemic blistering diseases may present with lesions in the anogenital region of napkin-wearing children. These include neonatal herpes simplex, hand, foot and mouth disease, chronic bullous dermatosis of childhood, bullous mastocytosis, incontinentia pigmenti, epidermolytic hyperkeratosis and epidermolysis bullosa. Diagnosis is based on the morphology of the lesions, their

Table 8.4: Differential diagnosis of diaper dermatitis

Common	Less common	Rare

Irritant contact dermatitis (Fig. 8.1)
• Glazed erythema ± scale →
  punched out erosions
• Favors convex surface, often spares
  folds
• Prolonged contact with urine/feces
  (especially if diarrhea), friction
• Over time pseudoverrucous papules
  can develop
 	
Candidiasis (Fig. 8.4)
• Intense erythema with
  desquamation/superficial erosions
  and peripheral scale/collarettes
• Satellite pustules
• Favors folds, genitalia
• Yeast/pseudohyphae on KOH
  preparation
• ± Recent antibiotic use, thrush
 	
Seborrheic dermatitis (Fig. 8.5)
• Well-demarcated, salmon-colored
  to red, moist or scaly patches/
  plaques
• Favors folds
• Involvement of other flexural sites,
  scalp
	Bacterial infections
	Bullous impetigo
	• Flaccid bullae, vesiculopustular,
	  superficial shiny red erosions
	  with a collarette of scale
	• Grain stain
	*Streptococcal perianal dermatitis
	and intertrigo* (Fig. 8.6)
	• Sharply demarcated, bright red
	  erythema
	• Usually no satellite lesions
	• Perianal area, skin folds
	• Pain, itch, foul odor
	• ± Pharyngitis in patient or family
	  members
	
	Psoriasis
	• Well-demarcated erythematous
	  plaques
	• Shiny in folds, scaly on convex
	  surfaces
	• Psoriasiform lesions elsewhere,
	  ± family history
	
	Allergic contact dermatitis*
	• Consider if fails to respond to
	  usual therapy
	• 'Holster' distribution if reaction
	  to rubber additives in diaper
	  elastics
	• May affect folds if reaction to
	  components of baby wipes or
	  topical preparations
	
	Atopic dermatitis (AD)
	• Excreations, lichenification
	• Favors skin at diaper margins
	  and convex surfaces
	• Other relative sparing of the
	  diaper area
	• Marked pruritus
	• Other pruritic eczematous
	  lesions in usual sites of AD
		• Acrodermatitis enteropathica,
		  other forms of 'nutritional
		  dermatitis' (Fig. 8.7)
		• Langerhans cell histiocytosis
		  (LCH) (Fig. 8.8)
		• Other infections (e.g.
		  congenital syphilis,
		  dermatophytosis; Fig. 8.9)
		• Granular parakeratosis
		• Early Kawasaki disease
		• Systemic blistering diseases
		  (*see* text)
		• HIV
		• Miliaria
		• Bullous impetigo
		• Child abuse
		Differentials of pseudoverru-
		cous papules and plaques:
		• Crohn's disease
		• Condyloma acuminatum
		• LCH
		• Granuloma gluteale
		  infantum

*Potential allergens include sorbitan sesquioleate (an emulsifier in diaper balms), fragrances, disperse dyes, rubber additives (e.g. mercaptobenzothiazole), preservatives in baby wipes, and diaper components.

distribution outside the napkin area and other diagnostic criteria. An erythematous, desquamating perineal eruption is as an early sign of Kawasaki disease and may have to be differentiated from IDD. Miliaria is commonly concentrated in the napkin area in hot tropical areas but other typical areas of involvement like the face, neck and axilla would also be involved. Miliaria crystallina is more commonly seen in the newborn while in older

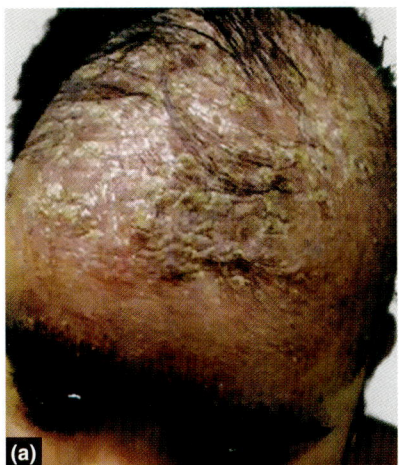

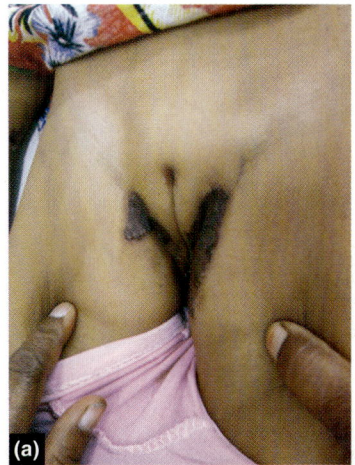

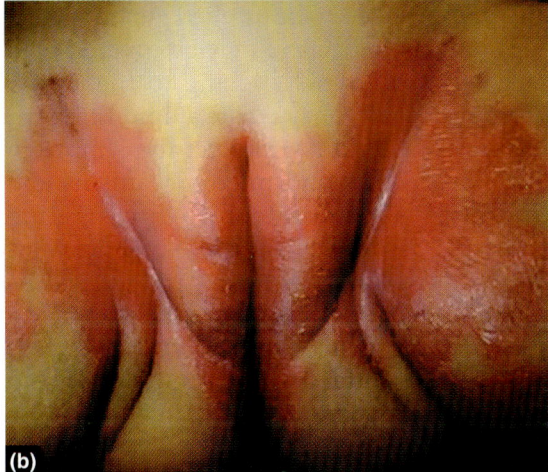

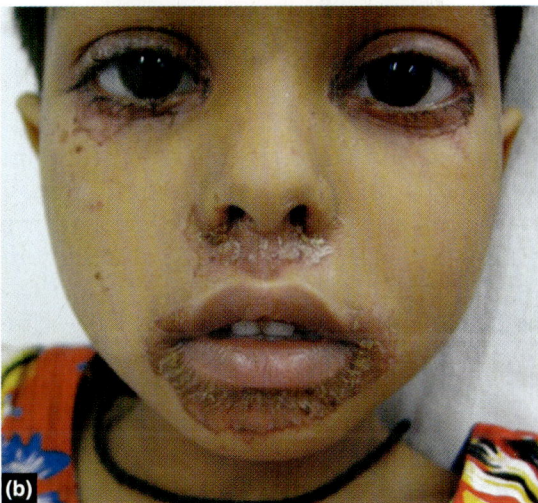

Fig. 8.5a and b: (a) Cradle cap; (b) Seborrheic dermatitis with greasy scales affecting the inguinal region

Fig. 8.7a and b: Periorifacial eczematous papulo-squamous rash (Zn deficiency)

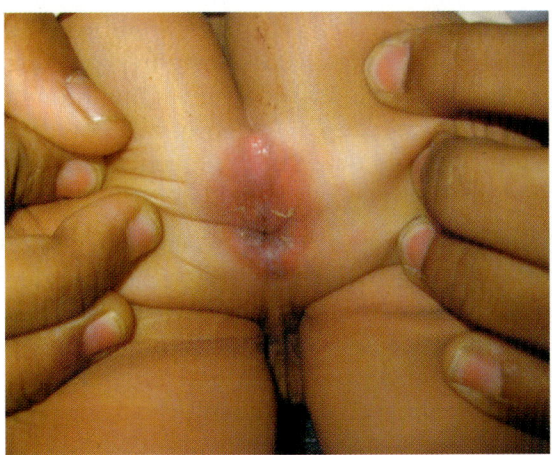

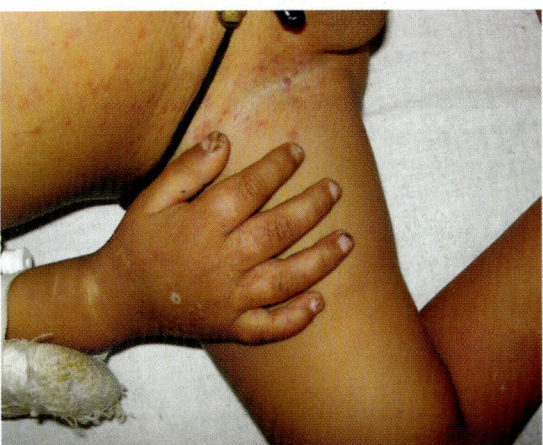

Fig. 8.6: Streptococcal perianal dermatitis

Fig. 8.8: Purpuric papules seen in LCH

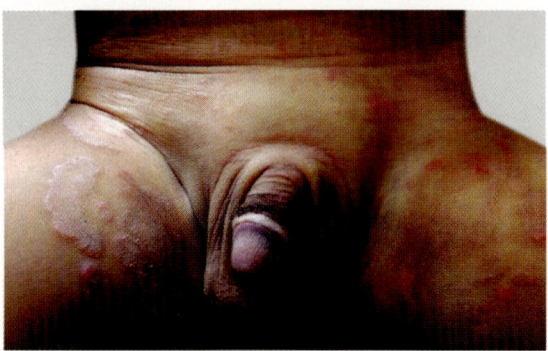

Fig. 8.9: Dermatophytosis affecting the diaper area

infants, miliaria rubra (or pustulosa) is more common. Although uncommon nowadays, congenital syphilis can present with raised, moist, warty lesions (condylomata lata) lesions in the anogenital region along with moist eroded areas. A generalized papulosquamous rash as seen in secondary syphilis will point to the diagnosis. Bullous impetigo may present as superficially eroded areas in the diaper area. It is especially common in newborns as a result of colonization of the umbilicus with *Staphylococcus aureus*. The maculopapular and vesicular lesions of varicella can sometimes be more florid in areas of pre-existing skin inflammation and thus may more profusely involve the diaper area. Child abuse should be considered where the skin of the buttocks is red and blistered in a 'dunking' pattern, and especially if the lateral aspects of the feet are affected. This pattern follows lowering a child into scalding hot water holding his/her feet.

Pseudoverrucous papules and nodules may be mistaken for cutaneous Crohn disease, granuloma gluteale infantum, condyloma acuminatum or Langerhans cell histiocytosis.

A descriptive algorithm is given in Table 8.4 which covers the common differentials of diaper dermatitis.

MANAGEMENT

The basic regime to be followed in treatment of IDD can be remembered by the Mnemonic **ABCDE:**

A for air or time without diaper, **B** for barrier cream, **C** for cleansing/corticosteroids, **D** for diaper to be used, **E** for education of the parents (Boiko et al).

Aeration of the skin possibly when the infant is sleeping or just after urination and defecation provides respite from the frictional and irritant effects of the wet diaper fabric.

Barrier preparations, such as generic preservative free zinc oxide ointment or paste, are effective for preventing and even treating mild IDD. Barrier creams may include petrolatum, cod liver oil, dimethicone, lanolin, white soft paraffin and titanium oxide (Ward et al). These need to be applied generously at each diaper change and may be covered with petrolatum to avoid sticking to the diaper (Borowski et al). They create a lipid film over the surface of skin to protect the skin from friction, irritants and micro-organisms and their lipids penetrate into the stratum corneum, assuming the role of endogenous lipids and preventing excessive water loss (Atherton et al, Shin et al). Ointments and pastes are more effective than oils, creams and lotions as the latter do not adhere that well to denuded skin and may contain preservatives. Topical vitamin A has been shown to be ineffective for prevention or treatment of IDD (Davies et al, Bosch-Banyeras et al). Products containing fragrances and additives such as vitamins, boric acid, camphor, phenol, salicylates and baking soda should be avoided. Corn starch is effective in protecting from frictional injury and preventing growth of *Candida albicans* (Leyden et al). Powders should be used with care to prevent aspiration pneumonitis and talc should be avoided.

Cleansing: Avoidance of harsh scrubbing or over cleansing should be stressed taking due care to ensure that no urine or fecal residue is left in creases and folds. When using a disposable diaper, minimal cleansing is required after urination. Gentle cleansing with warm water and a mild cleanser should be carried out if the diaper area is soiled. Any residual adherent barrier paste does not need to be wiped off at each diaper change except after defecation for which mineral oil on a cotton- ball may be used. Cleansing agents with a high pH can adversely affect the skin barrier and use of syndets that have near physiologic pH is recommended (Lund et al, Blume-Peytavi et al, Klunk et al). Present day wipes are alcohol-free soft cloth like wipes with low abrasion potential and non-ionic surfactants (Odio et al, Manzini et al). Use of disposable wipes does not have any adverse effect on transepidermal water loss, skin pH, erythema or microbial flora as compared to cotton wool and water (Lavender et al) and is safe even in infants with atopic dermatitis (Ehretsmann et al). Wipes should not be used on eroded or ulcerated skin. Allergic contact dermatitis has been reported to the preservative methylisothiazolinone present in disposable wipes (Chang et al).

Diaper: The risk of IDD is dependent on type of diaper worn, length of time the diaper is worn and the frequency of diaper change. Ideally, diaper should be changed after every urination and defecation. This would mean changing the diaper every 1–2 hours in neonates with high wetting frequency and every 3–4 hours in other infants during daytime and at least once during the night. A diaper slightly larger than the infants size is preferable to minimize effect of frictional and irritant factors. Early diapers had a cellulose fluff and impenetrable outer cover to prevent leakage of fluids that led to increased humidity and skin maceration. Present day disposable diapers have an absorbent gelling material (AGM) core containing cross-linked sodium polyacrylate polymers that can absorb more than 80 times its weight in liquid and outermost layer made of polypropylene that is permeable to air and vapor but impermeable to fluids (Table 8.3). The AGM core binds water in a gel matrix away from the skin reducing skin wetting, mixing of urine and feces and achieving better pH control and is less likely to cause IDD as compared to conventional disposable or cloth diapers (Akin et al, Campbell et al, Davis et al). However, such superabsorbent diapers can also lead to IDD, if left in place for too long. Cloth diapers are not advisable for infants with IDD as they increase skin wetness and allow mixing of urine and feces.

Corticosteroid use: In cases with severe symptoms or persisting symptoms despite conservative therapy, hydrocortisone 1% cream can be applied sparingly to the affected area before barrier cream for not more than 2 weeks unless under supervision of a dermatologist. Mid-to-high potency steroids should never be used in the diaper area as they can lead to atrophy, candidiasis, granuloma gluteale infantum and significant systemic absorption due to presence of moisture, occlusive diapers and higher body surface area to volume ratio in infants. Tacrolimus and other calcineurin inhibitors can be used as steroid sparing agents (Patel et al). Antifungal creams, such as clotrimazole, ketoconazole and miconazole, may be used when there is superinfection with *Candida* or in any IDD that lasts longer than a few days and requires at least mild topical steroids to control infection. Application should be continued till at least 1 week after clearance of the eruption.

Bibliography

1. Adalat S, Wall D, Goodyear H. Diaper dermatitis-frequency and contributory factors in hospital attending children. Pediatr Dermatol 2007;24:483–8.

2. Akin F, Spraker M, Aly R, Leyden J, Raynor W, Landin W. Effects of breathable disposable diapers: reduced prevalence of Candida and common diaper dermatitis. Pediatr Dermatol 2001;18:282–90.

3. Atherton DJ. A review of the pathophysiology, prevention and treatment of irritant diaper dermatitis. Curr Med Res Opin 2004;20:645–9.

4. Atherton DJ. Understanding irritant napkin dermatitis. Int J Dermatol 2016 Jul;55 Suppl 1:7–9.

5. Berg RW, Buckingham KW, Stewart RL. Etiologic factors in diaper dermatitis: The role of urine. Pediatr Dermatol 1986;3:102–6.

6. Bluestein J, Furner BB, Phillips D. Granuloma gluteale infantum: Case report and review of the literature. Pediatr Dermatol 1990;7:196–8.

7. Blume-Peytavi U, Cork MJ, Faergemann J Szczapa J, Vanaclocha F, Gelmetti C. Bathing and cleansing in newborns from day 1 to first year of life: recommendations from a European round table meeting. J Eur Acad Dermatol Venereol 2009; 23: 751–759.

8. Boiko S. Treatment of diaper dermatitis. Dermatol Clin 1999;17:235–40.

9. Borkowski S. Diaper rash care and management. Pediatr Nurse 2004; 30:467–70.

10. Bosch-Banyeras JM, Catala M, Mas P, Simon JL, Puig A. Diaper dermatitis. Value of vitamin A topically applied. Clin Pediatr 1988;27:448–50.

11. Campbell RL, Bartlett AV, Sarbaugh FC, Pickering LK. Effects of diaper types on diaper dermatitis associated with diarrhea and antibiotic use in children in day-care centers. Pediatr Dermatol 1988;5:83–87.

12. Chang MW, Nakrani R. Six children with allergic contact dermatitis to methylisothiazolinone in wet wipes (baby wipes). Pediatrics 2014;133: e434–e438.

13. Coughlin CC, Eichenfield LF, Frieden IJ. Diaper dermatitis: Clinical characteristics and differential diagnosis. Pediatr Dermatol 2014;31 Suppl 1:19–24.

14. Coughlin et al, Scheinfeld et al, Shin et al, Humphrey et al, Morris et al. Transfer for original Chapter.

15. Davies MW, Dore AJ, Perissinotto KL. Topical vitamin A, or its derivatives, for treating and preventing napkin dermatitis in infants. Cochrane Database Syst Rev 2005:19;4:CD004300.

16. Davis JA, Leyden JJ, Grove GL, Raynor WJ. Comparison of disposable diapers with fluff absorbent and fluff plus absorbent polymers: effects on skin hydration, skin pH, and diaper dermatitis. Pediatr Dermatol 1989;6:102–8.

17. Ehretsmann C, Schaefer P, Adam R. Cutaneous tolerance of baby wipes by infants with atopic dermatitis, and comparison of the mildness of baby wipe and water in infant skin. J Eur Acad Dermatol Venereol 2001;15 (Suppl 1):16–21.

18. Humphrey S, Bergman JN, Au S. Practical Management Strategies for Diaper Dermatitis. Skin Therapy Letter 2006;11:1–6.

19. Jordan WE, Lawson KD, Berg RW, Franxman JJ, Marrer AM. Diaper dermatitis: frequency and severity among a general infant population. Pediatr Dermatol 1986;3:198–207.

20. Keswick BH, Seymour JL, Milligan MC. Diaper area skin microflora of normal children and children with atopic dermatitis. J Clin Microbiol 1987;25:216–221.

21. Klunk C, Domingues E, Wiss K. Update on diaper dermatitis. Clin Dermatology 2014;32:477–87.

22. Lavender T, Furber C, Campbell M, et al. Effect on skin hydration of using baby wipes to clean the napkin area of newborn babies: Assessor-blinded randomised controlled equivalence trial. BMC Pediatr 2012;12:59.

23. Leyden JJ. Cornstarch, Candida albicans, and diaper rash. Pediatr Dermatol 1984;1:322–5.

24. Liu N, Wang X, Odio M. Frequency and severity of diaper dermatitis with use of traditional Chinese cloth diapers: observations in 3- to 9-month-old children. Pediatr Dermatol 2011;28:380–6.

25. Lund C. Prevention and management of infant skin breakdown. Nurs Clin North Am 1999;34:907–920.

26. Manzini BM, Ferdani G, Simonetti V, Donini M, Seidenari S. Contact sensitization in children. Pediatr Dermatol 1998;15:12–17.

27. Morris A, Rogers M, Fischer G, Williams K. Childhood psoriasis: a clinical review of 1262 cases. Pediatr Dermatol 2001;18:188–98.

28. Murat-Susiae S, Husar K. Differential diagnosis of skin lesions in the diaper area. Acta Dermato venerol Croat 2007;15:108–12.

29. Odio M, Friedlander SF. Diaper dermatitis and advances in diaper technology. Curr Opin Pediatr 2000;12:342–346.

30. Patel RR, Vander Straten MR, Korman NJ. The safety and efficacy of tacrolimus therapy in patients younger than 2 years with atopic dermatitis. Arch Dermatol 2003;139:118–46.

31. Pratt AG, Reed WT Jr. Influence of the type of feeding on pH of stool, pH of skin and the incidence of perianal dermatitis in the newborn infant. J Pediatr 1955;46:539–43.

32. Rattet JP, Headley JL, Barr RJ. Diaper dermatitis with psoriasiform ID eruption. Int J Dermatol 1981; 20:122–5.

33. Scheinfeld N. Diaper dermatitis: a review and brief survey of eruptions of the diaper area. Am J Clin Dermatol 2005;6:273–81.

34. Shin HT. Diagnosis and management of diaper dermatitis. Pediatr Clin North Am 2014;61:367–82.

35. Shin HT. Diaper dermatitis that does not quit. Dermatol Ther 2005;18:124–35.

36. Thiboutot DM, Beckford A, Mart CR, Sexton M, Maloney ME. Cytomegalovirus diaper dermatitis. Arch Dermatol 1991;127:396–8.

37. Ward DB, Fleischer AB, Feldman SR, Krowchuk DP. Characterization of diaper dermatitis in the United States. Arch Pediatr Adolesc Med 2000; 154: 943–946.

38. Yan AC, Honig PJ. Clinical Features and Differential Diagnosis of Napkin Dermatitis. In Irvine A, Hoeger P, Yan A eds. Harper's textbook of pediatric dermatology 3rd ed. Blackwell Publishing Ltd, UK, 2011.

9

Atopic Dermatitis

Kabir Sardana, Ananta Khurana, Khushbu Mahajan, Aniket Bhole

DEFINITION AND INTRODUCTION

Atopy is a familial tendency to develop certain diseases (rhinoconjunctivitis, asthma bronchiale, eczema) on the basis of hypersensitivity of skin and mucous membranes against environmental agents, associated with increased IgE production and/or altered nonspecific reactivity and epithelial barrier dysfunction (Fig. 9.1).

Atopic dermatitis (AD) is an acquired, chronic, inflammatory, pruritic skin disease of unknown origin that usually starts in early infancy (an adult-onset variant is recognized) with remissions and exacerbations; it is characterized by pruritus, eczematous lesions, xerosis (dry skin), and lichenification (thickening of the skin and an increase in skin markings).

It is frequently associated with abnormalities in skin barrier function, allergen sensitization, and recurrent skin infections.

AD is a complex genetic disease with underlying epithelial barrier defect involving skin as well as mucosa hence is often accompanied by other atopic disorders such as allergic rhinoconjunctivitis and asthma. These conditions may appear simultaneously or develop in succession. AD has a predilection for infants and young children, while asthma favors older children and pollen allergy predominates in adolescents. This characteristic age-dependent sequence is referred to as the "atopic march" (Asher et al, Williams et al) (Fig. 9.2).

EPIDEMIOLOGY

Since the 1960s, there has been a more than threefold increase in the prevalence of AD worldwide (Eichenfield LF et al). Prevalence rates in different geographical regions vary from as low as 1% to as high as 20% with higher prevalence in developed countries than developing countries. In general, the prevalence of AD in rural areas and low income countries is significantly lower than in their

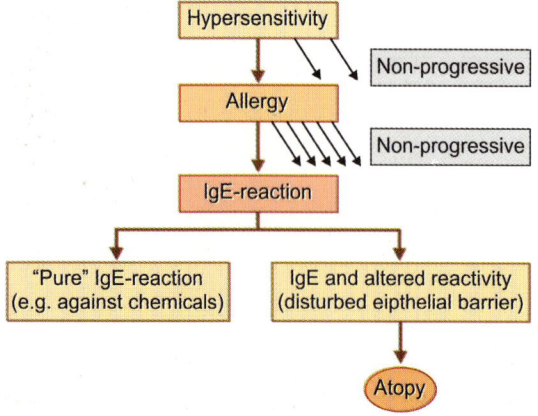

Fig. 9.1: Atopy as subgroup of IgE-mediated allergic reactions

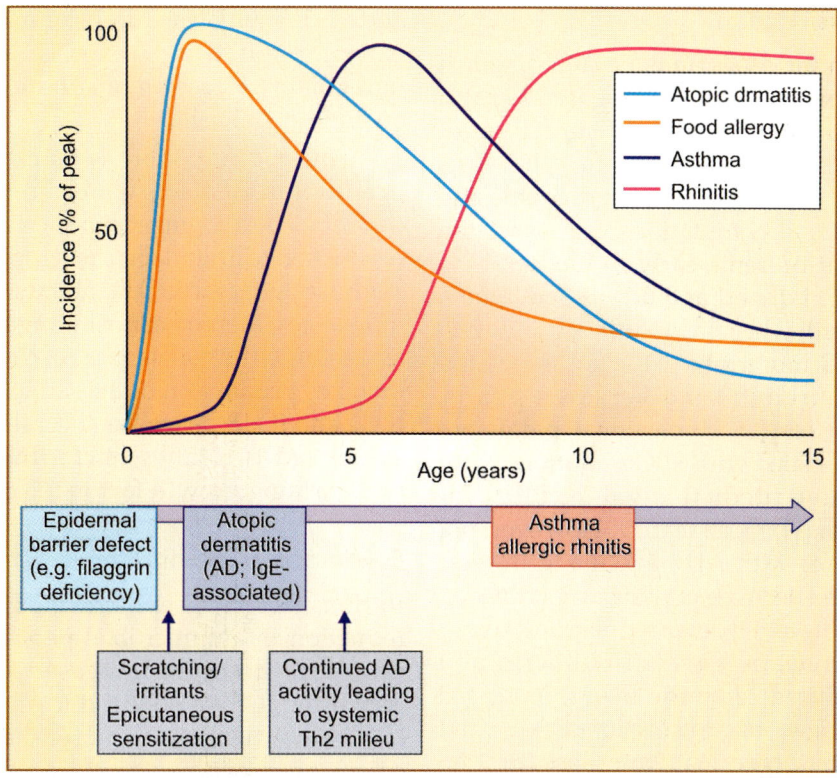

Fig. 9.2: A depiction of the atopic march

urban and high income counterparts, suggesting the importance of lifestyle and environment in expression of atopic disease. Factors traditionally associated with increased prevalence of AD include higher socioeconomic status, higher level of education, evolution of smaller families and increased urbanization (DaVeiga SP).

This observation supports the hygiene hypothesis, that allergic diseases might be prevented by "infection in early childhood transmitted by unhygienic contact with older siblings" (Strachan DP).

Prevalence of AD in Indian subcontinent is 3–4.2% and in general prevalence is increasing based on hospital data (Kanwar AJ).

PATHOGENESIS

Research in the last decades has led to change the view in genomic and immunologic mechanisms that drive cutaneous inflammation.

They have highlighted the critical role of the epidermal-barrier function and the immune system.

Large body of evidence now suggests that AD may be a disease of primary barrier failure, including defective stratum corneum permeability and antimicrobial defences which results in sustained and epicutaneous allergen penetration, leading to immune system activation and the resultant inflammation and pruritus that are typical of AD. The inappropriate activation of immune system results in further barrier disruption (Fig. 9.3) (Elias PM et al).

1. Genetics

Eighty percent of identical twins show concordance for AD. A child is at increased risk of developing AD, if either parent is affected.

2. Barrier Dysfunction

Mutations in the filaggrin gene (FLG), which encodes a protein that aggregates keratin filaments during terminal differentiation of the epidermis, are responsible for ichthyosis vulgaris and represent a major predisposing factor for AD. FLG mutations are associated with AD that presents early in life, tends to persist into childhood and adulthood, and is associated with wheezing in infancy and with asthma. FLG mutations are also associated with allergic rhinitis and keratosis pilaris, independent of AD. Hyperlinear palms are strongly associated with FLG mutations, with a 71% positive predictive value (PPV) for marked palmar hyperlinearity. However, not all the patients with AD have filaggrin gene defect. Marked decrease in skin barrier function also occurs due to the downregulation of other cornified envelope genes (involucrin and loricrin), reduced ceramide levels, increased levels of endogenous proteolytic enzymes, and enhanced transepidermal water loss (Bratton DL et al, Toda M et al).

This barrier dysfunction leads to increased allergen penetration into skin and increased microbial colonization and predisposes the affected individual to food allergies and respiratory allergies.

3. Defects in Adaptive and Immune Response Genes

Genetic defects responsible for immunological dysregulation are responsible for antigen presentation, cell-mediated and humoral immune response and cell signalling in skin, e.g. CD-14, IL-4, IL-5, IL-13, toll-like receptors, etc.

4. Immune Dysregulation

AD patients often demonstrate immunologic features. T helper 2 (*Th2*) cytokines (e.g. IL-4, IL-5, IL-13) predominate in *acute AD* lesions while *Th1* cytokines (IL-12 and IFN-γ) predominate in *chronic AD* lesions.

Acute AD is associated with the production of T helper 2 (Th2) type cytokines, notably IL-4 and IL-13, which mediate immunoglobulin isotype switching to IgE synthesis and upregulate expression of adhesion molecules on endothelial cells.

In chronic AD, there is an increase in the production of IL-5, which is involved in eosinophil development and survival. Increased production of granulocyte macrophage colony-stimulating factor in AD inhibits apoptosis of monocytes, thereby contributing to the persistence of AD. The maintenance of chronic AD also involves production of the Th1-like cytokines IL-12 and IL-18, as well as several remodeling-associated cytokines, including IL-11 and transforming growth factor-1 (Toda M et al).

5. Microbial Colonization in AD

Various factors, as epidermal barrier defects, reduction in antimicrobial peptides, toll-like receptors defects, decreased neutrophils recruitment to the skin and increased IgE levels, contribute to increased microbial colonization and recurrent infections of skin.

Staphylococcus aureus colonization of the skin occurs in >90% of AD patients (Cho SH et al). *S. aureus* contributes to sensitization and inflammation in AD via several mechanisms such as TLR-2 recognition of *S. aureus* cell wall components (e.g. lipoteichoic acid, peptido-glycan) which stimulates an inflammatory response, via staphylococcal superantigens that amplify, AD via multiple pathways (Cardona ID et al). This may contribute to corticosteroid resistance by inducing the competing β isoform of the glucocorticoid receptor. Staphylococcal enterotoxins A-D (SEA-D) can provoke IgE-mediated sensitization, which also correlates with disease severity (Bunikowski R et al).

Malassezia is colonized in 100% AD patients and *Malassezia* spp are capable of activating mast cells, and inducing the *Malassezia* specific IgEs thereby contributing to the inflammation in AD. Patients with AD lesions on head, neck and upper trunk tend to respond to anti-*Malassezia* measures (Barker JN et al).

Summary of Pathogenesis

An overview of the pathogenetic steps can be summarized in following steps (Fig. 9.3):

1. Th2 immune response in the initiation phase with consequent increased IgE production. It precedes a chronic phase in which Th0 cells (cells that share some activities of both Th1 and Th2 cells) and Th1 cells are predominant.

2. Abnormal skin-barrier function that causes "dry" skin. It is the result of epidermal-barrier components (filaggrin mutation, protease inhibitor deficiency, etc.) and/or abnormal lipid metabolism. Microbial colonization with pathogenic organisms, such as *Staphylococcus aureus* and *Malassezia furfur*.

3. Strong psychosomatic factors that influence the autonomic nervous system and an increased production of inflammatory mediators.

4. Pruritus which induces scratching that, as a vicious circle, increases pruritus.

A conglomerate view can be summarized as in Fig. 9.3 below, which highlights three phases.

The **first phase**, the *nonatopic* form of AD (when sensitization has not occurred yet) is the result of genetically determined epidermal-barrier dysfunction and the effect of environmental factors.

The **second phase** is when patients (60–80%) become sensitized as a consequence of the interaction between the genetic predisposition for IgE-mediated sensitization, the allergen exposition, and *Staphylococcus aureus* enterotoxin products **(atopic form of AD)**.

In the **last phase**, which can occur also in early life, the release of structural proteins due to tissue damage by scratching and molecular mimicry, with *Staphylococcus aureus* proteins, triggers an IgE response to self-proteins **(autoreactivity)**. The presence of auto-IgE has been shown to be associated a worse prognosis (higher severity and higher risk of becoming chronic).

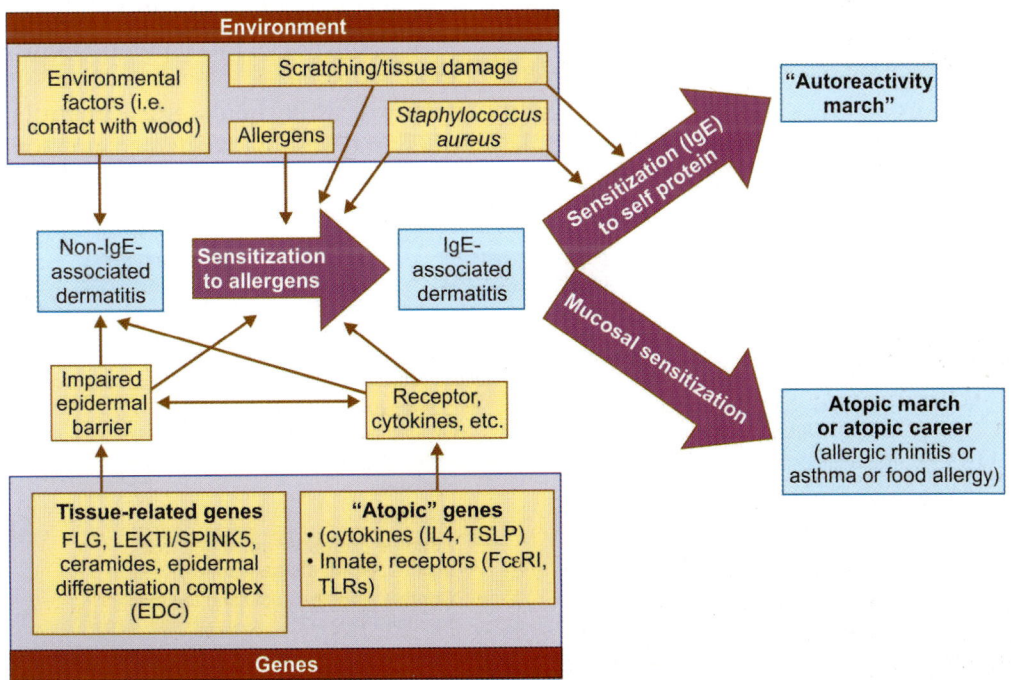

Fig. 9.3: A depiction of the interaction of the various factors that predict the onset and continuation of AD. FLG: Filaggrin; LEKTI: Lympho-epithelial Kazal-type-related inhibitor or SPINK-5: Serine Peptidase Inhibitor Kazal type 5; TSLP: Thymic stromal lymphopoietin

Triggers

Various environmental and other factors are known to worsen AD (Fig. 9.4).

Some of them are:

1. Changes in *temperature*: Atopic patients do not tolerate sudden changes in temperature. Lying under warm blankets, entering a warm room, and experiencing physical stress all intensify the desire to scratch. A sudden lowering of temperature, such as leaving a warm shower, promotes itching. Patients should be discouraged from wearing clothing that tends to trap heat.

2. *Sweating:* Sweating induces itching, particularly in the antecubital and popliteal fossae, to a greater extent in atopic patients than in other individuals.

3. Decrease in *humidity*

4. Contact with *irritants* as wool, chemicals, cosmetics, soaps, cigarette smoke.

5. *Aeroallergens* such as house dust mite, pollen, molds, pet dander, human dander.

   Spring and summer flare, often in association with hay fever, can be related to exposure to grass and tree pollens. This pattern is often associated with a facial distribution in the older child. Flares of the dermatitis may be associated with the introduction of a new trigger factor into the environment or even a new environment such as building works, shifting houses, and so the trigger factor history should be reviewed frequently.

6. *Food allergens* (eggs, peanuts, milk, fish, soy, wheat). Food allergy (FA) should be considered in infants, young children, and selected older children diagnosed with moderate to severe AD.

   Certain foods can provoke exacerbations of AD and other cutaneous signs and symptoms (Box 9.1). Many patients who react to food are not aware of their hypersensitivity. Foods can provoke allergic and nonallergic reactions. The *most common* offenders are *eggs, peanuts, tree nuts, sesame seeds, milk, fish, soy,* and *wheat*. Urticaria, an exacerbation of eczema, gastrointestinal or respiratory tract symptoms, or anaphylactic reactions may be signs of a food-induced reaction. Preservatives, colorants, and other low-molecular weight substances in foods may be offenders, but there are no tests for these substances.

   Cow's milk, hen's eggs, peanuts, tree nuts, and sesame seeds account for most food-induced allergic reactions in young

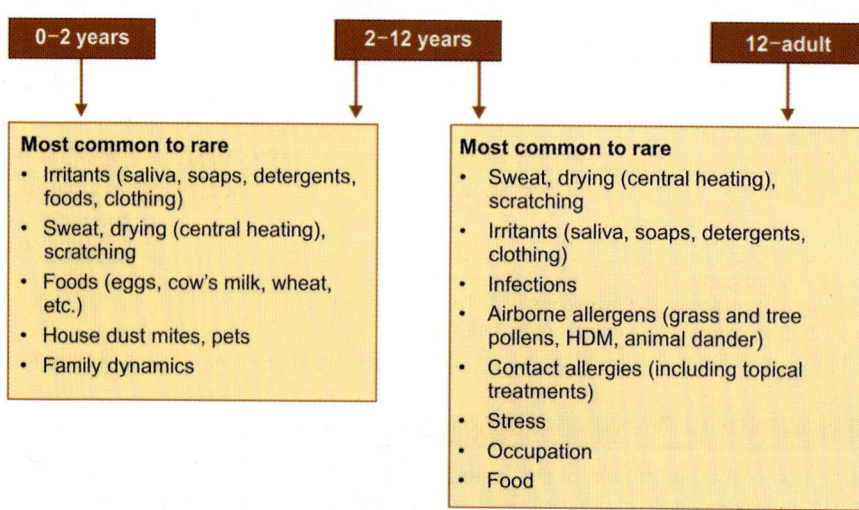

Fig. 9.4: Overview of age related triggers of AD

Box 9.1: Symptoms of food-induced allergic cutaneous reactions	
Immediate symptoms	Delayed symptoms
Erythema	Erythema
Pruritus	Flushing
Urticaria	Pruritus
Morbilliform eruption	Morbilliform eruption
Angioedema	Angioedema
	Eczematous rash

Box 9.2: Classification of water hardness	
Class	Hardness as $CaCO_3$ (in mg/l)
Soft	Below 75
Moderately hard	75–150
Hard	150–300
Very hard	Above 300

children, and kiwi allergy has been increasingly reported. Wheat and soy allergies, although frequently suspected, are rarely confirmed. Hen's eggs and cow's milk are the most common causes of food allergies among children throughout the world. Egg allergy has typically been thought to resolve in 66% of children by 5 years of age and in 75% of children by 7 years of age, but may last longer. Allergies to peanuts, tree nuts, and sesame seeds are infrequently outgrown.

In adults. Shellfish, fish, peanuts, and tree nuts are the most common causes of food allergies

7. Emotional stress
8. Hormones (menstrual cycle and pregnancy)
9. Water

We will focus on this aspect that is probably ignored and its dire necessity makes it a persistent cause of flares in India.

The hardness of water is an issue in many parts of India and possibly a missed factor in AD flares. In India, we may be using filters to drink water but the water used for bathing remains the same. The quality of water specifically its "hardness" is known to have a deleterious effect on AD.

The principal natural sources of hardness in water are sedimentary rocks and seepage and runoff from soils. In general, hard waters originate in areas with thick top soil and limestone formations. Ground water is generally harder than surface water. Total hardness is normally expressed as the total concentration of Ca^{2+} and Mg^{2+} in mg/l, equivalent $CaCO_3$. Calcium (Ca^{2+}) and magnesium (Mg^{2+}) are the important parameters for total hardness. The classification of water hardness is given in Box 9.2.

Perkin et al found that high domestic water $CaCO_3$ levels is associated with an increased risk of AD in infancy. The influence of increased total chlorine levels, however, was not confirmed. Chaumont et al also showed that exposure to hard water and infant swimming can lead to an increase in the prevalence of childhood eczema. They propounded the plausible theory that hard water may cause a breach of the epidermal barrier by detergents or salts in hard water and by chlorine-based oxidants in swimming pool water. These studies were predated by a study published in Lancet (McNally NJ), wherein exposure to hard water in the home was proposed to increase the risk of eczema in children of primary-school age. A study published in JID (Danby et al) studied the effect of hard water in AD patients with and without FLG mutations. The skin of each participant was washed with sodium lauryl sulfate (SLS) in water of varying hardness and chlorine concentration, rinsed and covered with chambers to determine the effects of surfactant residues. Sites washed with hard water exhibited significantly increased SLS deposits. These deposits increased transepidermal water loss and caused irritation, particularly in AD patients carrying FLG mutations. Also water softening by ion-exchange mitigated the negative effects of hard water.

Contrary to this, Font-Ribera et al did not find an association between eczema and water hardness at home or bathing exposure during the first four years of life. It has been felt that an intervention trial is required to see whether installation of a domestic device to decrease $CaCO_3$ levels around the time of birth can reduce the risk of AD. Though water hardness may be just one aspect, as it is a continuous insult, it does trigger attacks in patients of AD. Baby cleansers can bind free Ca^{2+} and reduce the effective water hardness of bath water, thus possibly this may help in preventing the irritant potential of hard water (Walters RM).

In a study published on hard water and quality of water (Central Water Commission, New Delhi, India) in Dwarka subcity in Delhi, it was found that the total hardness of the study area was found in the range of 144 to 3808 mg/l. The highest value of 3808 mg/l was observed in ground water source of Dwarka Sector 8 while the minimum value of 144 mg/l was seen in Dwarka Sector 4. In fact, in the majority of sectors, the water hardness was beyond the maximum permissible limit (300 mg/l). The important point is that if such is the state in the capital, this issue could be seen in other parts of the country and can impact the aggravation of eczema, including AD.

CLINICAL FEATURES

Stages of AD

Atopic dermatitis has been conventionally divided into *three* stages: Infantile AD, occurring from 2 months to 2 years of age; childhood AD, from 2 to 10 years; and adolescent/adult AD. In each stage, patients may develop acute, subacute and chronic eczematous lesions, all of which are intensely pruritic and often excoriated. AD typically begins during infancy. Approximately 50% of patients develop this illness by the first year of life and an additional 30% between the ages of 1 and 5 years. Between 50 and 80% of patients with AD develop allergic rhinitis or asthma later in childhood. Many of these patients outgrow their AD as they are developing respiratory allergy.

According to the classification of Wuthrich, it is possible to distinguish *five subgroups* based on the age of onset: Previous to 2 years (the so-called early-onset AD) (60% of cases), between 2 and 6 years, between 6 and 14 years, between 14 and 20 years, and later than 20 years (the so-called late onset).

The early onset is characterized by an increased risk of development of high levels of total and specific IgE (also known as atopic march or atopic career). The presence of high level of IgE is connected to the risk for AD of becoming chronic.

As reported in a recent paper by Garmhausen et al. (2013), the dermatitis is often chronic, and it is possible to individualize five most common groups according to the onset and course of AD. These five groups, which cover the 85% of the clinical course of AD, differentiate each other for the onset (one group for each of the five Wuthrich's groups) and for some clinical characteristics (i.e. the development of IgE is higher in those with early onset). It is worthy to know that in these five groups, the disease persists up to the adulthood with a chronic course.

On the basis of the presence of IgE, one classification distinguishes an IgE-associated form of AD (called "extrinsic" AD) from a non-IgE-associated form (called "nonatopic" or "intrinsic" or "atopiform" AD). This division might imply that extrinsic and intrinsic forms are two different diseases. As depicted previously (Fig. 9.3), the absence of IgE-mediated sensitization may be only a transient factor, and there is a need to reconcile these divergent hypotheses and to better describe the two "forms" and the different courses. In fact, a few patients with "intrinsic" AD will never produce high level of IgE, and they will not develop the atopic march. In these patients, allergen avoidance does not make sense. On the other hand, it is important to recognize which patients become sensitized (extrinsic AD) because they will benefit from allergen avoidance. Patients with *extrinsic AD* typically have:

a. An elevated **IgE level**
b. Harbor **FLG mutation** with a disruptive barrier
c. Exhibit an **early** onset
d. A **Th2**-dominant response.

On the other hand, *intrinsic AD* patients exhibit different features:

a. Do **not** show an elevated **IgE** level
b. Do **not** harbor **FLG** mutation
c. Exhibit an **adult** onset
d. Associated with more **Th17** and **Th22** immune activation than extrinsic AD patients

In all stages, pruritus is the hallmark. Itching often precedes the appearance of lesions; thus the concept that AD is **"the itch that rashes."** Pruritus may be intermittent throughout the day but is usually worse in the early evening and night. Its consequences are scratching, prurigo, papules, lichenification, and eczematous skin lesions.

Acute lesions predominate in infantile AD and are characterized by edematous, erythematous papules and plaques that may exhibit vesiculation, oozing and serous crusting.

Subacute eczematous lesions display erythema, scaling and variable crusting.

Chronic lesions, which typify adolescent/adult AD, present as thickened plaques with lichenification as well as scale; prurigo nodularis like lesions can also develop. Perifollicular accentuation, and small, flat-topped papules (papular eczema) are particularly common in individuals with darkly pigmented skin. In any stage of AD, the most severely affected individuals may evolve to a generalized exfoliative erythroderma. All types of AD lesions can leave postinflammatory hyper-, hypo- or (in more severe cases) depigmentation upon resolution.

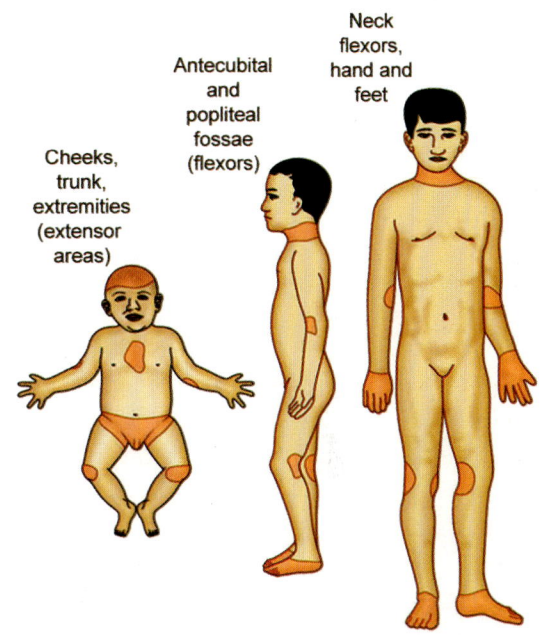

Fig. 9.5: Distribution of atopic eczema across various ages

At all stages of AD, patients usually have dry, lackluster skin. A depiction of the sites of involvement in different age groups is given in Fig. 9.5.

Infantile Phase (Birth to 2 Years)

The age of onset is usually between the age of 2 and 6 months, but usually not until after 2 months. The distribution is given in Fig. 9.6. Eczema in infancy usually begins as erythema and scaling of the cheeks (Fig. 9.7a to d).

The eruption may extend to the scalp, neck, forehead, wrists, extensor extremities, and buttocks. The diaper area is usually spared. There may be significant exudate; secondary effects from scratching, rubbing, and infection include crusts, infiltration, and pustules, respectively. Worsening of AD is often observed in infants after immunizations and viral infections. Partial remission may occur during the summer, with relapse in winter.

Childhood Atopic Dermatitis (2–12 Years)

During childhood, lesions tend to be less exudative. The classic locations are the

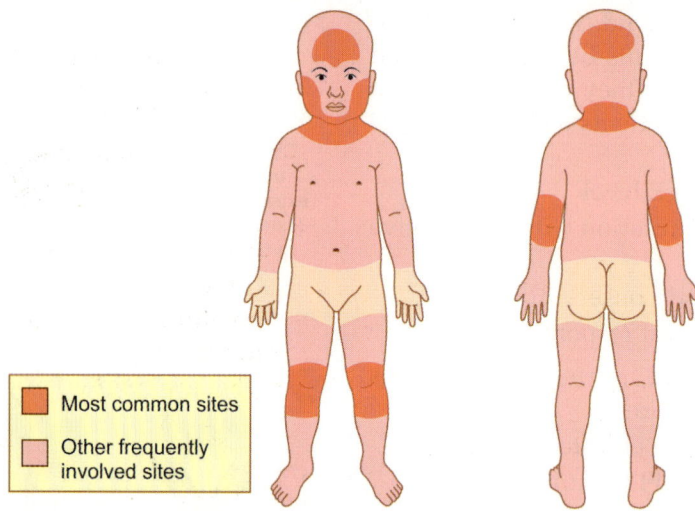

Most common sites

Other frequently
involved sites

Fig. 9.6: A depiction of sites affected in infantile AD

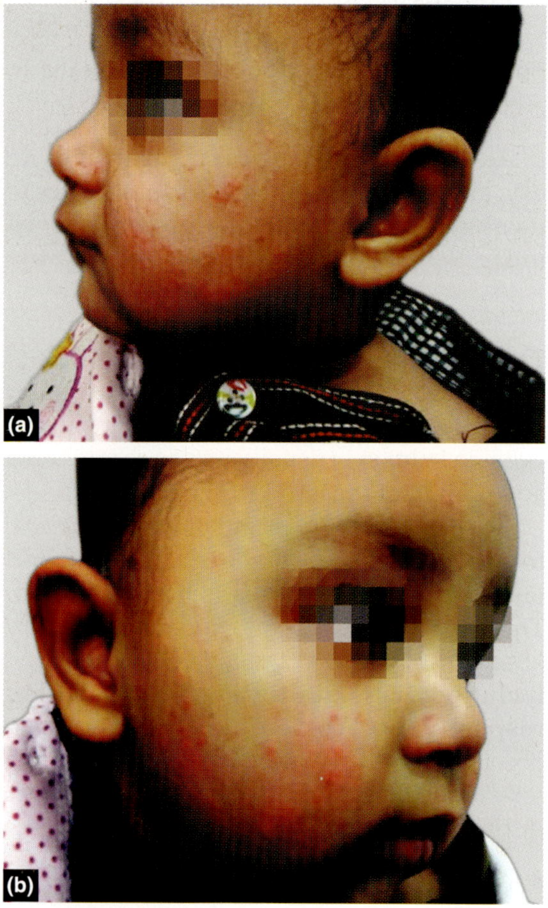

Fig. 9.7a and b: Eczematous papules on the cheek in a child will AD

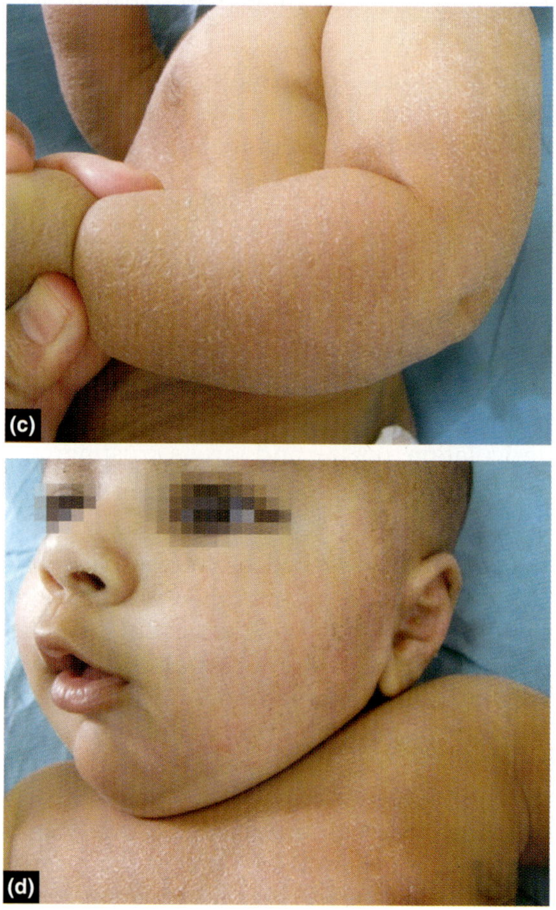

Fig. 9.7c and d: Infantile AD with involvement of cheek with diffuse scaling on the trunk

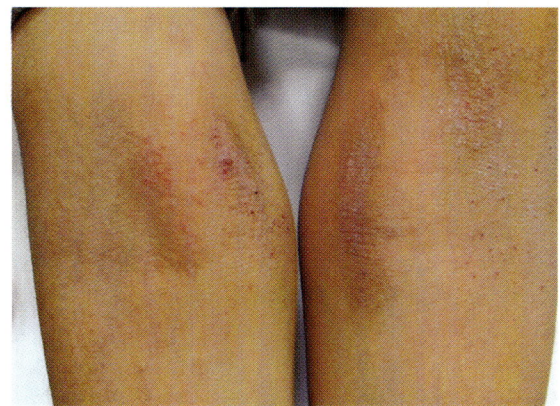

Fig. 9.8a: Childhood AD with involvement of the antecubital fossa

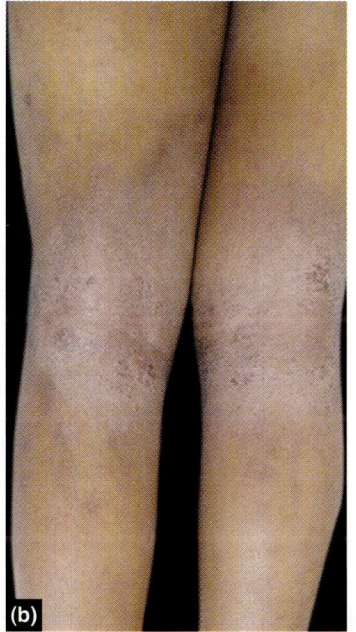

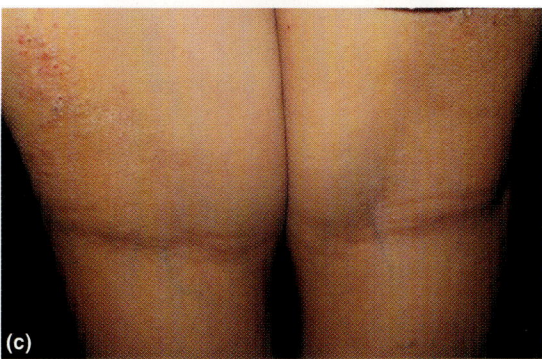

Fig. 9.8b and c: Involvement of the popliteal fossa in AD

antecubital and popliteal fossae, flexor wrists, (Fig. 9.8a to c) eyelids, face, and around the neck. Scratching induces lichenification and may lead to secondary infection. A vicious cycle may be established, the itch-scratch cycle, as pruritus leads to scratching, and scratching causes secondary changes that in themselves cause itching. Severe AD involving a large percentage of the body surface area can be associated with growth retardation. Restriction diets and steroid use may exacerbate growth impairment.

Atopic Dermatitis in Adolescents and Adults

AD often subsides as the patient grows older, leaving an adult with dry skin that is prone to itching and inflammation when exposed to exogenous irritants. Chronic hand eczema may be the primary manifestation of many adults with AD. AD may begin after age of 18 years in only 6–14% of patients diagnosed with AD. In adolescents, the eruption often involves certain sites (Fig. 9.9) including antecubital and popliteal fossae (Fig. 9.10), front and sides of the neck, forehead, and area

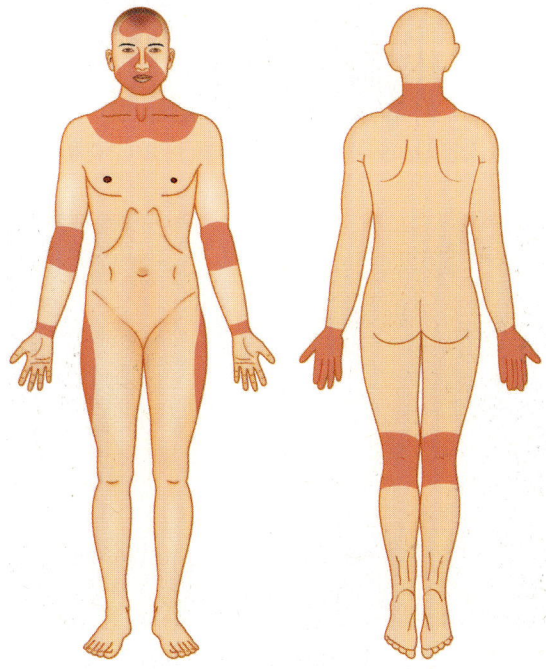

Fig. 9.9: Distribution of AD in adults

around the eyes (Fig. 9.11). In older adults, the distribution is generally less characteristic, and localized dermatitis may be the predominant feature, especially hand, nipple, or eyelid eczema. In elderly, like infants, extensors are more commonly involved.

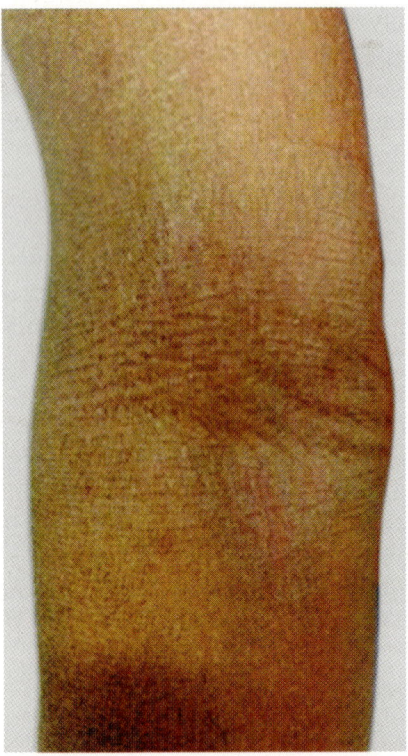

Fig. 9.10: Involvement of flexures in an adult case of AD

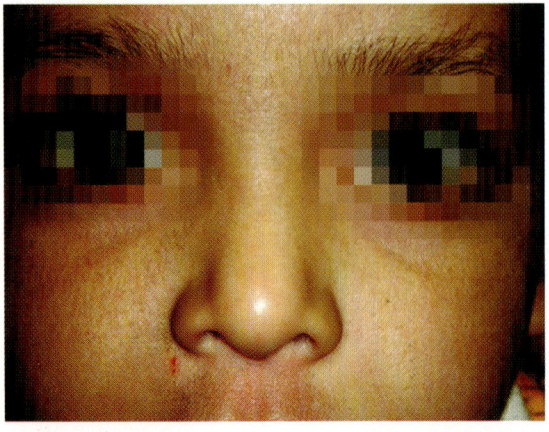

Fig. 9.11: A case of AD with periorbital erythema consequent to frequent rubbing by the patient

Regional Variants and Associated Features

Several regional variants of AD can occur in isolation or together with the classic age-related patterns of involvement (Fig. 9.12). The associated features are depicted in Fig. 9.13. It must be emphasized that these associated features are not diagnostic. An array of depictive clinical finings are listed in Fig. 9.14a to 9.14n.

Face and neck (Fig. 9.14a) is a frequent site for various associated findings in AD either alone or in association with classical features of AD.

Chronic scratching may lead to loss of lateral one-third of the eyebrow (Fig. 9.14b).

A linear transverse fold just below the edge of the lower eyelids, known as the Dennie-Morgan fold, is widely believed to be indicative of AD (Fig. 9.14c).

In atopic patients with eyelid dermatitis (Fig. 9.14d), increased folds and darkening under the eyes (allergic shiners) is common. Eyelid eczema along with lichenification of periorbital skin may be seen in AD patients.

Eczema of the lips is common in AD patients, especially during the winter. It is characterized by dryness ("chapping") of the vermilion lips, sometimes with peeling and fissuring, and may be associated with angular cheilitis. Patients try to moisten their lips by licking, which in turn, may irritate the skin around the mouth, resulting in so-called lip-licker's eczema (Fig. 9.14e).

The less involved skin of atopic patients is frequently dry and slightly erythematous and may be scaly.

Juvenile plantar dermatosis presents with erythema, scale and fissuring on the balls of the feet and plantar aspect of the toes in children with AD, especially during the winter.

Frictional lichenoid eruption has a predilection for atopic children (especially boys) and presents as multiple small, flat topped, pink to skin-colored papules on the elbows and (less often) knees and dorsal hands

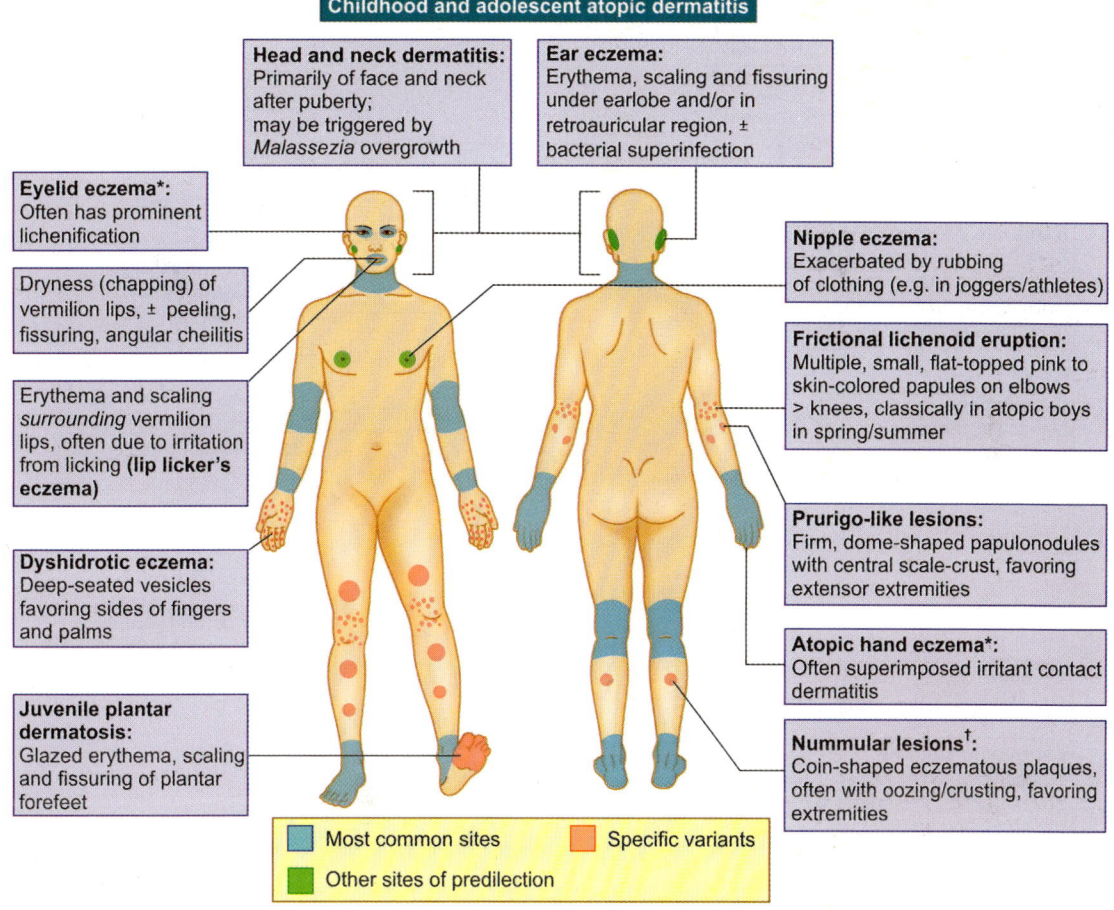

Fig. 9.12: Distribution patterns of atopic dermatitis (AD) and regional variants

*May be the only manifestation of AD in adults.
†Nummular eczema may occur outside the setting of AD

(Fig. 9.14g). It classically occurs in the spring or summer, pruritus is variable, and the histologic findings are nonspecific (Sardana K).

Sometimes patient may just have hyperlinear palms and soles (Fig. 9.14 n).

Keratosis pilaris (KP) consists of horny follicular lesions of the outer aspects of the upper arms, legs, cheeks, and buttocks and is often associated with AD. It affects >40% of patients with AD and ~15% of the general population. The keratotic papules on the face may be on a red background, a variant of KP called keratosis pilaris rubra faceii.

Nummular eczema, and nipple eczema may be seen in children and adults wth AD.

Diagnostic Criteria

Several authors and groups have suggested guidelines to assist in establishing the clinical diagnosis of AD.

The criteria proposed by Hanifin and Rajka (Table 9.1) in 1980 are considered to be the 'gold standard' for the clinical diagnosis of AD (Marenholz I et al).

UK working party criteria (Table 9.2) are a simple set of one major and five minor criteria designed for use in population-based surveys (Williams HC et al). These criteria are extensively validated and found to be similar to the Hanifin and Rajka criteria in terms of sensitivity and specificity.

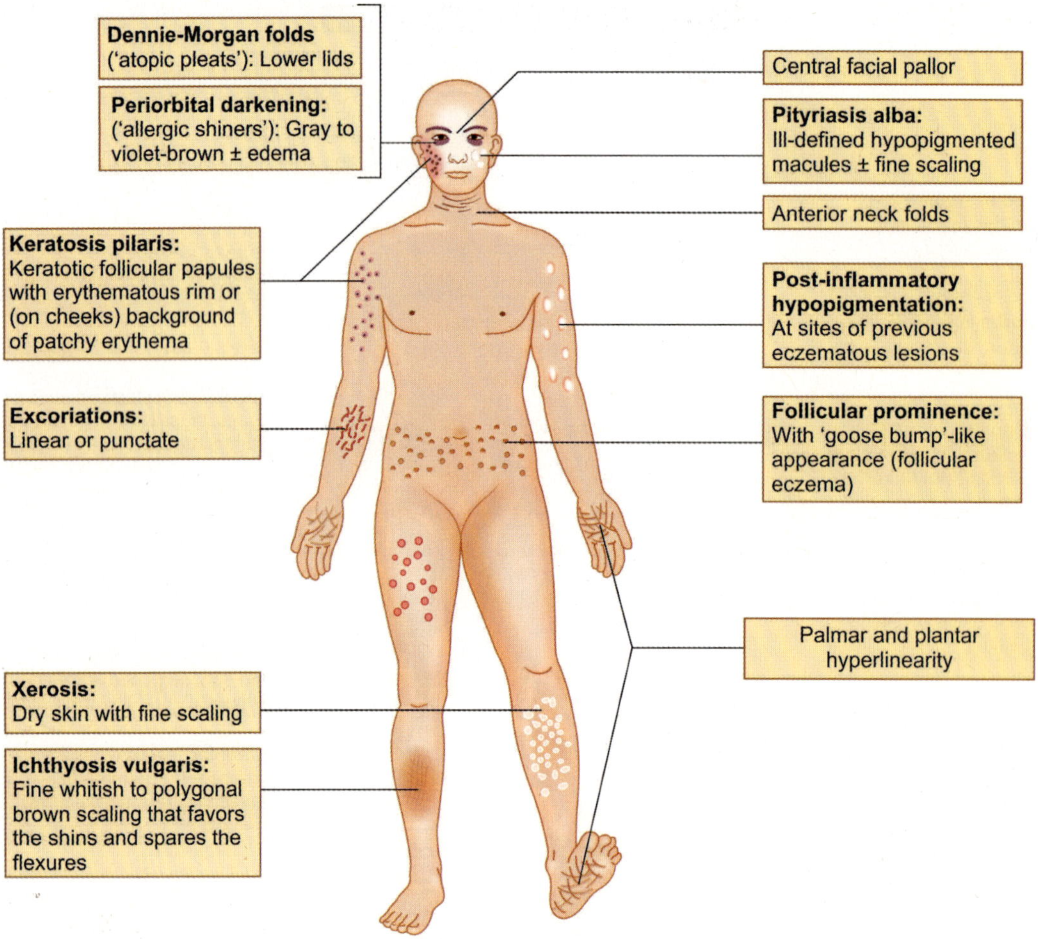

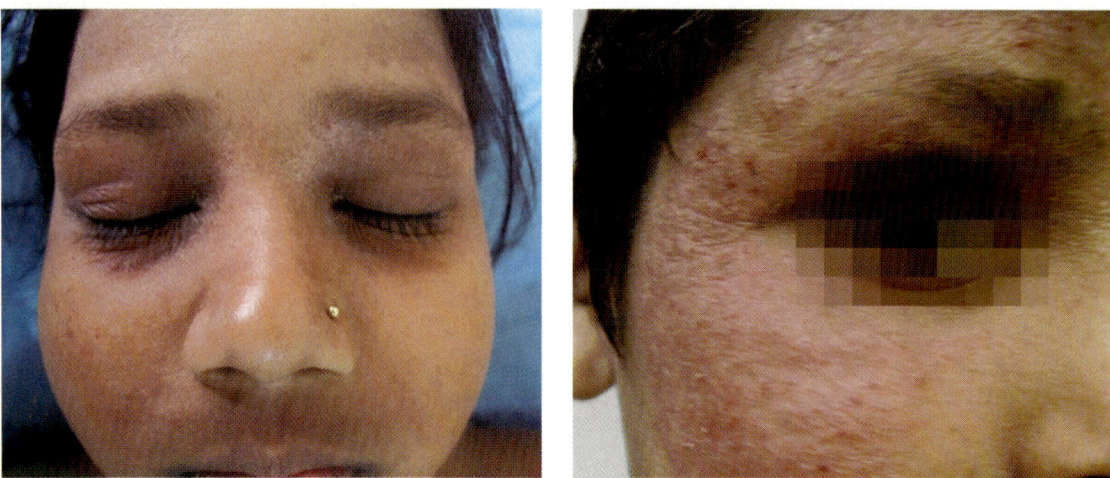

Dennie-Morgan folds ('atopic pleats'): Lower lids

Periorbital darkening: ('allergic shiners'): Gray to violet-brown ± edema

Keratosis pilaris: Keratotic follicular papules with erythematous rim or (on cheeks) background of patchy erythema

Excoriations: Linear or punctate

Xerosis: Dry skin with fine scaling

Ichthyosis vulgaris: Fine whitish to polygonal brown scaling that favors the shins and spares the flexures

Central facial pallor

Pityriasis alba: Ill-defined hypopigmented macules ± fine scaling

Anterior neck folds

Post-inflammatory hypopigmentation: At sites of previous eczematous lesions

Follicular prominence: With 'goose bump'-like appearance (follicular eczema)

Palmar and plantar hyperlinearity

Fig. 9.13: A depiction of the associated features of atopic dermatitis

Fig. 9.14a: Head and neck dermatitis. Note the marked periocular involvement and the loss of eyebrows (right)

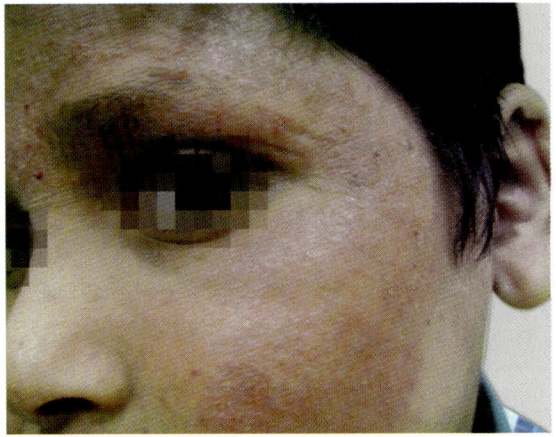

Fig. 9.14b: Hertoghe's sign

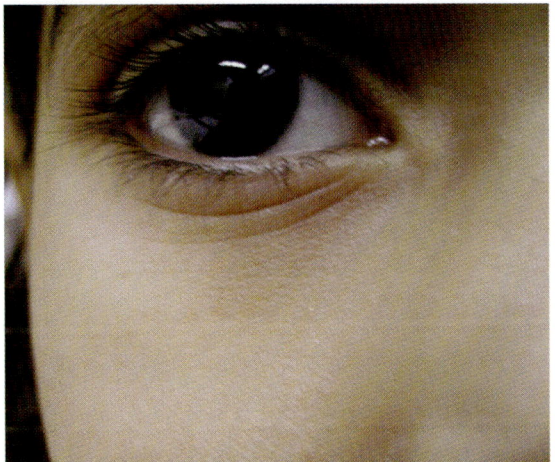

Fig. 9.14c: Dennie-Morgan folds

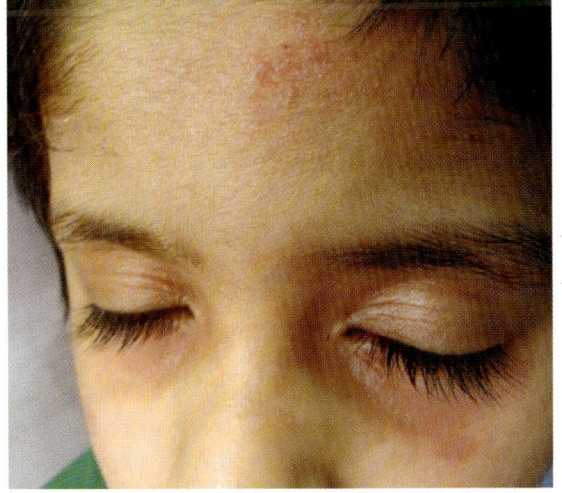

Fig. 9.14d: Eyelid eczema

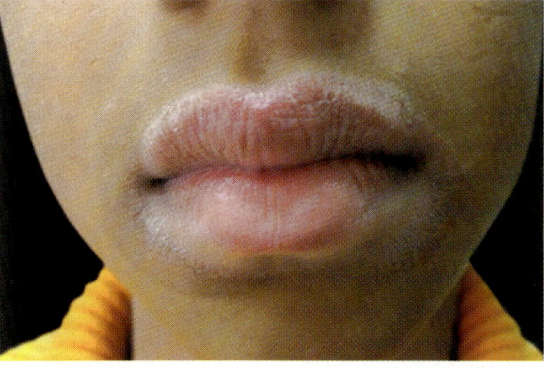

Fig. 9.14e: Lip licker's eczema

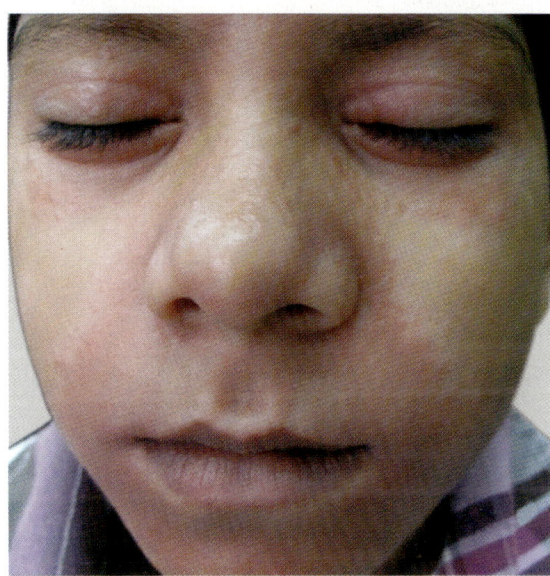

Fig. 9.14f: Periorifacial eczema involving the nose, eyelide and mouth is a rare feature of AD

Validated scores to assess the severity of AD include the EASI (Eczema Area Scoring Index), SCORAD (SCORing Atopic Dermatitis) and POEM (Patient-Oriented Eczema Measure) [Ricci G et al]. The most relevant is the SCORAD and is detailed in Fig. 9.15. Here different skin lesions are semiquantitatively evaluated from 0 (absent) to 3 (maximal). The subjective complaints are registered on a visual analog scale (VAS) from 0 to 10 by the patient (or the parents, respectively). AD with an objective SCORAD higher than 40 is generally regarded as "severe," whereas below 20 can be regarded as "mild."

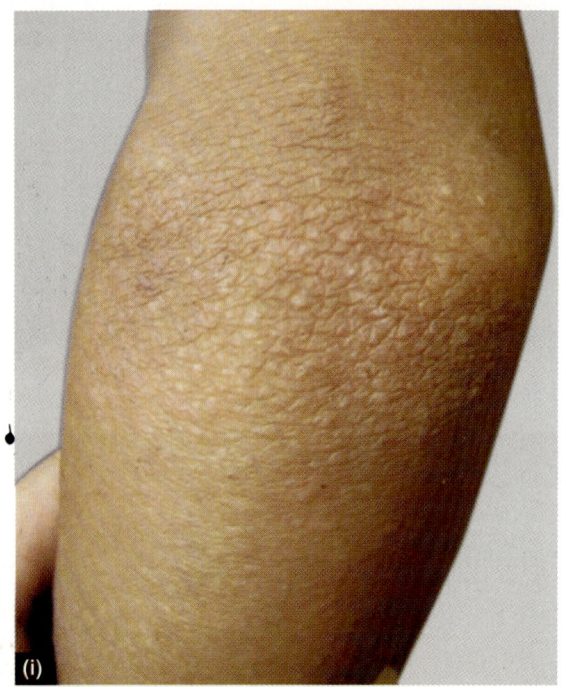

(i)

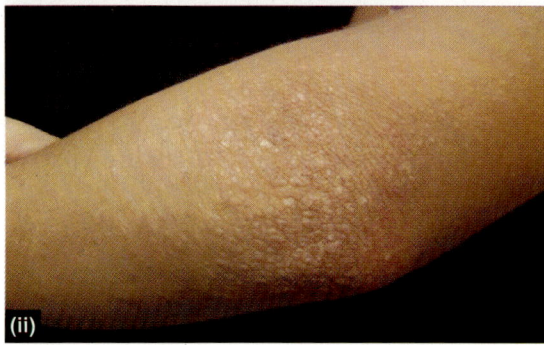

(ii)

Fig. 9.14g (i and ii): Frictional lichenoid eruption: small, flat topped, pink to skin-colored papules on elbows more than knees

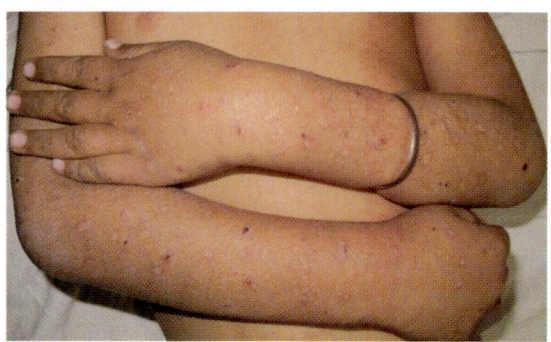

Fig. 9.14h: Prurigo simplex. Excoriated papules with crusting

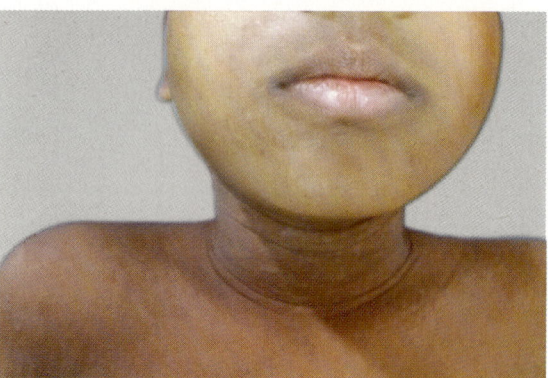

Fig. 9.14i: Anterior neck folds

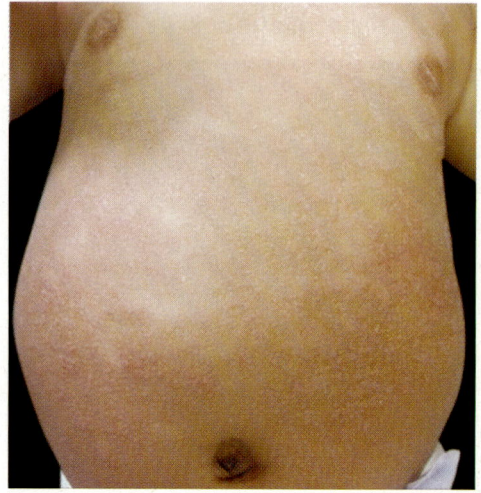

Fig. 9.14j: Follicular prominence; the so-called "Follicular eczema"

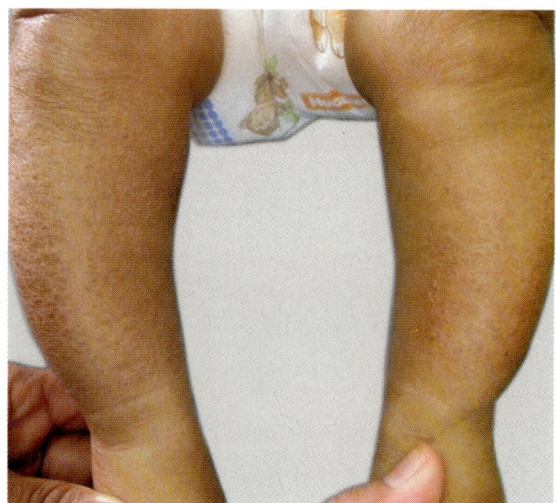

Fig. 9.14k: Ichthyosis

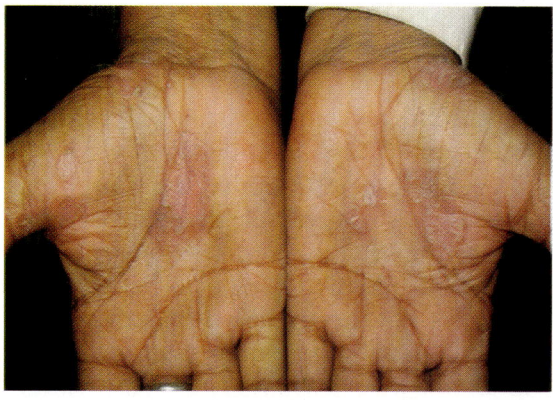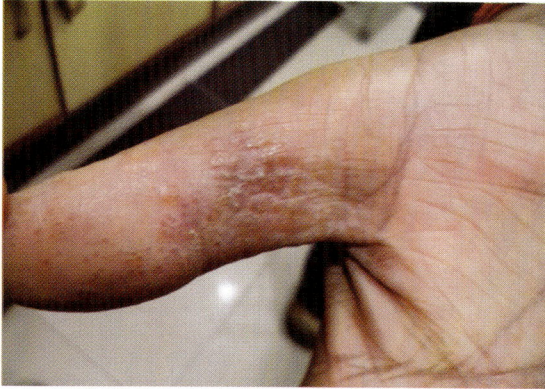

Fig. 9.14l: Hand eczema (left hyperkeratotic eczema right pompholyx)

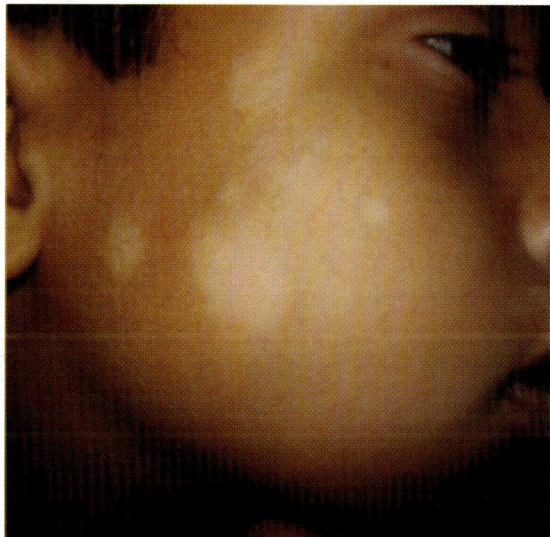

Fig. 9.14m: Pityriasis alba

Table 9.1: Hanifin and Rajka criteria
Major criteria
Must have three of the following:
1. Pruritus
2. Typical morphology and distribution
• Flexural lichenification in adults
• Facial and extensor involvement in infancy
3. Chronic or chronically relapsing dermatitis
4. Personal or family history of atopic disease (e.g. asthma, allergic rhinitis, atopic dermatitis).
Minor criteria
Must also have three of the following:
1. Xerosis
2. Ichthyosis/hyperlinear palms/keratosis pilaris
3. IgE reactivity (immediate skin test reactivity, RAST test positive)
4. Elevated serum IgE
5. Early age of onset
6. Tendency for cutaneous infections (especially *Staphylococcus aureus* and HSV).
7. Tendency to nonspecific hand/foot dermatitis
8. Nipple eczema
9. Cheilitis
10. Recurrent conjunctivitis
11. Dennie-Morgan infraorbital fold
12. Keratoconus
13. Anterior subcapsular cataracts
14. Orbital darkening
15. Facial pallor/facial erythema

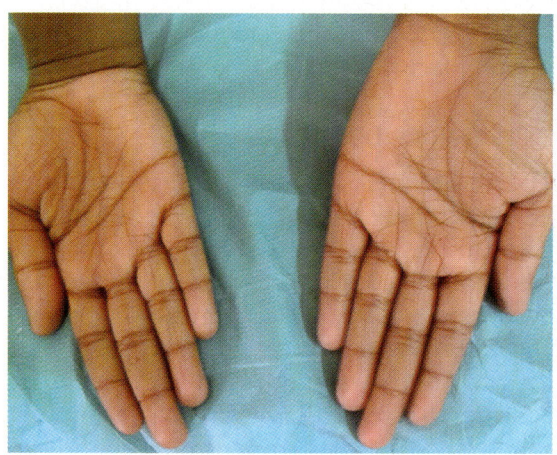

Fig. 9.14n: Hyperlinear palms

(Contd.)

Table 9.1: Hanifin and Rajka criteria (*Contd.*)

16. Pityriasis alba
17. Itch when sweating
18. Intolerance to wool and lipid solvents
19. Perifollicular accentuation
20. Food hypersensitivity
21. Course influenced by environmental and/or emotional factors
22. White dermatographism or delayed blanch to cholinergic agents

RAST: Radioallergosorbent assay; *HSV:* Herpes simplex virus.

Table 9.2: UK working criteria

Itchy skin condition (or parental report of scratching or rubbing in a child) plus three or more of the following features:

1. *Onset* under age of 2 years (not used if child <4 years)
2. A *history* of flexural involvement (including cheeks in <10 years)
3. A *history* of asthma or hay fever (or a history of atopic disease in siblings and parents, if the child is under 4 years).
4. A *history* of generally dry skin in the last year.
5. *Visible* flexural dermatitis.

Complications

Ocular Complications

Up to 10% of patients with AD develop cataracts, either anterior or posterior subcapsular. The spectrum of atopic eye disease also includes chronic manifestations such as atopic keratoconjunctivitis (typically in adults) and vernal keratoconjunctivitis (favors children living in warm climates). Atopic keratoconjunctivitis is usually bilateral and can have disabling symptoms that include itching, burning, tearing, and copious mucoid discharge.

Infections

Patients with AD are predisposed to the development of skin infections because of factors including an impaired skin barrier and modified immune milieu. Bacterial and viral infections represent the most common complications of AD. Patient with AD with secondary bacterial infections is frequently associated with weeping and crusting of skin lesions, retro- and infra-auricular and perinasal fissures, folliculitis, and adenopathy.

Eczema herpeticum represents rapid dissemination of a herpes simplex viral infection over the eczematous skin of AD patients. It initially develops as an eruption of vesicles, but affected individuals more often present with numerous monomorphic, punched-out erosions with hemorrhagic crusting. It is often associated with fever, malaise and lymphadenopathy, and complications may include superinfection with *S. aureus* or *S. pyogenes* as well as herpetic keratoconjunctivitis and meningoencephalitis.

Patients with AD are also predisposed to the development of widespread molluscum contagiosum.

Superficial fungal infections are also more common in atopic individuals and may contribute to the exacerbation of AD.

Erythroderma

Patients with extensive skin involvement may develop exfoliative dermatitis. This is associated with generalized redness, scaling, weeping, crusting, systemic toxicity, lymphadenopathy, and fever. Although this complication is rare, it is potentially life-threatening. In some cases, the withdrawal of systemic glucocorticoids used to control severe AD may be a precipitating factor for exfoliative erythroderma.

DIFFERENTIAL DIAGNOSIS

The differential diagnosis of AD is broad and includes other chronic dermatoses, infections, infestations and malignancies as well as metabolic, genetic (e.g. primary immunodeficiencies) and autoimmune disorders. Depending upon the age of the patient and the clinical presentation, such entities may be considered prior to diagnosing AD, especially when the history, morphology and/or distribution of the skin lesions are atypical.

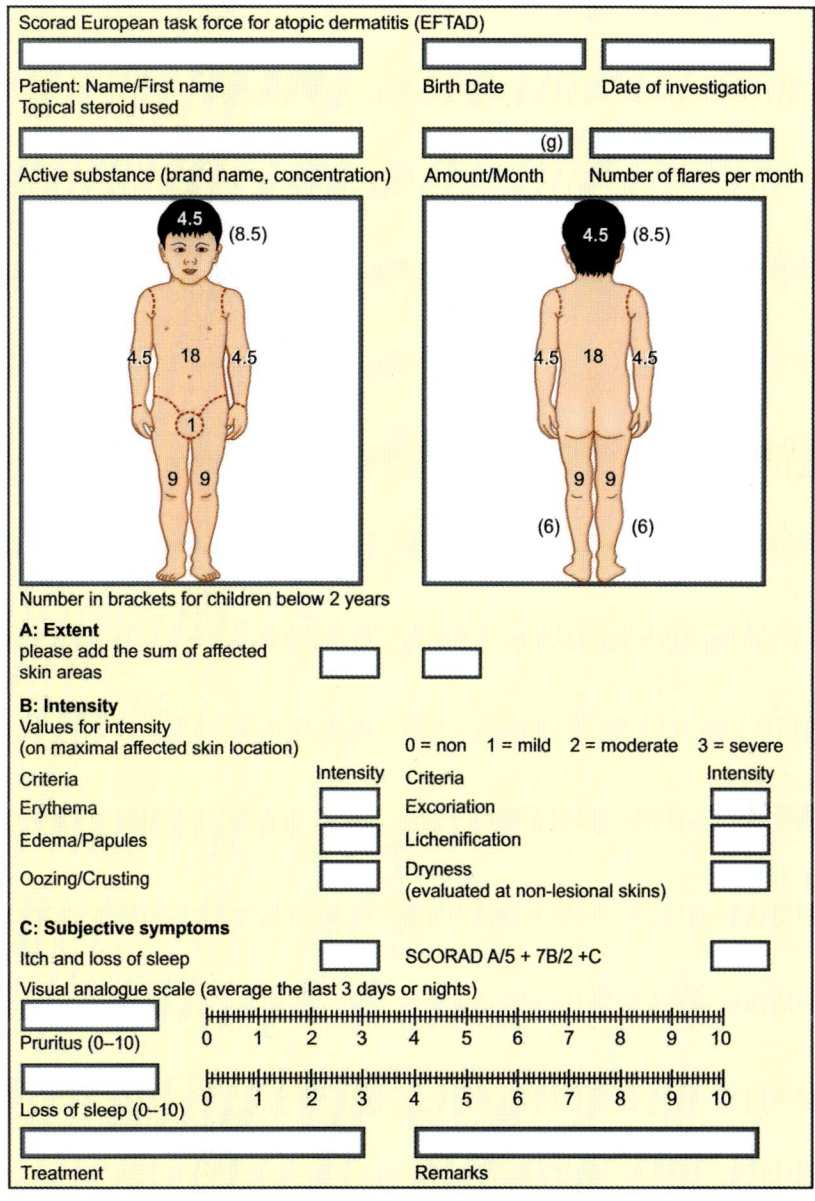

Fig. 9.15: SCORAD scoring panel (maximum score is 104)

In children, common conditions that can mimic AD are scabies, seborrheic dermatitis, contact dermatitis and psoriasis.

Rerely, immunodeficiency disorders mimic AD such as agammaglobulinemia, Wiskott-Aldrich syndrome, hyper-IgE (Job's syndrome), Omenn's syndrome, and Leiner's syndrome.

Other conditions that can mimic AD are acrodermatitis enteropathica, ataxia-telangiec-tasia, dermatitis herpetiformis, Langerhans cell histiocytosis, Hurler syndrome and phenylketonuria.

INVESTIGATION

Laboratory testing is *not* needed in the routine evaluation and treatment of uncomplicated AD. Serum IgE levels are elevated in approximately 70–80% of AD patients. The majority of patients with AD also have peripheral blood eosinophilia.

Classical tests for IgE-mediated hypersensitivity are skin prick test and RAST (radioallergosorbent test for specific IgEs in the blood). The atopy patch test is one of the recently described tests in AD and is preferred for aeroallergen testing.

Food allergy (FA) testing. Testing and interpretation of these tests are performed by allergy specialists. Skin-prick testing (SPT) is used to assist in the identification of foods that may be provoking IgE-mediated food-induced allergic reactions, but the SPT alone cannot be considered diagnostic of FA. The history and physical examination are important. Intradermal testing should not be used to make a diagnosis of FA. The routine use of measuring total serum IgE level should not be utilized to make a diagnosis of FA. Skin-prick testing has a sensitivity of 90% and a specificity of 50%. IgE testing has a high sensitivity but a low specificity. In some patients, food challenges are required to establish allergy or tolerance.

Histopathology is not diagnostic and similar findings are observed in other eczematous dermatoses such as allergic contact dermatitis. The histology of AD varies with the stage of the lesion, with many of the changes induced by scratching.

TREATMENT

Parental and patient education is very important in the management of AD.

Because AD is a chronic relapsing disease, the classic approach to therapy is targeting acute flares with short-term treatment regimens, i.e. reactive management. Based on recent insights into the underlying skin barrier defect and its relationship to inflammatory processes in the skin and other organs, a proactive approach that includes long-term maintenance therapy is now recommended (Wollenberg A et al). (*see* page 140)

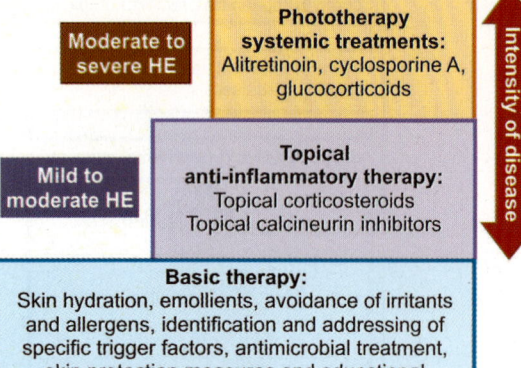

Fig. 9.16: A depiction of the treatment of AD based on severity

Multipronged approach that incorporates education about the disease state, skin hydration, pharmacologic therapy, and the identification and elimination of flare factors such as irritants, allergens, infectious agents, and emotional stressors, constitutes successful treatment.

Management strategy should be adapted to the severity of the disease. Mild cases are typically controlled by continuous use of emollients and intermittent use of a low-potency topical corticosteroid for flares, moderate AD may also require proactive maintenance with anti-inflammatory agents. In more severe and refractory cases, the use of phototherapy and systemic drugs may be necessary to control the disease.

A summary of the existing protocol is given in Fig. 9.16. Novel drugs are discussed in the next section, page 145.

General Measures

Elimination of Aggravating Factors

A number of environmental aggravating factors have been identified in AD. Careful history in determining specific aggravating factors and further avoidance of exposure to such triggering factors may help in avoiding exacerbations. Couselling regarding modification of lifestyle may help in avoiding triggers. Some important lifestyle modification measures are detailed in Table 9.3.

Table 9.3: Lifestyle modification and measures to avoid trigger factors in AD

Avoiding aeroallergens

1. Frequent wet mopping of floors and surfaces
2. Avoid pets
3. Avoid carpets/rugs
4. Plastic covering of mattresses

Clothing

1. Avoid woollen or synthetic clothing
2. Use cotton clothing which covers exremities

Food allergens

1. Advise exclusive breastfeeding till 6 months of age.
2. Elimination diet should not be routinely advised unless it is confirmed by oral food challenge tests.

Bathing and detergent contact

1. Use of mild soaps, preferably syndets, with pH around 6.
2. Avoidance of frequent or lengthy bathing. Ideal duration is **5 min**. In care of a flare, hard water may be a issue.
3. Soap should be applied only to intertriginous sites (groin and axillae).
4. Liberal use of emollients to moist skin after bathing to trap moisture.
5. Topical medications should be applied first to the affected areas of skin, with emollient applied afterwards to the non-affected areas of skin.

Environmental control

Temperature:
1. Maintain cool, stable temperatures
2. Do not overdress
3. Limit number of bed blankets
4. Avoid sweating

Humidity: Humidify the house in winter

Airborne allergens and dust:
1. Do not have rugs in bedrooms
2. Vacuum drapes and blankets
3. Use plastic mattress covers
4. Wet-mop floors

(Contd.)

Contd...

5. Avoid aerosols
6. Ventilate cooking odors
7. Avoid cigarettes
8. Have only artificial plants
9. Minimize animal dander—no cats, dogs, rodents, or birds
10. Change geographic location; sudden improvement may occur

This aspect of avoidance of irritants is very crucial as mistakes are made by clinicians in choosing strong and possibly risky drugs before they even tried to start with simple avoidance of irritants and skin care. We have seen patients on cyclosporine when simple avoidance of trigger factors like soaps and the use of hard water is the culprit. A leaflet is depicted (Fig. 9.17) which explains the importance of many so-called trivial things. Of course this leaflet cannot replace the dialogue which is very time-consuming and practically not achievable in the average office time of a practicing physician (J. Ring) (Fig. 9.17).

Barrier Repair

Critical role of an impaired skin barrier in the pathogenesis of AD underscores the importance of a continuous basic therapy with emollients, even in periods and sites in which AD is not active.

Galenics is the art to bring effective substances together with the desired vehicles into the correct mixture so that they reach the respective tissue. It is the most important aspect of topical dermatotherapy. In principle, there are different physicochemical characteristics of topical preparations which can be classified according to their nature with the so-called phase triangle according to Polano (Fig. 9.18) as: Solid phase (e.g. powder), lipid phase (lipids of various origin) and fluid phase (e.g. aqueous or alcoholic solutions). By the

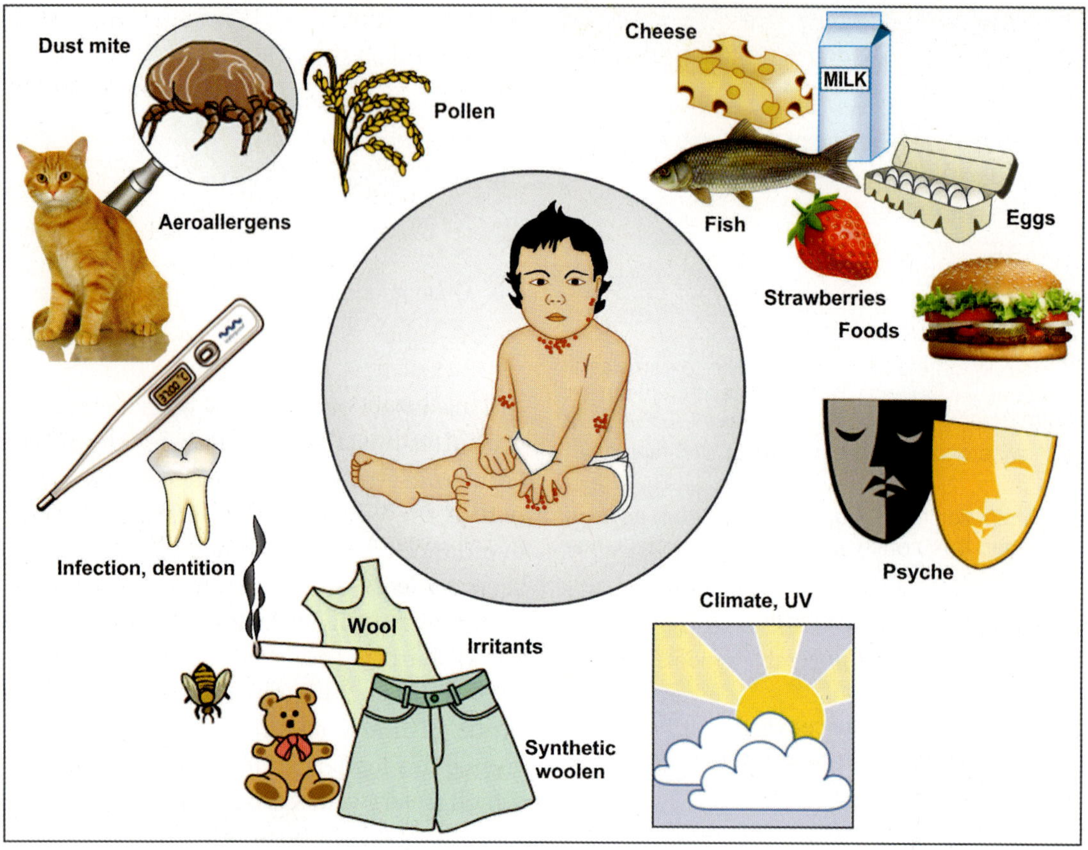

Fig. 9.17: Individual trigger factors of eczema flares patient information infographic

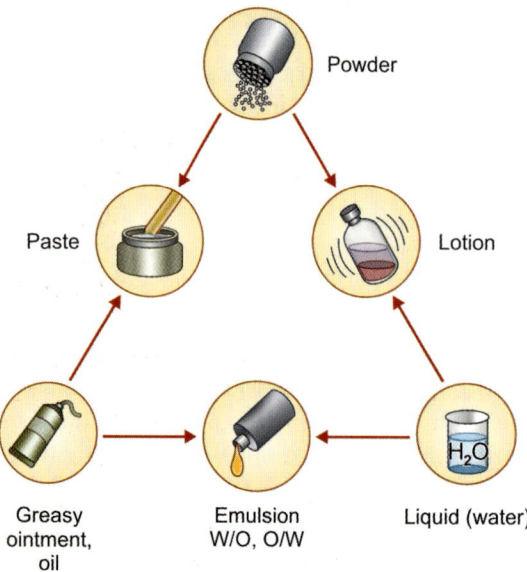

Fig. 9.18: Phase triangle according to Polano for selection of vehicle in topical dermatotherapy (Ring, 2005)

mixture of these three different basic conditions, a variety of preparations with very different characteristics with regard to efficacy and acceptability can be derived.

The contents of topical therapeutics can be of animal, plant, or mineral origin and show their effect already in the upper layers of the epidermis. It has to be considered that fatty materials form an occlusive film over the skin surface which prevents the loss of humidity but also the exchange of substances occurring normally through the skin barrier. This can be a disadvantage in very acute inflammatory conditions so that too greasy ointments should not be given in acute stages. The dermatological paradox describes that the opposite of moist is not "dry," but "fat"; a very moist preparation like an aqueous solution will—by increasing evaporation—lead to further dryness of the skin, while the application of a greasy ointment will contain humidity and moisture in the upper skin layers.

The secret of every topical preparation is how to bring water and fat together to form a suitable emulsion. This amphiphilic system can be regarded on a spectrum between pure fatty constituents like petrolatum or paraffin and pure solutions like water or alcohol and is characterized according to their nature constituent as either water-in-oil (W/O) or oil-in-water (O/W) emulsion. Creams are oil-in-water emulsions, while ointments in the dermatological terminology are water-in-oil emulsions. The larger the aqueous part of an emulsion, the more emulsifiers have to be used, which means that these are rather complex systems containing more substances than a rather fatty ointment with only petrolatum. The best protection of the skin can be achieved by water-in-oil emulsions which form a fatty film on the skin surface and provide protection also in occupational context (itchy hand dermatitis).

Ointments (e.g. petrolatum) and water-in-oil creams are more occlusive and tend to cause less burning and stinging than oil-in-water creams and lotions. However, the greasiness of an ointment is not acceptable to all patients.

Emollients should be applied twice daily to the entire cutaneous surface. Emollients containing particular combinations of lipids that are normally present in the stratum corneum (e.g. cholesterol, fatty acids, ceramides) may optimize barrier repair. Potentially allergy-provoking ingredients, such as perfumes, lanolin and herbal extracts, should be avoided.

Cost vs quantity: As the amount required is usually high, the cost may restrict their use thus there is a trade off between the high-quality emollients (i.e. sterile and low in contact allergens) with a high cost versus the low quality (glycerol, urea plus sodium chloride, and white petrolatum with liquid paraffin) emollients. It is more **logical** and enormously more **practical** to give a cheaper emollients as that way consistent compliance is achieved.

Site: In the selection of the right galenics, several aspects have to be considered, namely (Fig. 9.19):
• The tissue inflammation which tells you how deep the effective substance should penetrate
• The type of inflammation, whether infectious or noncontagious
• The duration, i.e. chronicity
• The individual skin type (dry skin, sebostasis, or greasy skin)
• The localization (extensor sides versus flexures or intertriginous areas)

The intertriginous areas where skin touches skin, like in the anogenital area or the axilla, are not a good place for too fatty topicals. Here powders or pastes should be preferred (Fig. 9.19).

Allergen Avoidance

The role of allergen avoidance in AD management is still controversial. Patients with moderate to severe AD can benefit from a diet eliminating those foods that have elicitated clinical early or late reactions upon controlled oral provocation tests.

Regarding the aeroallergens, the most **important** in atopy are the following:
• House dust
• House dust mite
• Pollen (tree/grass/weed)
• Animal dander (cat/dog)
• Mold

It is generally believed that they should be avoided because they have been shown to elicit eczematous skin lesions. Especially patients who will develop sensitization will benefit from avoidance strategies.

House dust mite avoidance strategies have been proved to have positive effects on the course of the disease. House dust mites live in a complex ecosystem consisting of air

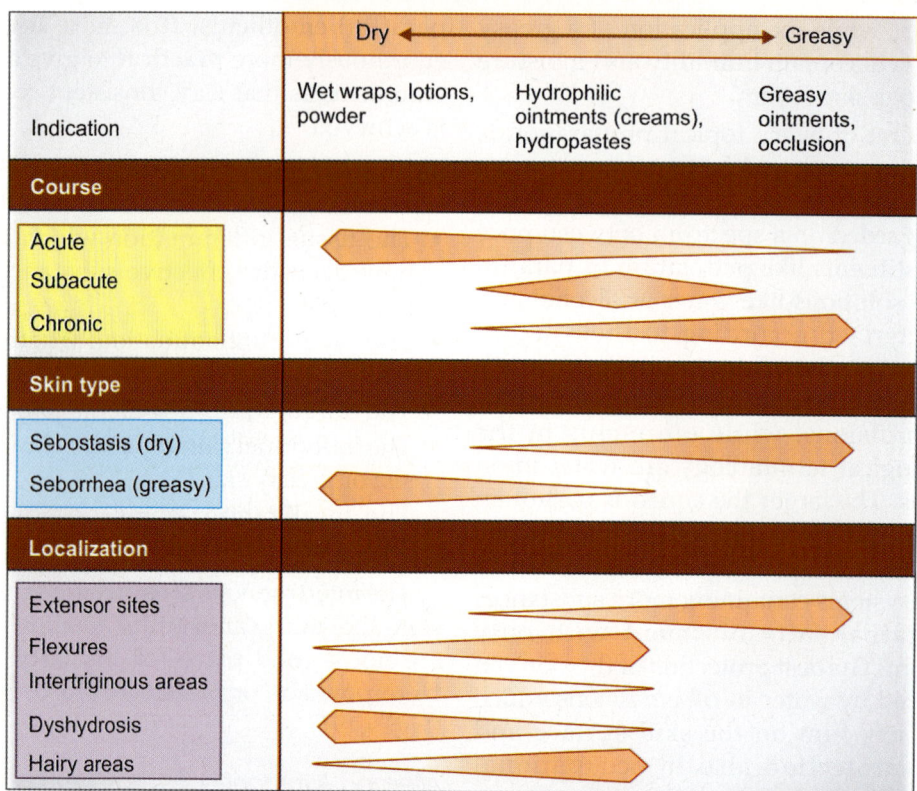

| Indication | Dry ← → Greasy | | |
	Wet wraps, lotions, powder	Hydrophilic ointments (creams), hydropastes	Greasy ointments, occlusion
Course			
Acute			
Subacute			
Chronic			
Skin type			
Sebostasis (dry)			
Seborrhea (greasy)			
Localization			
Extensor sites			
Flexures			
Intertriginous areas			
Dyshydrosis			
Hairy areas			

Fig. 9.19: Selection of vehicle according to disease acuity, localization, and individual skin type (from Ring and Fröhlich (1995))

humidity, temperature, and organic materials. Contacts with these allergens can be prevented with the use of dust mite-proof covers for mattresses and pillows, wet-mopping floors, and avoiding rugs (especially in bedrooms).

In spring- and summer time, pollen exposure as well as dusty ambience may exacerbate AE; thus, pollen avoidance measures have to be recommended.

Lastly, in selected highly sensitized patients, an allergen-specific immunotherapy (ASIT) may have positive therapeutic implications in AD and its associated allergic respiratory diseases. The best evidence so far is available for ASIT with house dust mite allergens.

Among food allergens, several studies have emphasized the etiological role of food allergens in AD exacerbation in infancy. Common implicated food allergens are cow's milk, hen's egg, wheat, soy, tree nuts, peanuts, fish, and apple. It is accepted that the importance of food allergens rapidly decreases with increasing age. The longest and scientifically best investigated dietary recommendation for primary allergy prevention consists of exclusive breastfeeding over at least 4 months (Fig. 9.20). When breastfeeding is not possible, application of hypoallergenic infant formula is recommended; partially hydrolyzed whey preparations as well as extensively hydrolyzed casein products have been shown in large clinical trials to yield the best effects. Regular intake of fish also as early as during pregnancy and lactation may have beneficial effects as well as a Mediterranean diet and a general diversity of foods. The role of introduction of solid food seems to be less important, and it can be started after the fourth month of life. Recent studies have shown that being overweight is associated with a higher

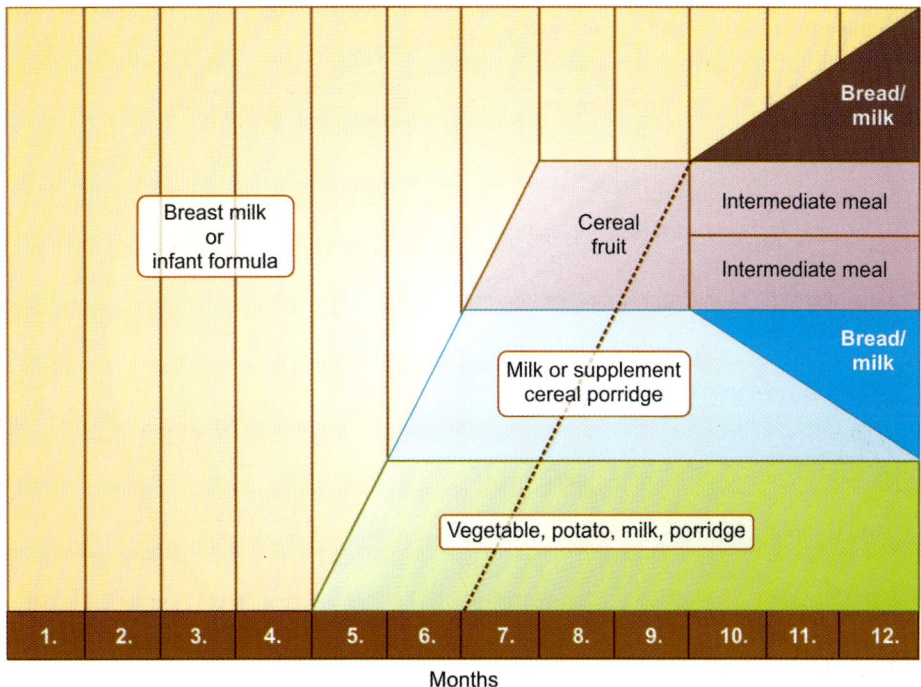

Fig. 9.20: Dietary schedule for healthy nutrition in the first year of life (ideal scenario for AD patients)

risk of asthma; therefore, avoidance of high-calorie diets has also been included in recommendations for allergy prevention.

It is important that the diet in the first year of life contains all the necessary elements and vitamins and a certain degree of diversity according to general nutrition recommendations (Fig. 9.20).

Specific Therapy

Topical Anti-inflammatory Drugs

Topical steroids (TCS) with emollients: Topical steroids are used in the management of AD in both adults and children and are the mainstay of anti-inflammatory therapy. They suppress production of several transcription factors, which leads not only to reduced expression of proinflammatory cytokines but also to inhibition of cell growth and decreased synthesis of collagen and other structural proteins (explaining side effects such as skin atrophy). They are typically introduced into the treatment regimen after failure of lesions to respond to good skin care and regular use of moisturizers alone. In most body sites, once-daily application of a corticosteroid is almost as effective as more frequent applications, at lower cost and with less systemic absorption. In *infants,* low-potency steroid ointments, such as hydrocortisone, desonide, are preferred. In *older children and adults,* medium-potency steroids, such as fluticasone, mometasone, are often used, except on the face, where milder steroids or calcineurin inhibitors are preferred. Proactive, intermittent use of TCS as maintenance therapy (2–3 *times per week*) on areas that commonly flare is recommended to help prevent relapses while reducing the need for topical corticosteroids, and is more effective than the use of emollients alone (Fig. 9.21).

If an atopic patient worsens or fails to improve after the use of topical steroids and moisturizers, the possibility of allergic contact dermatitis to a preservative or the corticosteroids must be considered. The incidence of reported side effects from TCS use is low;

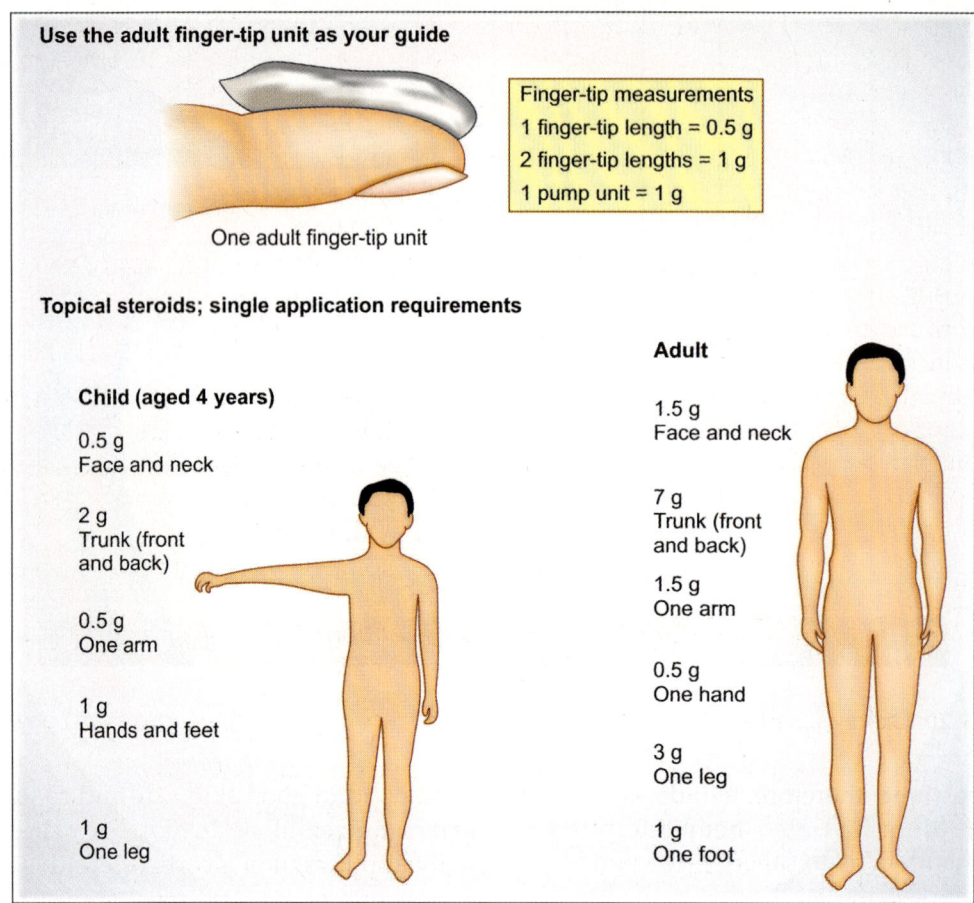

Fig. 9.21: Important aspects of topical steroid use in AD

however, long-term use may cause potential complications which include purpura, telangiectasia, striae, focal hypertrichosis, and acneiform or rosacea-like eruptions. Many of these side effects will resolve after discontinuing TCS use, but may take months.

The patient should be instructed to not stop the treatment too early and to be educated in the correct use of TCS for a long period. In fact, with *subclinical* to *mild* disease activity, a small amount of topical corticosteroids from once to thrice weekly (considering a monthly amount in the mean range of *15 g in infants, 30 g in children, and up to 60–90 g in adolescents/adults*), together with a correct use of emollients, generally allows a good and long-term maintenance therapy (Fig. 9.21).

The use of emollients on the entire body with reactive and proactive anti-inflammatory treatments is advised. The emollient should be applied first, about *15 min before* the topical anti-inflammatory treatments. Patients with acute and erosive lesions sometimes do not tolerate standard topical application. In these cases, *wet wraps* should be used. They are also protective to persistent scratching, and they decrease the itch by cooling the skin.

Topical calcineurin inhibitors (TCIs): US food and drug administration (FDA) approval for the treatment of AD: Tacrolimus 0.03% and 0.1% ointment (for "moderate to severe" disease) and pimecrolimus 1% cream (for "mild to moderate" disease). These agents suppress T cell activation and modulate the secretion of cytokines and other proinflammatory mediators. Their efficacy in the treatment of AD has been proven in clinical trials in adults and children at least 2 years of age (and, for pimecrolimus, infants ages 3–23 months, although it is not approved for this group).

The anti-inflammatory efficacy of 0.1% tacrolimus ointment is similar to a corticosteroid with intermediate activity, which is more active than 1.0% pimecrolimus cream. The use of pimecrolimus is inexplicable as it is actually inferior than tacrolimus and its use over tacrolimus defies any pharmacological logic, but that it still sells speaks volumes of the marketing skills of the industry than the clinicians understanding of its efficacy.

The major side effect of both medications is burning at the site of application; they are not associated with cutaneous atrophy. Burning of the skin or a feeling of warmth is a side effect of these compounds. It starts about 5 min after each application and may last up to 1 h. These side effects usually disappear after a few days of treatment.

Topical calcineurin inhibitors are particularly useful on the face (eyelids, perioral skin), intertriginous sites, and the anogenital area. These are areas prone to steroid atrophy, when steroid allergy is a consideration, or when systemic steroid absorption is a concern.

Recent randomized controlled studies have shown that the **proactive application** of tacrolimus ointment (e.g. twice weekly as maintenance) can prevent flares of AD without increasing the overall amount of medication used. Also adding mid-week use of tacrolimus ointment to the topical corticosteroid weekender approach (2/week) has been used to improve control of severe AE.

Treatment of Bacterial Infections

Topical or oral antibiotics should be reserved for cases with frank evidence of secondary infection, which may worsen eczema through action of superantigens.

Bleach bathes which reduce staphylococcal colonization have rapidly become a mainstay in AD patients. Tepid bath with ¼ cup of standard household bleach (6%) diluted in 20 gallons of water used twice a week dramatically improves AD on the trunk and extremities, but less so on the face.

Intranasal application of *mupirocin* is beneficial in reducing nasal carriage of staphylococci.

Phototherapy

All forms of phototherapy, like PUVA, narrow band UVB, broadband UVB, UVA1 are effective in treatment of AD and are mainly used for long-term maintenance treatment, along with topicals.

UV sources have an immunomodulatory and antimicrobial effect (reducing the colonization of *S. aureus*), and they increase the vitamin D balance.

UVB mainly acts by inhibiting antigen presentation by Langerhans cells, T cell activation and cytokine production by keratinocytes.

Phototherapy is usually a part of a wider treatment plan in adults and much less in children. Phototherapy should be avoided in children under the age of 12 years and in those patients who reported a worsening of their dermatitis during sun exposure.

1. **NBUVB** is preferable to PUVA especially in children due to its better tolerability and safety profile.
2. **Narrowband UVB** is to be preferred to broadband UVB. Studies have shown that medium-dose UVA1 has similar efficacy as narrowband UVB.
3. Topical steroid and emollients can be combined but *not tacrolimus*.
4. In case of *acute eczema* exacerbation, **UVA1** should be the suggested UV source.

Systemic Treatment

Systemic anti-inflammatory treatment should be restricted to severe, refractory cases of AD that do not respond adequately to intensive topical therapy. Of note, no systemic medications besides corticosteroids have been **FDA-approved** for treatment of AD.

In general, *systemic corticosteroids* should be used only to control acute exacerbations. In patients requiring systemic steroid therapy, short courses **(<3 weeks)** are preferred. If repeated or prolonged courses of systemic corticosteroids are required to control the AD, phototherapy or a steroid-sparing agent should be considered. Systemic steroids are not a preferred agent in children with AD due to their side effect profile and rebound flare on withdrawal.

Cyclosporine A (CSA) is one of the most commonly used systemic agents for AD as it is shown to be safe and effective in both children and adults, although probably tolerated *better* in children. Oral cyclosporine 3–5 mg/kg/day typically leads to rapid improvement of skin disease and associated pruritus in patients with AD, and its efficacy has been established in randomized controlled trials.

Dose: An initial daily dose between 3 and 5 mg/kg/day, divided upon two single doses, is recommended. When a satisfactory clinical response is achieved, a dose reduction of 0.25–0.5 mg/kg/day every 2 weeks is recommended.

Virtually all patients respond rapidly with a reduction in eczema severity by approximately 55% at 6–8 weeks. In the UK, cyclosporine is *licensed* for an *8-week course*. If the dose can be reduced down to or below 2.5 mg/kg and regular monitoring of renal function and blood pressure are satisfactory, cyclosporine may be continued for up to 1 year.

Low-dose cyclosporine may be used 'off label' in severe and refractory disease in children and is the commonest first line systemic agent prescribed in Europe.

Cyclosporine treatment has to be performed over longer time periods, since after withdrawal, severe "rebound" reactions can occur. Due to its side effects (*see* below), a maximal treatment duration of **2 years** is recommended.

Side effects: It is very useful to gain rapid control of severe AD. Potential long-term side effects, especially nephrotoxicity, require careful monitoring, with attempts to transition the patient to a potentially less toxic agent when possible. The combination with UV therapy should be avoided; the patient should be educated to a proper photo protection in summertime due to the increased risk of cutaneous malignancies.

Azathioprine can be an effective treatment for moderate to severe AD in children and adults, with modest benefit. It is used in dose of 2.5–3.5 mg/kg/day along with other treatment modalities simultaneously. It works slowly (12 weeks).

Other immunosuppressive agents that can be used are mycophenolate mofetil and methotrexate. **Methotrexate** appears as efficacious as azathioprine. Time to maximal effect is approximately 10 weeks.

Biologicals are discussed in detail in the next section, page 145.

For moderate to severe AE, cyclosporine is used to gain control of acute flares but with a short duration of therapy. For patients with resistant moderate to severe AE with *chronic* and more *stable* disease, both azathioprine and methotrexate may be considered as first line options although further comparative studies are recommended. For the rare patients with **chronic resistant disease** unresponsive or intolerant of azathioprine and methotrexate, myclophenolate mofetil is used as third line.

Anti-Itch Agents

Antihistamines are frequently used but pruritus of AD is notoriously resistant to antihistamines especially nonsedating ones. If prescribed, sedating antihistamines are used nightly to break "itch scratch cycle" (not "as needed"). Diphenhydramine, hydroxyzine, and doxepin can all be efficacious.

Box 9.3: Anti-itch measures in atopic dermatitis

General principles	• Cleansing, bathing, practices use of emollients/basic therapy. • Elimination of provocative factors: avoidance strategies (i.e. too long and hot bathing, contact with irritant substances or allergens, hard water, etc.)
Anti-inflammatory therapy	• TCS and TCI • CsA • Phototherapy
Topical agents	Creams/lotions containing urea, camphor, menthol, topical polidocanol or N-palmitoylethanolamine
Systemic agents	• Opioid receptor antagonists (e.g. naltrexone) • Sedative anti histamines

*see Table 9.5.

Studies on the second-generation, nonsedating antihistamines, i.e. loratadine, cetirizine, or fexofenadine, demonstrated no or only a weak relief of pruritus. But second-generation antihistamines have the advantage that they are efficacious in the relief of the symptoms of common mucosal comorbidities such as allergic asthma and rhinoconjunctivitis.

A summary of the anti-itch measures is given in **Box 9.3**.

TREATMENT PLAN

As all patients of atopic dermatitis are different, an individualized approach is needed depending on the severity of AD, thus in mild cases, topical emollients and mild steroids may suffice, but this may not apply to all cases of AD. Another treatment approach is given below which is known as the *proactive approach*.

Thus the *reactive* approach (Fig. 9.22a) has been combined with the *proactive* approach (Fig. 9.22b), which is defined as a predefined, long-term, low-dose treatment with anti-inflammatory drugs that have to be applied to the previously affected areas (Wollenberg et al). This is based on the fact that the chronic and relapsing nature of AD can be halted by targeting the normal-looking, nonlesional AD skin which is not normal at all, but is characterized by a clinically meaningful barrier function defect and a subclinical eczematous skin reaction.

Proactive approach has the advantage of control of the subclinical disease with minimal

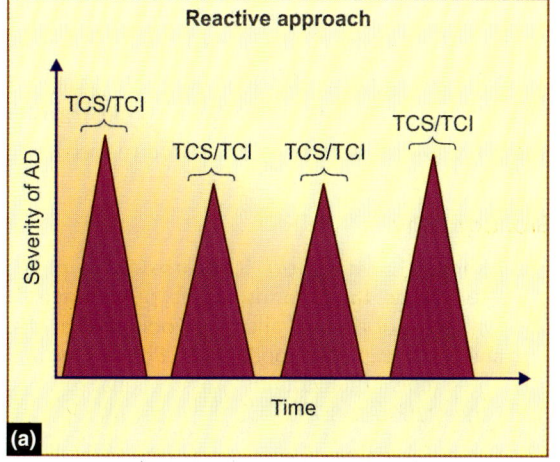

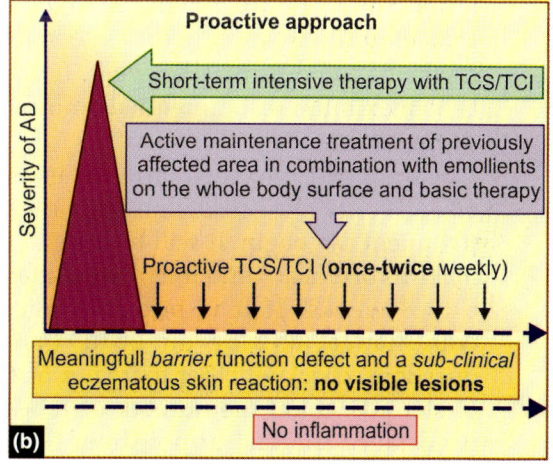

Fig. 9.22a and b: A depiction of the reactive proactive approach of the treatment of AD. (a) Depicts 'as-when' use of TCS/TI, while (b) shows a concurrent maintenance regimen with occasional intensive therapy. (TCS = Topical steroids, TCI = Topical calcineurin inhibitors) see text above

use of anti-inflammatory drugs and is safe and reduces relapses.

Proactive treatment indicated in forms with flare-ups that follow on quickly one after another or when symptoms are permanent (this means when lesions reappear as soon as anti-inflammatory treatment is stopped). It entails using anti-inflammatory treatment routinely (even in the absence of lesions) on the areas that are usually affected, 2 to 3 times a week, over a long period of time (several weeks or even months). This method leads to a clear reduction in the number of flare-ups in the medium term and a decrease in the amount of anti-inflammatory used when compared to a standard reactive treatment regimen. If a flare-up develops during maintenance treatment, the same principles as for the acute phase treatment are applicable while the flare-up is being treated.

This treatment plan consists of two steps:

a. A short *"acute"* phase of treatment (*1 to 2 weeks*), the purpose of which is to obtain the fullest clinical remission as quickly as possible. This phase is based on the once a day usage of a topical steroid, that is suitable in terms of potency and pharmaceutical form, for the patient according to their age and lesion sites. The treatment is stopped *without* gradual tapering off as soon as erythema and pruritus disappear. There is no maximum recommended amount during acute phase treatment.

If the acute phase treatment is as effective as expected, maintenance treatment can begin. It will be assessed in terms of efficacy and tolerability after 6 to 8 weeks. If it is not effective, compliance may be an issue (ask questions, check whether there is a fear of steroids, count the number of tubes used since the last appointment). If adherence is satisfactory, the second line treatment must be started, including potent steroids, phototherapy or systemic agents. This method is called the early *reactive treatment*. This is indicated in cases of AD with flare-ups that are spaced several weeks apart.

b. A *"maintenance"* phase, the purpose of which is to maintain remission in the long term. This phase consists of:

   • Daily usage of emollients;

   • Usage of a topical steroid or even topical tacrolimus following one of two different regimens. Topical steroids are often prescribed as a **first line** treatment for maintenance. Topical tacrolimus is offered as a **second line** treatment where topical steroids have failed or as a first line treatment if there is a contraindication to topical steroids or in certain high-risk sites (especially the face).

Proactive therapy should be carried out in children and in adults. Long-term studies (up to 4 years) have been performed either with **tacrolimus** (0.03% and 0.1%) or with corticosteroids (i.e. *fluticasone propionate* cream and ointment and *methylprednisolone* cream). In **adults**, long-term treatment with *0.1% tacrolimus* ointment appears to be as effective as a corticosteroid regimen for the trunk and extremities and more effective in the face and neck area.

It is believed that initiation of these measures at a very early stage of the disease might even have a beneficial effect also on respiratory symptoms and serum IgE (atopic march).

Bibliography

1. Asher MI, Montefort S, Bjorksten B, et al. Worldwide time trends in the prevalence of symptoms of asthma, allergic rhinoconjunctivitis, and eczema in childhood: ISAAC Phases One and Three repeat multicountry crosssectional surveys. Lancet 2006;368:733–43.

2. Barker JN, Palmer CN, Zhao Y, Liao H, Hull PR, Lee SP, Allen MH, Meggitt SJ, Reynolds NJ, Trembath RC, McLean WH. Null mutations in the filaggrin gene (FLG) determine major susceptibility

to early-onset atopic dermatitis that persists into adulthood. J Invest Dermatol 2007 Mar;127(3): 564-7. Epub 2006 Sep 21.

3. Bratton DL, et al. Granulocyte macrophage colony-stimulating factor contributes to enhanced monocyte survival in chronic atopic dermatitis. J Clin Invest 1995;95:211.

4. Bunikowski R, Mielke M, Skarabis H, et al. Prevalence and role of serum IgE antibodies to the Staphylococcus aureus-derived superantigens SEA and SEB in children with atopic dermatitis. J Allergy Clin Immunol 1999; 103:119–24.

5. Chaumont A, Voisin C, Sardella A, Bernard A. Interactions between domestic water hardness, infant swimming and atopy in the development of childhood eczema. Environ Res 2012 Jul;116:52–7.

6. Cho SH, Strickland I, Boguniewicz M, Leung DY. Fibronectin and fibrinogen contribute to the enhanced binding of Staphylococcusaureus to atopic skin. J Allergy Clin Immunol 2001 Aug;108(2):269–74.

7. Danby SG, Brown K, Wigley AM, Chittock J, Pyae PK, Flohr C, Cork MJ. The effect of water hardness on surfactant deposition following washing and subsequent skin irritation in atopic dermatitis patients and healthy controls. J Invest Dermatol 2017 Sep 12.

8. DaVeiga SP. Epidemiology of atopic dermatitis: a review. Allergy Asthma Proc 2012 May-Jun;33(3): 227-34. doi: 10.2500/aap 2012.33. 3569.

9. Eichenfield LF, Ellis CN, Mancini AJ, Paller AS, Simpson EL. Atopic dermatitis: epidemiology and pathogenesis update. Semin Cutan Med Surg 2012 Sep;31(3 Suppl):S3-5. doi: 10.1016/j.sder.2012.07.002.

10. Elias PM, Hatano Y, Williams ML. Basis for the barrier abnormality in atopic dermatitis: outside-inside-outside pathogenic mechanisms. J Allergy Clin Immunol 2008 Jun;121(6):1337-43. doi: 10.1016/ j.jaci.2008. 01.022. Epub 2008 Mar 7.

11. Font-Ribera L, Gracia-Lavedan E, Esplugues A, Ballester F, Jiménez Zabala A, Santa Marina L, Fernández-Somoano A, Sunyer J, Villanueva CM. Water hardness and eczema at 1 and 4 y of age in the INMA birth cohort. Environ Res 2015Oct;142: 579–85.

12. Garmhausen D, Hagemann T, Bieber T, Dimitriou I, Fimmers R, Diepgen T, Novak N. Characterization of different courses of atopic dermatitis in adolescent and adult patients. Allergy 2013;68(4): 498–506.

13. J. Ring, Atopic Dermatitis: Eczema. Springer International Publishing Switzerland 2016.

14. Kanwar AJ, De D. Epidemiology and clinical features of atopic dermatitis in India. Indian J Dermatol 2011;56:471–5.

15. Katayama I, Kohno Y, Akiyama K, et al. Japanese Guidelines for atopic dermatitis. Allergol Int 2011;60:205–20.

16. Marenholz I, Kerscher T, Bauerfeind A, Esparza-Gordillo J, Nickel R, Keil T, Lau S, Rohde K, Wahn U, Lee YA. An interaction between filaggrin mutations and early food sensitization improves the prediction of childhood asthma. J Allergy Clin Immunol 2009 Apr;123(4):911-6. doi: 10.1016/j.jaci.2009.01.051.

17. McNally NJ, Williams HC, Phillips DR, Smallman-Raynor M, Lewis S, Venn A,Britton J. Atopic eczema and domestic water hardness. Lancet 1998 Aug 15;352(9127):527-31. Pub Med PMID: 9716057.

18. Perkin MR, Craven J, Logan K, Strachan D, Marrs T, Radulovic S, Campbell LE, MacCallum SF, McLean WH, Lack G, Flohr C. Enquiring About Tolerance Study Team. Association between domestic water hardness, chlorine, and atopic dermatitis risk in early life: A population-based cross-sectional study. J Allergy Clin Immunol 2016 Aug;138(2):509–16.

19. Proudfoot LE, Powell AM, Ayis S, et al. The European treatment of severe atopic eczema in Children Taskforce (TREAT) survey. Br J Dermatol 2013;169(4):901.

20. Ricci G, Dondi A, Patrizi A. Useful tools for the management of atopic dermatitis. Am J Clin Dermatol 2009;10:287–300.

21. Sardana K, Goel K, Garg VK, Goel A, Khanna D, Grover C, Khurana N. Is frictional lichenoid dermatitis a minor variant of atopic dermatitis or a photodermatosis. Indian J Dermatol 2015 Jan-Feb;60(1):66–73.

22. Strachan DP. Hay fever, hygiene, and household size. BMJ 1989;299:1259.

23. Superantigens in atopic dermatitis: implications for future therapeutic strategies. Am J Clin Dermatol 2006;7:273–9.

24. Toda M, et al. Polarized in vivo expression of IL-11 and IL-17 between acute and chronic skin lesions. J Allergy Clin Immunol 2003;111:875.

25. Tokura Y. Extrinsic and intrinsic types of atopic dermatitis. J Dermatol Sci 2010 Apr;58(1):1–7.

26. Walters RM, Anim-Danso E, Amato SM, Capone KA, Mack MC, Telofski LS, Mays DA. Hard water softening effect of a baby cleanser. Clin Cosmet Investig Dermatol 2016 Oct 11;9:339–45.

27. Williams HC, Burney PG, Hay RJ, Archer CB, Shipley MJ, Hunter JJ, Bingham EA, Finlay AY, Pembroke AC, Graham-Brown RA, et al. The UK Working Party's Diagnostic Criteria for Atopic Dermatitis. I. Derivation of a minimum set of discriminators for atopic dermatitis. Br J Dermatol 1994 Sep;131(3):383–96.

28. Williams HC. Clinical practice. Atopic dermatitis. N Engl J Med 2005;352:2314–24.

29. Wollenberg A, Bieber T. Proactive therapy of atopic dermatitis-an emerging concept. Allergy 2009;64:276–8.

A CRITICAL OVERVIEW OF NOVEL THERAPIES FOR ATOPIC DERMATITIS

During the past decade, the underlying molecular basis for AD has been increasingly understood, particularly with a focus on **barrier dysfunction**, cutaneous and systemic **immune abnormalities**, and the role of the **microbiome**, allowing development of more targeted therapies.

Although debate has focused on whether AD pathogenesis is primarily **"inside-out"** (primary role of the immune system) versus **"outside-in"** (primary role of the epidermal barrier), it is now clear that the barrier, immune system, and microbes are all interconnected, with each abnormality progressively exacerbating another until successful intervention is introduced. In addition, the underlying basis for itch at the peripheral and central nervous system levels is an active area of investigation.

Though there are numerous novel therapies, it is important to understand that these supplant and do not replace the basic bulwark of therapies. They can be divided into 3 categories: topical products, monoclonal antibodies (mAbs) or small-molecule inhibitors.

The Barrier and Th2 Response

The skin provides a barrier that protects from the external environment. This barrier is comprised of epidermal proteins of the stratum-corneum, stratum granulosum, and tight junctions, as well as epidermal lipids, such as ceramides. When this barrier is impaired, external stimuli (e.g. irritants, bacteria, and dust mite and food protein allergic triggers) can more easily induce inflammation.

This remains the critical component determining AD and several studies have demonstrated that skin barrier dysfunction is a critical component of AD (Egawa G). High transepidermal water loss, a measure of barrier dysfunction, at 2 days of age is associated with a 7.1-fold higher increased risk

of having AD by 1 year of age than having low transepidermal water loss (Kelleher M).

In addition, having an inherited deficiency in epidermal barrier proteins (notably filaggrin [FLG] increases the risk of AD and allergic disorders, presumably by attenuating the skin barrier, facilitating the interaction of external antigens with skin-resident immune cells and driving the cutaneous inflammation that leads to systemic immune responses (Egawa G).

These observations suggest that maintaining skin barrier function is important for the effective management of AD. However, even **without** FLG mutation, FLG expression in adults with AD is decreased, implicating factors associated with disease chronicity. The Th2 cell responses intercalate with the barrier defect (Box 9.4).

The Immunological Pathway of AD

AD has been considered an immunological disorder, but in recent times the focus has shifted to Th2 cells the concept of other cells like Th1, Th2, Th9, Th17, and Th22 cells with complex cross talks is also known to play a rule in AD. A depiction of the same is seen in Fig 9.23. It also lists the important aspects of the immunological pathways which are in turn targets for novel therapies. These are listed in Box 9.5.

The problem with all such checkpoints is the relative emphasis of each of them. It is not possible to target all of them, and hence every new research throws up novel agents and

---

Box 9.4: Th2 and its effect on barrier

Th2 cytokines (IL-4 and IL-13) downregulate the production of:
1. FLG and keratins
2. Cornified envelope components (loricrin and involucrin),
3. Cell adhesion molecules (desmogleins and zonula occludens)
4. Ceramide lipids.

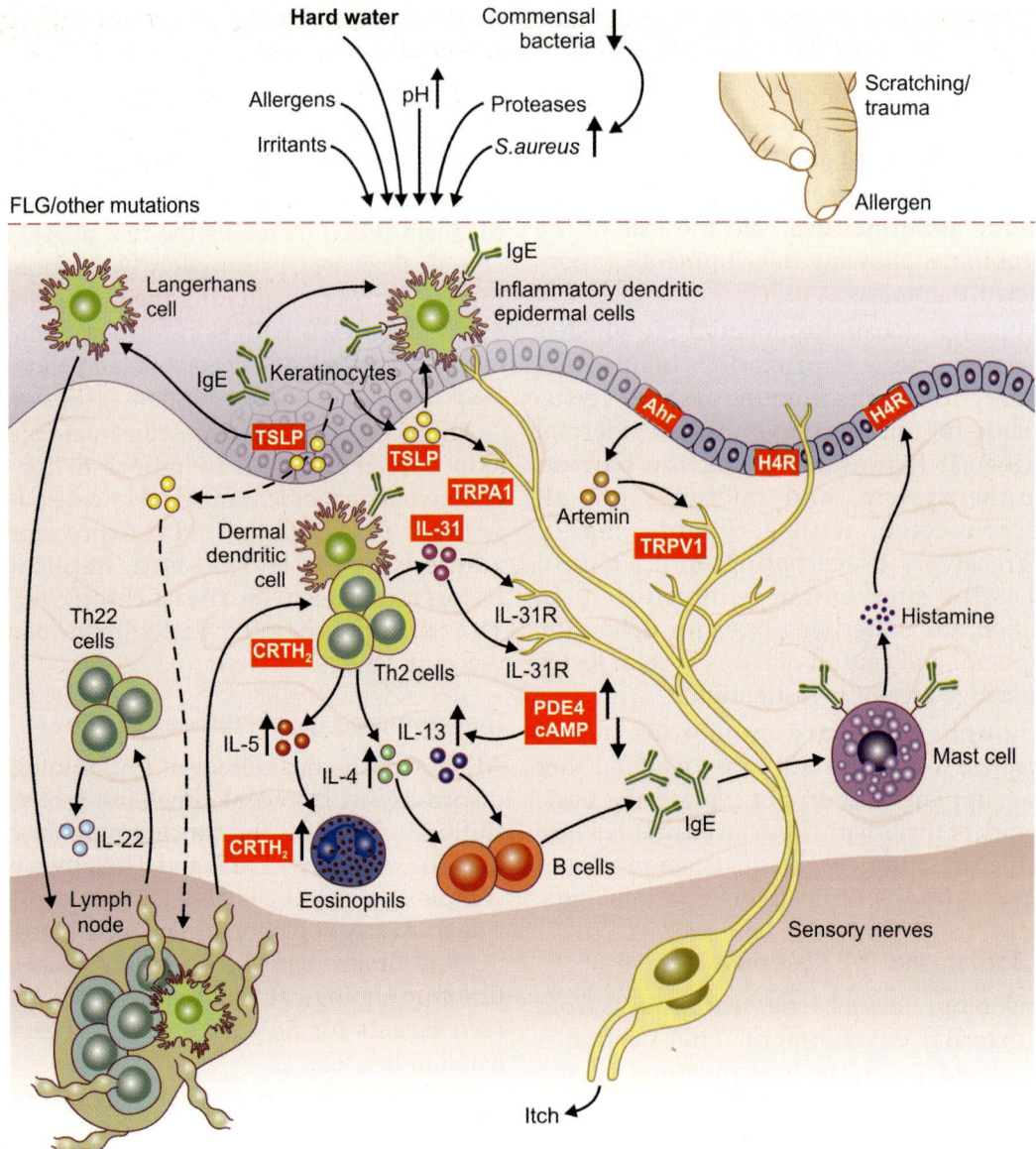

Fig. 9.23: Interplay of the epidermis and immune system in patients with AD demonstrates the targets for new therapy. Barrier defects promote the ingress of epicutaneous antigens that interface with epidermal Langerhans cells and dermal dendritic cells, leading to immune activation, particularly of the Th2 and Th22 signaling pathways. CRTh2, a prostaglandin D_2 receptor on a variety of inflammatory cells, promotes Th2 cell migration into the skin. Th2 cytokines (i.e. IL-4, IL-3, and IL-5) lead to IgE class-switching and induce peripheral eosinophils and mast cells. Increases in PDE4 also increase Th2 cytokine expression. Th22 cells produce IL-22, which induces epidermal hyperplasia and is prominent in patients with chronic disease. Th2 and Th22 cytokines also contribute to the impaired expression of barrier proteins and barrier impairment, which is thought to increase the risk of infection. *S. aureus* is increased and bacterial diversity is decreased with flares. The Th2 cytokine IL-31 is upregulated and associated with causing itch but not inflammation. TSLP production by keratinocytes not only induces a Th2 response but is also thought to induce itch by directly stimulating transient receptor potential A1 (TRPA1) receptors in cutaneous sensory neurons. Newer targets are AhR and H4R, which is expressed on both keratinocytes and Th2 cells and regulates IL-31 expression

Box 9.5: Check points in the cytokine and immuno-logical pathway of AD

AhR	Aryl hydrocarbon receptor
TSLP	Thymic stromal lymphopoietin
CRTh2	Chemoattractant receptor-homologous molecules expressed on Th2 lympho-cytes
IL	IL-4 and IL-13
	IL-5
	IL-31 and IL-31 receptor A
PDE4	Phosphodiesterase 4
Ig	IgE
H4	Histamine receptor type 4
NK1R	Neurokinin 1 receptor

targets. Ultimately clinical trials decide the ultimate utility of these novel drugs. It is pertinent to point out that the research seems to be moving upstream, from IgE, which is the target of most therapies today and has now moved towards IL4 and PDE5. A summary of the various checkpoints and the agents is given below.

1. AhR (Agonist of the Aryl Hydrocarbon Receptor)

What is it?: In the skin, AhR is a ubiquitously expressed, ligand-activated transcription factor, acting as a receptor for xenobiotics. In human AD skin AhR expression is increased (Kim HO), and its increased expression and activation by coal tar restores FLG expression in FLG-haploinsufficient keratinocytes and interferes with the Th2 cytokine signaling.

Agent: The first is the topical used of **tar** (van den Bogaard EH). The other agent, AhR agonist **tapinarof** (GSK2894512; formerly, WBI-1001; in China, benvitimod).

2. TSLP (Thymic Stromal Lymphopoietin)

What is it?: Thymic stromal lymphopoietin (TSLP) is known as a keratinocyte-derived cytokine that leads to conditioning of skin-derived dendritic cells, ultimately generating

a strong Th2 response (VerstraeteK). Moreover, in animal models, TSLP has been reported to be key in the mechanisms underlying the atopic march. TSLP, which is regulated in keratinocytes by the ORAI1/NFAT calcium-signaling pathway, also directly communicates with a subset of transient receptor potential A1 (TRAPA1) positive cutaneous sensory neurons to promote pruritus.

Agent: Currently, **tezepelumab**, an anti-TSLP antibody, has completed phase 1 trials.

3. CRTh2 (Chemoattractant Receptor-Homologous Molecules Expressed on Th2 Lymphocytes)

What is it?: Mast cells have been speculated to be a potential source of PGD2 in AD skin. A prostaglandin D2 (PGD2) receptor (chemo-attractant receptor-homologous molecules expressed on Th2 lymphocytes [CRTh2]) was found to be expressed on inflammatory Th2 cells (Mitson-Salazar A), type II innate lymphoid cells, eosinophils, and basophils.

Agents: A series of proof-of-concept (PoC) studies have been initiated with 2 different representatives of a new class of compounds (OC000459 and fevipripant/QAW039); posted results from QAW039 suggest lack of significant efficacy (NCT01785602).

3. Interleukins

IL-4 and IL-13

What is it?: IL-4 and IL-13 are the 2 most important cytokines involved in regulation of IgE synthesis, as well as in generating "atopic inflammation." Recent evidence has also suggested that the shared receptor subunit for IL-4 and IL-13 (IL-4Ra) on sensory neurons can mediate chronic pruritus through Janus kinase (JAK) signaling (Oetjen I).

Agent: **Dupilumab,** a biologic targeting IL-4Ra, has recently been approved in the United States for therapy of moderate-to-severe forms of AD. In the pivotal set of phase 3 studies, dupilumab led to an improvement of at least 75% from baseline to week 16 in the Eczema Area and Severity Index (EASI) score is 48% on every other week dupilumab and 50% on every week dupilumab U/S 13% subjects receiving placebo (P <.001 for both active arms) (Simpson EL).

Other targets include, IL-4 or IL-13. Trials for AD have been completed for **pitrakinra**, an antagonist of IL-4, and **tralokinumab** and **lebrikizumab**, both biologics targeting IL-13.

IL-5

What is it?: This cytokine should have been the potential point of inhibition as IL-5 attracts eosinophils within the inflamed tissue and thus represents an ideal target to inhibit the migration of eosinophils, which play a key role in subsets of patients with asthma and eosinophilic esophagitis, although their role in AD is unclear.

Agent: **Mepolizumab** is an anti-IL-5 biologic, which has been approved recently in the United States and European Union for severe eosinophilic asthma. This compound did not fulfill the efficacy parameters, but another study is being planned.

IL-31 and IL-31 receptor A

What is it?: In human subjects and mice, IL-31 is predominantly produced by Th2 cells, and its receptor, IL-31 receptor A, is expressed on C-fibers (Dillon SR). It is known to primarily mediate itch in AD.

Agent: Monthly injections of an anti-IL-31 receptor A antibody (CIM331; **nemolizumab**) significantly inhibited pruritus in patients with moderate-to-severe AD in a phase 2 clinical trial; significant improvement in pruritus was seen by 3 days; the effect on AD severity by week 12 was low (Ruzicka T).

4. PDE4

The intracellular cyclic-AMP level is regulated by phosphodiesterase 4 (PDE4) activity and in turn modulates the generation of either proinflammatory (high level of PDE4) or anti-inflammatory (low level of PDE4) cytokines by immune cells. Increased PDE4 levels have been reported in cells from atopic subjects, and targeting PDE4 by specific inhibitors is thought to reduce the secretion of proinflammatory mediators in patients with AD (Zane LT).

Agents: The topical boron-based PDE4 inhibitor **crisaborole** has been approved recently by the US Food and Drug Administration in the United States for patients with mild-to-moderate AD aged 2 years and greater (Paller AS).

In the pivotal set of phase 3 studies, crisaborole-treated children and adults achieved the primary end point (clear/almost clear with ≥2-grade improvement) more often than vehicle-treated patients with AD (32. 8% vs 25. 4% [P 5. 038] in one study and 31. 4% vs 18. 0% [P <.001] in the other) (Palller AS).

Although the systemic PDE4 inhibitor apremilast has been tried. It did **NOT** meet the primary end point.

5. IgE

IgE is considered a hallmark of atopic diseases, including AD. Patients with AD with "normal total IgE levels" are known to have relevant amounts of allergen-specific IgE (oligo-sensitized), as determined by using RAST or chip technology. However, the anti-IgE biologic omalizumab did not show efficacy in PoC studies in adults (Bangert C).

5. Histamine Receptor Type 4

What is it?: Histamine levels are increased in patients with AD and assumed to be involved in the generation of inflammatory reactions. The histamine receptor type 4 (H4R) is expressed on keratinocytes and Th2 cells, and H_4 stimulation leads to IL-31 production in human subjects. The role of histamine as an itching-inducing mediator is well known, but the effect of medications that target classical anti-H_1 and anti-H_2 receptors in managing itch in patients with AD has always been disappointing (Apfelbacher CJ). But our own experience has been that a combination of olopatadine with hydroxyzine tends to help in recalcitrant itch, probably due to the H_4 effect of the former and the sedative effect of the latter.

Agents: Oral administration of an H_4R antagonist (JNJ-39758979) to patients with AD significantly reduced pruritus but was terminated because of agranulocytosis. ZPL-389, an H_4R antagonist, has completed phase 2 clinical trials for AD with promising results (Werfel T).

Olopatidine is another drug with an H_4 receptor action and has been used in Japan for AD.

6. Th22 Cytokine Levels

Several case reports and case series have suggested the efficacy of the IL-12/IL-23p40 antibody **ustekinumab**, which regulates Th1 and Th17 pathways, in improving the severity of AD. A recent double-blind, randomized trial with 60 patients of an anti-IL-22 **(fezakinumab)** mAb (NCT01941537) showed significant improvement only in the severely affected patients with AD (Guttman-Yassky E).

In addition, Th17 increases (which can contribute to increase in IL-22) have been described in some adults with AD, particularly in Asian patients (Noda S), and in affected children with recent-onset disease who are 5 years of age and less, (Esaki H) although Th2 cytokine level increases still predominate. In addition, TSLP has been shown to induce IL-17A through a CXCR2-dependent mechanism, and anti-IL-17A mAb suppressed AD-like skin lesions in mice (Mizutani N). As a result, the Th17 inhibitor **secukinumab** is also currently being studied in adults with AD (NCT02594098).

7. JAK Inhibitors

JAK-signal transducer and activator of transcription (STAT) is an intracellular signaling pathway on which many different proinflammatory cytokines (e.g. IL-4, IL-5, IL-13,

and IL-31) elicit their pathophysiologic functions (Villarino AV).

In a mouse model of AD, the topical JAK inhibitor **JTE-052** decreased IL-4 and IL-13 signaling and improved skin barrier function. In a phase 2a trial, the mean percentage change from baseline at week 4 in EASI score was significantly greater (P <.001) for topical **tofacitinib** (81.7%) than for vehicle (29.9%) (Bissonnette R).

Oral JAK inihibitors are being also tried that include baricitinib (JAK1/2 inhibitor), PF-04965842 (JAK1 inhibitor), and upadacitinib (JAK1 inhibitor).

Summary

One important and relevant aspect is that with so many drugs under research why is it that very few have achieved the status of approved drugs. There are many cases of failure with these drugs which cannot be glossed over. In fact it is uncommon for the erudite speakers at various forums of AD to discuss why a certain drug fails in AD. I have seen patients failing cyclosporine, a drug considered to have magical effects on AD. The reason, which is probably know to the researchers, which are a few and never speak in forums, is that there is a variation in the cytokine mileu among patients of AD, which may affect the ultimate therapeutic effect of these drugs. This can explain possibly why a disorder where IgE levels are high fails to respond to omazilu-mab!

A lot is still unknown about AD which will determine the future of effective therapeutics, this includes

a. To what extent activation of immune pathways in addition to Th2 signaling contribute to AD pathogenesis.

b. Whether there are subphenotypes that respond selectively to more targeted topical and systemic medications.

c. Whether new medications directed against targets thought to drive AD will prove to be effective and without significant risk.

ITCH OF AD AND ITS MANAGEMENT

Mechanism of pruritus (mediators, hyper-innervation, and chronicity): AD is characterized by chronic pruritus/itch that induces scratch behavior (Kabashima K). Scratch can serve as a physiologic self-protective mechanism to prevent the body from being hurt by harmful external agents but is well recognized to damage skin and increase inflammation, which further exacerbates pruritus, leading to the "itch-scratch cycle."

Various mediators can cause itch (Table 9.4 and Fig. 9.24). Pruriceptive primary sensory nerves (C-fibers) transmit the pruritic signal induced by histamine-dependent and independent pruritogens (e.g. proteases, house dust mite proteases, endothelin-1, IL-4, IL-13, IL-31, and chloroquine) through afferent fibers from the epidermis or dermis to the spinal cord. Histamine released by immune cells activates 2 major histamine receptors: H_1R and H_4R. For histamine-independent pruritus, Mas-related G protein-coupled receptors and gastrin-releasing peptide receptor (GRPR) mediate the pruritic sensation in the C-fiber and dorsal spinal cord, respectively (Liu Q).

Receptor activation of pruritogens on peripheral nerve endings induces electrical firing, Ca influx, and activation of intracellular cell signaling pathways. Sprouting and thickening of epidermal nerve fibers are found in human and animal AD, (Tominaga M), which might explain the characteristic skin pruritus (alloknesis) produced by innocuous mechanical stimulation.

Artemin, which is secreted by dermal fibroblasts in response to substance P, has also received attention recently. Artemin leads to abnormal peripheral innervation and thermal hyperalgesia. Moreover, air pollutants have been found to act on keratinocytes to produce artemin, leading to epidermal hyper-innervation and hypersensitivity to pruritus (Kabashima K).

Another characteristic of pruritus in patients with AD is its chronicity. With chronic pruritus, scratching causes skin lesions, which in turn lead to activation of STAT3 in spinal dorsal horn astrocytes. Induction of lipocalin

Table 9.4: Major mediators of pruritus and their receptors on C-fibers		
Source	Mediators	Receptor on C fibres
Mast cells	Histamine	HR1, HR4
	Kallikreins, tryptase, trypsin, cathepsins, and other endogenous/exogenous proteases	PAR-2
Nerves	Substance P	NK1R
Eosinophils	Reactive oxygen	TRPA1
Fibroblasts	Artemin	GFR a 3
Keratinocytes	Nerve growth factor	Nerve growth factor receptor (TrkA and p75NTR)
	Semaphorin 3A	Neuropilin-1 (NRP1)
	TSLP	TSLP receptor
T cells	IL-31	IL-31 receptor
Endothelial cells	Endothelin (ET1, ET2)	ETA, ETB
	Acetylcholine	Ach receptor

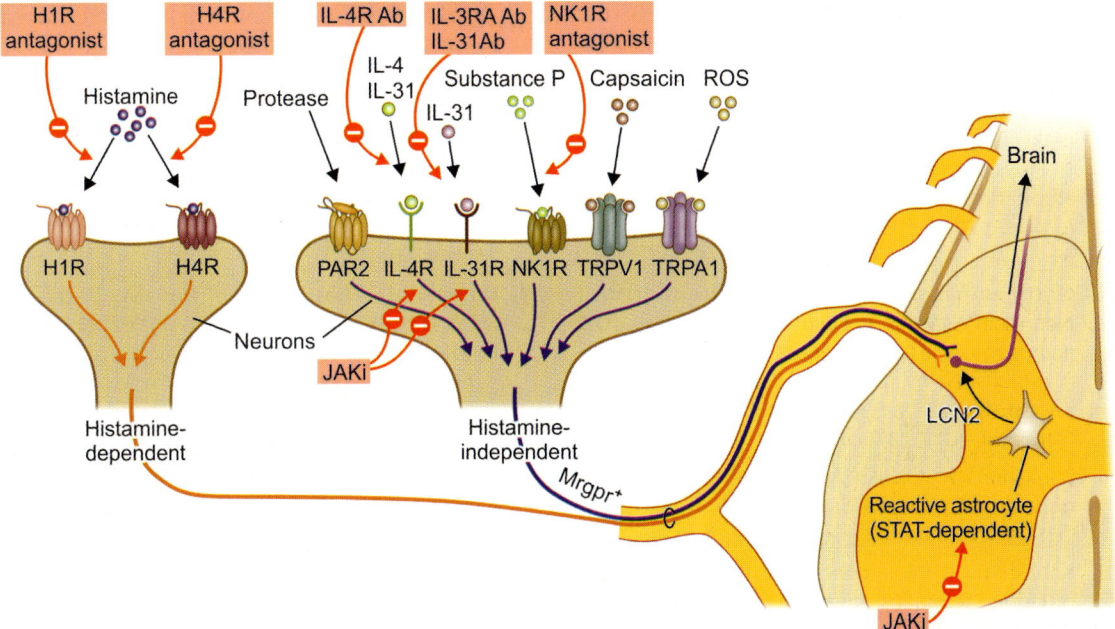

Fig. 9.24: Mechanisms of pruritus. Each of the proritogens involved in AD has its own specific receptor to induce itch. Both H1R[+] histamine-dependent and Mas-related G protein-coupled receptor (Mrgpr)[+] histamine-independent signaling pathways are thought to mediate pruritus in patients with AD. In the spinal dorsal horn, STAT3-dependent reactive astrocytes produce lipocalin 2 (LCN2), which sensitizes a pruritic processing neuronal network involving GRPR[+] neurons, leading to chronic pruritus. As shown in this figure, each antipruritic drug blocks individual pruritic pathway. IL-4, IL-13, and IL-31 elicit their functions through JAK-STAT signaling. (*PAR2*, Protease-activated receptor 2)

2 by astrocytes sensitizes a pruritus-processing neuronal network involving GRPR 1 spinal dorsal horn neurons, and thereby contributes to the vicious cycle of itching and scratching and to chronic pruritus (Fig. 9.24) (Shiratori-Hayashi M).

Trial Drugs

Monthly injections of an anti-IL-31 receptor A antibody (CIM331; nemolizumab) significantly inhibited pruritus in patients with moderate-to-severe AD in a phase 2 clinical trial. Use of nemolizumab was not associated with any serious adverse events (Ruzicka T). Nemolizumab also increased sleep efficiency and decreased the use of topical hydrocortisone butyrate in the phase 2 clinical trial.

Two NK1R antagonists (tradipitant, NCT02651714; and serlopitant, NCT02975206) are currently in phase II clinical trials for AD.

Bibliography

1. Apfelbacher CJ, van Zuuren EJ, Fedorowicz Z, Jupiter A, Matterne U, Weisshaar E. Oral H1 antihistamines as monotherapy for eczema. Cochrane Database Syst Rev 2013;(2):CD007770.

2. Bangert C, Loesche C, Jones J, Weiss D, Bieber T, Stingl G. Efficacy, safety and pharmacodynamics of a high-affinity anti-IgE antibody in patients with moderate to severe atopic dermatitis: a randomized, double-blind, placebo-controlled, proof-of-concept study [abstract]. Exp Dermatol 2016;25 (suppl 4):37.

3. Bissonnette R, Papp KA, Poulin Y, Gooderham M, Raman M, Mallbris L, et al. Topical tofacitinib for atopic dermatitis: a phase IIa randomized trial. Br J Dermatol 2016;175:902–11.

4. Dillon SR, Sprecher C, Hammond A, Bilsborough J, Rosenfeld-Franklin M, Presnell SR, et al. Interleukin 31, a cytokine produced by activated T cells, induces dermatitis in mice. Nat Immunol 2004;5:752–60.

5. Egawa G, Kabashima K. Multifactorial skin barrier deficiency and atopic dermatitis: essential topics to prevent the atopic march. J Allergy Clin Immunol 2016;138:350–8.

6. Esaki H, Brunner PM, Renert-Yuval Y, Czarnowicki T, Huynh T, Tran G, et al. Early-onset pediatric atopic dermatitis is Th2 but also Th17 polarized in skin. J Allergy Clin Immunol 2016;138:1639–51.

7. Guttman-Yassky E, Khattri S, Brunner PM, Neumann A, Malik K, Fuentes-Duculan J, et al. A pathogenic role for Th22/IL-22 in atopic dermatitis is established by a placebo-controlled trial with an anti-IL-22/ILV-094 mAb [abstract]. J Invest Dermatol 2017;137(suppl):S53.

8. Kabashima K, Otsuka A, Nomura T. Linking air pollution to atopic dermatitis. Nat Immunol 2016;18:5–6.

9. Kabashima K. New concept of the pathogenesis of atopic dermatitis: interplay among the barrier, allergy, and pruritus as a trinity. J Dermatol Sci 2013;70:3–11.

10. Kelleher M, Dunn-Galvin A, Hourihane JO, Murray D, Campbell LE, McLean WH, et al. Skin barrier dysfunction measured by transepidermal water loss at 2 days and 2 months predates and predicts atopic dermatitis at 1 year. J Allergy Clin Immunol 2015;135:930–5.

11. Kim HO, Kim JH, Chung BY, Choi MG, Park CW. Increased expression of the aryl hydrocarbon receptor in patients with chronic inflammatory skin diseases. Exp Dermatol 2014;23:278–81.

12. Liu Q, Tang Z, Surdenikova L, Kim S, Patel KN, Kim A, et al. Sensory neuron-specific GPCR Mrgprs are itch receptors mediating chloroquine-induced pruritus. Cell 2009;139:1353–65.

13. Mitson-Salazar A, Yin Y, Wansley DL, Young M, Bolan H, Arceo S, et al. Hematopoietic prostaglandin D synthase de?nes a proeosinophilic pathogenic effector human Th2 cell subpopulation with enhanced function. J Allergy Clin Immunol 2016;137:907–18.

14. Noda S, Suarez-Farinas M, Ungar B, Kim SJ, de Guzman Strong C, Xu H, et al. The Asian atopic dermatitis phenotype combines features of atopic dermatitis and psoriasis with increased Th17 polarization. J Allergy Clin Immunol 2015;136:1254–64.

15. Oetjen I, Mack M, Whelan T, Guo C, Yang L, Hamilton S, et al. Neuronal IL-4Ra and JAK1 signaling medicate chronic itch [abstract]. J Invest Dermatol 2017;137:S100.

16. Paller AS, Tom WL, Lebwohl MG, Blumenthal RL, Boguniewicz M, Call RS, et al. Efficacy and safety of crisaborole ointment, a novel, nonsteroidal phosphodiesterase 4 (PDE4) inhibitor for the topical treatment of atopic dermatitis (AD) in children and adults. J Am Acad Dermatol 2016;75:494–503.

17. Ruzicka T, Hani?n JM, Furue M, Pulka G, Mlynarczyk I, Wollenberg A, et al. Anti-interleukin-31 receptor a antibody for atopic dermatitis. N Engl J Med 2017;376:826–35.

18. Shiratori-Hayashi M, Koga K, Tozaki-Saitoh H, Kohro Y, Toyonaga H, Yamaguchi C, et al. STAT3-dependent reactive astrogliosis in the spinal dorsal horn underlies chronic itch. Nat Med 2015;21:927–31.

19. Simpson EL, Bieber T, Guttman-Yassky E, Beck LA, Blauvelt A, Cork MJ, et al. Two phase 3 trials of dupilumab versus placebo in atopic dermatitis. N Engl J Med 2016;375:2335–48.

20. Tominaga M, Ozawa S, Tengara S, Ogawa H, Takamori K. Intraepidermal nerve fibers increase in dry skin of acetone-treated mice. J Dermatol Sci 2007;48:103–11.

21. van den Bogaard EH, Bergboer JG, Vonk-Bergers M, van Vlijmen-Willems IM, Hato SV, van der Valk PG, et al. Coal tar induces AHR-dependent skin barrier repair in atopic dermatitis. J Clin Invest 2013;123:917–27.

22. Verstraete K, Peelman F, Braun H, Lopez J, Van Rompaey D, Dansercoer A, et al. Structure and antagonism of the receptor complex mediated by human TSLP in allergy and asthma. Nat Commun 2017;8:14937.

23. Villarino AV, Kanno Y, O'Shea JJ. Mechanisms and consequences of Jak-STAT signaling in the immune system. Nat Immunol 2017;18:374–84.

24. Werfel T, Asher A, Tsianakas A, Gupta B, Sarmiento R. A phase 2a proof of concept clinical trial to evaluate ZPL-3893787 (ZPL-389), a potent, oral histamine H-4 receptor antagonist for the treatment of moderate to severe atopic dermatitis (AD) in adults [abstract]. Allergy 2016;71:95.

25. Zane LT, Chanda S, Jarnagin K, Nelson DB, Spelman L, Gold LS. Crisaborole and its potential role in treating atopic dermatitis: overview of early clinical studies. Immunotherapy 2016;8:853–66.

10

Seborrheic Eczema

Ananta Khurana, Wai-Kwong Cheong, Chia-Chun Ang

INTRODUCTION

Seborrheic eczema or seborrheic dermatitis (SD) is a common dermatitis that affects both adults and infants (infantile SD/ISD). It is estimated to affect all ethnic groups and both genders, and can adversely affect the quality of life (Szepietowski JC et al, Manapajon A et al). The prevalence (beyond infancy) is highest in puberty and early adulthood, followed by a second peak around the age of 50 years. There is no proven relationship between ISD and adult-type SD, and it is established that infants with ISD do not develop classic SD more frequently.

There are several epidemiologic studies on SD looking at the prevalence and gender predilection in different population (Palamaras et al). The prevalence for adult SD ranges from 2.35% in Scotland (Ratzer), 4.05% in Greece (Palamaras et al), 4.3% in Iran (Baghestani et al), 6.9% in Australia (Plunkett et al) and 7% in Singapore (Goh et al). Infantile SD has a prevalence of 2.5% in Greece (Palamaras et al), 3.1% in Kuwait (Nanda et al), 4.3% in Turkey (Tamer et al) and 11.3% in India (Sardana et al).

A study conducted in an Indian pediatric population noted 13.42% of children below 5 years were affected by SD. This involved infants predominantly and was worse during winter (Banerjee S et al). Another study from India looking at scalp dermatoses in adults visiting a tertiary referral center reported 18.7% of their cohort with scalp SD (Pillai et al).

ETIOLOGY AND PREDISPOSING FACTORS

Seborrheic dermatitis is more commonly seen in adult patients with immunocompromised states like human immunodeficiency virus (HIV), organ transplant recipients and lymphomas (Mathes BM et al). Most cases of SD in HIV patients are diagnosed with CD4+ T lymphocyte counts between 200 and 500/mm^3, and decreased CD4+ counts are often associated with worse SD. Fewer cases occur when CD4+ T cells is more than 500/mm^3. SD is also associated with neurological disorders and psychiatric diseases, including Parkinson's disease, neuroleptic induced parkinsonism, tardive dyskinesia, traumatic brain injury, epilepsy, facial nerve palsy, spinal cord injury and mood depression. In temperate climates, SD can be worse in the winter months. It is also reported to be aggravated by hot climate (Manapajon A et al). Other diseases that have been reported to occur with SD include chronic alcoholic pancreatitis (Barba A et al), hepatitis C infections (Cribier B et al), malignancies (Clift DC), Down syndrome (Ercis M et al), Hailey-Hailey disease (Marren P et al) and cardiofacio-cutaneous syndromes (Gross-Tsur et al).

Drug-related SD is less commonly seen but should be suspected in patients who are exposed to drugs including erlotinib or sorafenib, recombinant interleukin-2, psoralen plus ultraviolet A (PUVA; especially as facial involvement) and isotretinoin (Naldi et al).

PATHOGENESIS

SD is postulated to arise from an interaction between yeasts from the *Malassezia* genus with the immune system (Hay RJ). Metabolites from the *Malassezia* such as malassezin and indole-3-carbaldehyde interact with the aryl hydrocarbon receptor and modulate immune responses to *Malassezia* (Gaitanis et al). The role of this yeast is indirectly shown by the resolution of SD after treatment with antifungal agents (Shuster S). Sebum lipids are essential for *Malassezia* proliferation, so a certain amount of sebum is always required in order to provide permissive conditions for SD development. SD is most common in puberty and adolescence, during periods of highest sebum production, and multiple studies have shown that a higher distribution of *M. globosa*, *M. furfur* and *M. restricta* colonies correlates with skin of lipid-rich anatomic locations and with greater disease severity. Dysregulation of sebum production plays a pivotal role in the progression of SD. Not only is there a change in quantity of sebum released, but also the quality of sebum changes. This sebum enriched condition of skin provides a conducive ambience for *Malassezia* to grow. Several reports suggest that triglycerides and squalene are reduced in the skin of patients with SD, but free fatty acids and cholesterol are present in copious amounts. Lipases secreted from colonizing *Malassezia* can initiate an inflammatory response by releasing oleic and arachidonic acid from the sebum lipids. Both of these unsaturated fatty acids have direct irritative and desquamative effects on keratinocytes. Furthermore, arachidonic acid, metabolized by cyclooxygenase, serves as a source of proinflammatory eicosanoids (particularly prostaglandins), leading to inflammation and subsequent damage of stratum corneum. In addition, these metabolites induce keratinocytes to produce proinflammatory cytokines such as IL-1α, IL-6, IL-8 and TNF-α, thus prolonging the inflammatory cycle. In addition, epidermal barrier integrity, neurogenic factors and emotional stress, genetic factors, nutritional factors and androgenic hormonal influence are postulated to play a role as well.

CLINICAL PHENOTYPES

Infantile SD (ISD) is seen in up to 70% of children within the first 3 months of life, but the lesions normally resolve spontaneously by the age of 8–12 months. It is thus a self-limited condition in this age group. In patients with a family history of atopy, a significant portion (30–40%) goes on to develop atopic dermatitis (Alexopoulos A et al). The relation between ISD, infantile psoriasis and atopic eczema entities is still not completely understood and is a matter of debate. Most infants with SD have mild disease with cradle cap, involvement of the eyebrows, forehead, retroauricular areas and nasolabial folds (Figs 10.1 to 10.3). An orangish hue is typical in the fair skinned. Commonly the lesions also develop in the neck folds, axillae, umbilicus, inguinal and intergluteal folds, in the so-called "bipolar" ISD. The differential diagnoses to consider include infantile atopic dermatitis, infantile psoriasis, Langerhans' cell histiocytosis, multiple carboxylase deficiency, intertrigo and tinea capitis (Table 10.1). It is noteworthy that many reports have demonstrated development of typical atopic dermatitis and psoriasis in infants previously seen as ISD. Typically, the inflammation resolves with transient hypopigmentation, which can be very pronounced in children with darker skin color. However, this is a post-inflammatory phenomenon (not due to the treatments applied), and always recovers within a few weeks.

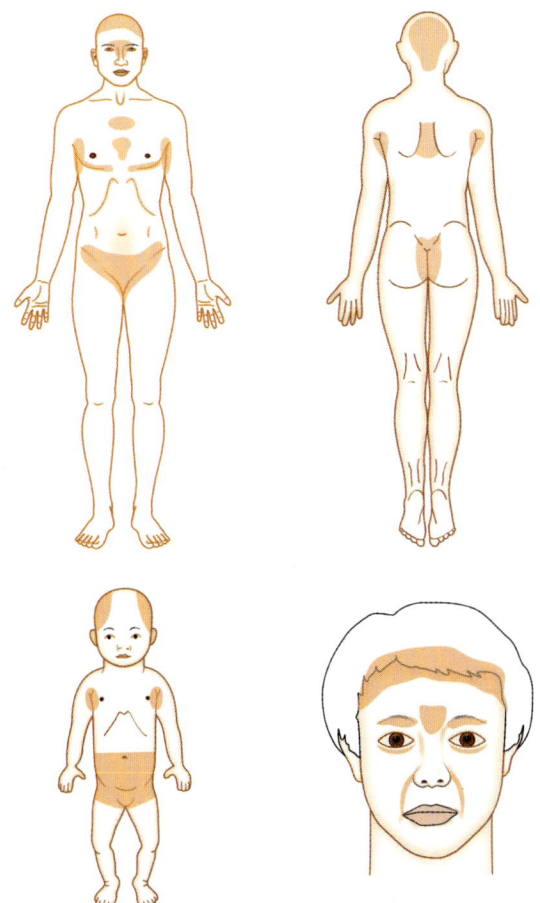

Fig. 10.1: Distribution of seborrheic dermatitis in adults and children

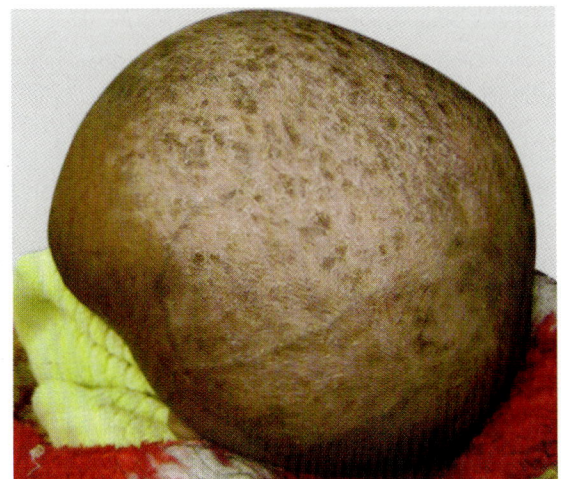

Fig. 10.2: Greasy scales on the scalp in a case of Cradle cap

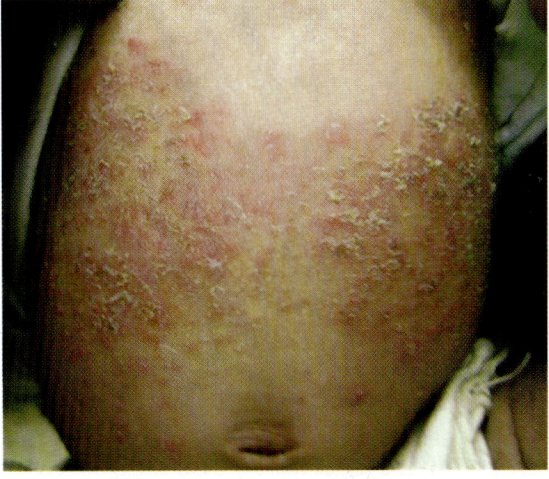

Fig. 10.3: ISD involving the trunk

In rare instances when infants present with SD-like erythroderma and failure to thrive, one has to consider other differential diagnoses including genodermatoses, primary immune deficiency (Leiner's disease), metabolic diseases or infection (Fraitag S et al). These infants require specialized investigations and management by dermatologists.

Adult SD affects areas with high sebaceous gland activity (Fig. 10.1). Mild SD on the scalp can present with dandruff. In severe cases of scalp SD, thick scales with matted hairs typical of pityriasis amiantacea can occur (Fig. 10.4). On the face, SD typically presents with persistent scaly, thin pink papules and plaques on the medial aspects of the eyebrows, nasolabial folds and periauricular areas and sometimes with overlying yellowish oily scales (Fig. 10.5). On the trunk (presternal and interscapular areas), SD presents with thin pink papules and plaques with fine scaling in a petaloid (described as circinate patches with a light-red scaling area in the center and darker red papules at their margin) (Fig. 10.6), or pityriasiform pattern. SD may also affect the axillae, submammary area, umbilicus and anogenital area. The common differentials for adult SD are mentioned in Table 10.1.

Various manifestations of SD are depicted in Figs 10.7 to 10.9.

In immunosuppressed patients, SD is often more extensive, intense, and refractory to treatment. It is considered an early skin presentation of AIDS in both children and adults. SD may also be a cutaneous sign of the immune reconstitution inflammatory

Table 10.1: Differential diagnoses of seborrheic dermatitis
Adults
Psoriasis vulgaris: Typical lesions in psoriasis are thicker and present as sharply delineated plaques with silvery white scales. It tends to extend beyond the scalp margin (Figs 10.10 and 10.11). Facial involvement less common.
Rosacea: Usually involves malar areas on the face, sparing the nasolabial folds, and does not show scaling. Associated flushing and telangiectasias (+)
SLE: Clear photodistribution, such as acute flares of bilateral malar rash, and may be associated with extracutaneous abnormalities. Nasolabial fold is generally spared.
Pemphigus foliaceus: Erythema with scale-crust first on head and neck and subsequently expands to chest and back. Immunofluorescence confirms the diagnosis (Fig. 10.12).
Pityriasis rosea: Abrupt onset, appearance of herald patch and resolution within weeks
Secondary syphilis: Peripheral lymphadenopathy, mucosal lesions and palmoplantar maculo-papules. Serology confirms the diagnosis
Nutritional deficiencies producing SD-like appearance: Pyridoxine, zinc, niacin and riboflavin
Drugs inducing SD-like dermatitis: Griseofulvin, ethionamide, buspirone, haloperidol, chlorpromazine, IL-2, interferon-α, methyldopa, psoralens
Pediatric age group
Diaper dermatitis: Occurs on convex skin surfaces in contact with diaper, such as lower abdomen, genitalia, buttocks and upper thighs. Spares skin folds.
Cutaneous Langerhans cell histiocytosis: Multisystem disease. Brown to purplish or purpuric macules and papules prone to coalesce on the scalp, retroauricular areas, axillae and inguinal folds. The lesions have a tendency to desquamate on the scalp and to erode and ulcerate in the folds. Possible lytic bone lesions, liver, spleen and lung involvement. Histology confirms diagnosis (Fig. 10.13)
Atopic eczema: Lesions usually do not appear until after 3 months of age and affect extensors prominently. ISD usually appears earlier and rarely affects extensor areas. However, the relationship is complex and a clear cut diagnosis is not always possible.
Psoriasis: Difficulty in infants where psoriasis is almost always a psoriasis of the folds (i.e. napkin or inverse psoriasis). It can be expected that some patients with ISD will develop a typical psoriasis years later.
Intertrigo: Young infants are especially susceptible because of their short necks and relative muscle weakness leading to a persistently flexed posture, all of which produce deep skin folds. Secondary candidal infections are relatively common, especially in the napkin area.
Multiple carboxylase deficiency: Can present in infancy with dermatological manifestations, including an eczematous scaly facial and/or periorificial rash. The eruption starts on the scalp, on the eyebrows and at the eyelid margins, extending later to the perioral, perianal areas and to other flexural sites. There may be associated blepharitis and keratoconjunctivitis causing photophobia. Neurological symptoms are prominent particularly convulsions, developmental delay, hypotonia and ataxia.
Tinea capitis: Rare in infancy; causes partial alopecia; confirmed by KOH/culture

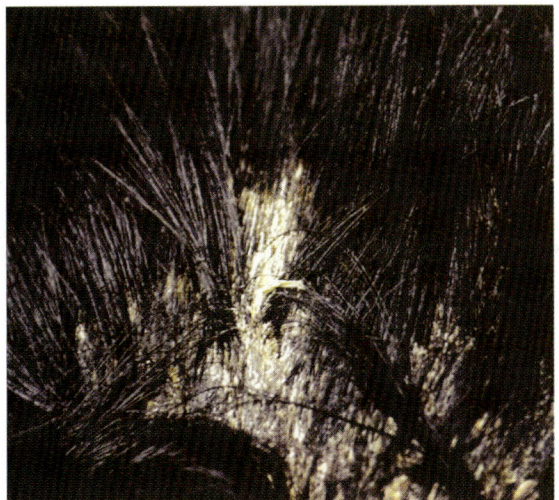

Fig. 10.4: Seborrheic dermatitis of the scalp in a 15-year-old male showing thick adherent scales typical of pityriasis amiantacea

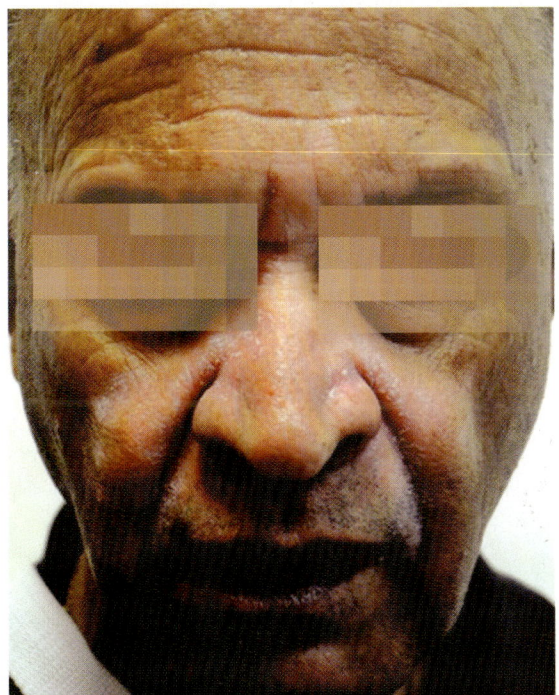

Fig. 10.5: Seborrheic dermatitis affecting the nasolabial folds and medial corners of the eyebrows

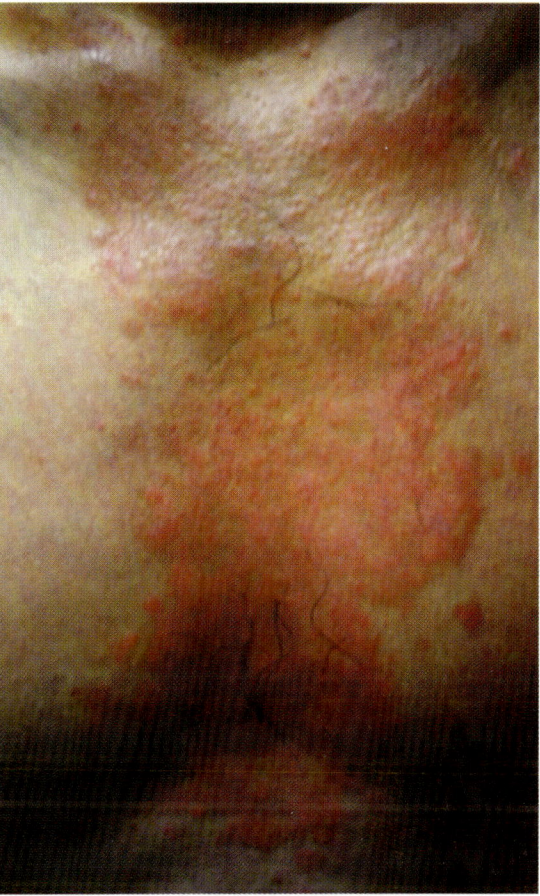

Fig. 10.6: Seborrheic dermatitis affecting the presternal area in a petaloid pattern

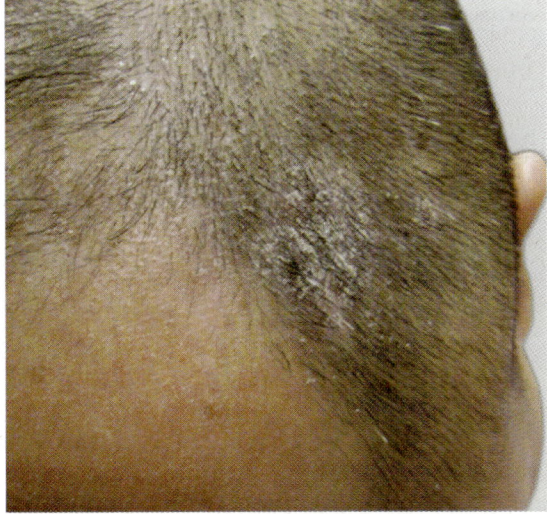

Fig. 10.7: Localized patch of adherent scaling

syndrome in patients with highly active antiretroviral therapy (HAART). However, there have also been reports of SD regression with HAART.

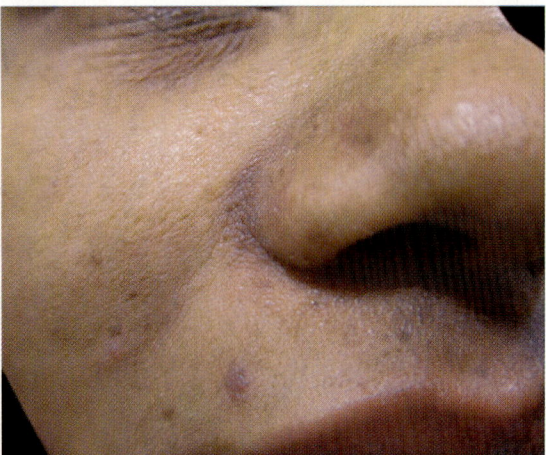

Fig. 10.8: Mild scaling in the perinasal area

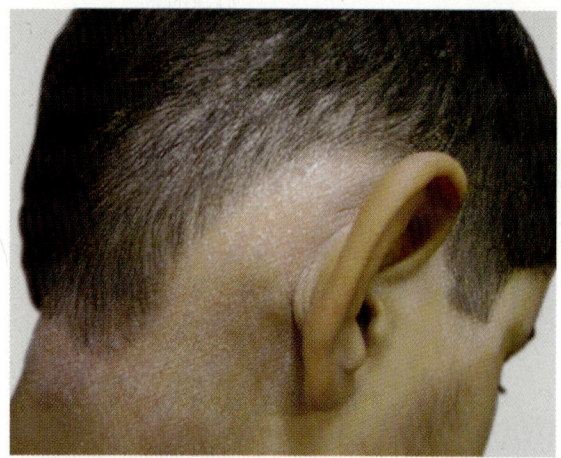

Fig. 10.11: This case has diffuse scaling the morphology is suggestive of pityriasis sicca

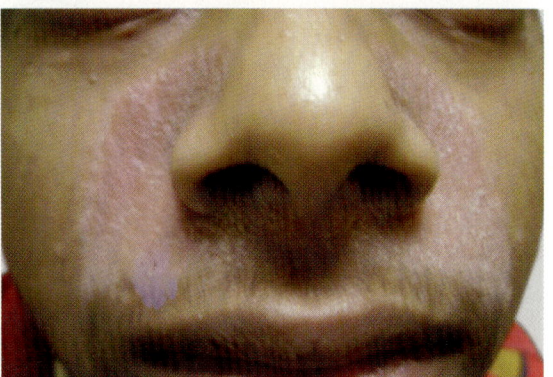

Fig. 10.9: Marked erythema and scaling in the perinasal area labeled as psoriasis by an alternative practitioner!

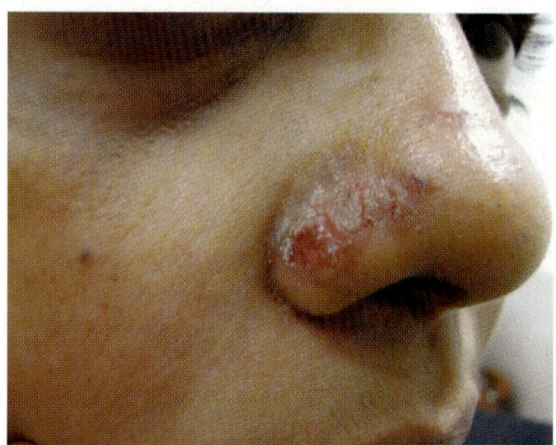

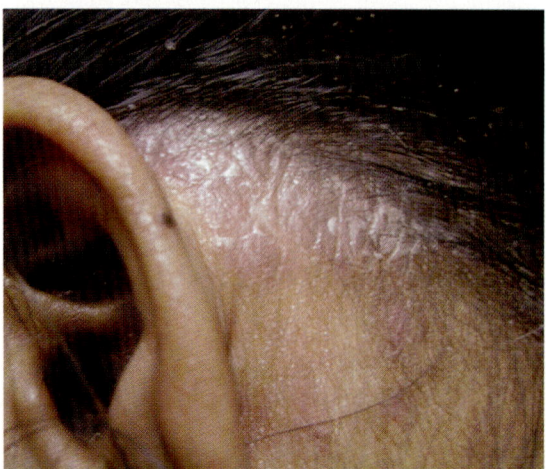

Fig. 10.10: Silvery white scale in a plaque extending beyond the scalp margin (psoriasis)

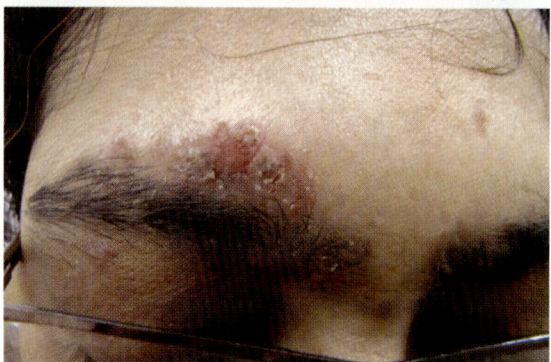

Fig. 10.12: This case was "successfully treated" numerous times by topical steroids for SD. A close look reveals the erosions underlying the crusts. Thumb rule "more crusts and less scales" it is likely to be Pemphigus foliaceus (Dsg 3 and I ELISA +; Bx: pemphigus foliaceus)

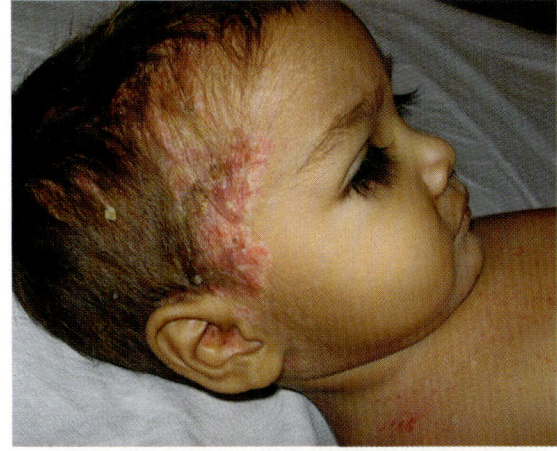

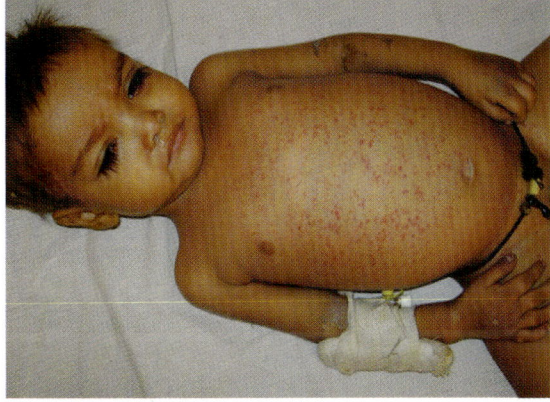

Fig. 10.13: The purpuric lesions interspersed with the scaly papules and enlarged liver and spleen (LCH)

INVESTIGATIONS

SD is usually a clinical diagnosis. The differentials (enlisted in Table 10.1) may pose diagnostic difficulties in some cases and histopathology may be required. Histologically, the development of SD can be divided into two stages. In the acute and sub-acute stages, SD shows superficial perivascular and perifollicular inflammatory infiltrates, composed mainly of lymphocytes and histiocytes in association with spongiosis and psoriasiform hyperplasia, and can be coupled with parakeratosis around follicular opening ("shoulder parakeratosis"). Neutrophils can also be found in the scale crust at the margins of follicular ostia. On the other hand, in chronic

lesions, marked psoriasiform hyperplasia and parakeratosis can be present with dilation of the venules of surface plexus which resembles psoriasis. However, in psoriasis, parakeratosis is often associated with thinning or loss of the granular layer due to accelerated keratinocyte differentiation.

Recently, dermoscopic features of scalp SD have been defined and mainly include twisted red loops and comma vessels. These may help to differentiate it from its close clinical differential scalp psoriasis, which shows atypical red vessels, red dots and globules, signet ring vessels, structureless red areas and hidden hairs.

When infants present with SD and other atypical features (e.g. poor response to treatment, recurrent severe flares, failure to thrive), further evaluation becomes essential.

TREATMENT

The treatment of SD should be tailored to the location and severity of SD in the individual patients, bearing in mind that SD is a chronic condition with frequent recurrences in adults, while it is self-limiting in infantile group.

ISD: In mild cases, such as with only a 'cradle cap', no treatment is required. However, vegetable (olive, sweet almond) or mineral (liquid paraffin) oils may be useful in removing excess scale. They can be massaged into the scalp prior to bathing. Following this, regular washing of the scalp with a mild baby shampoo and gentle combing to loosen scales is often enough. For more refractory cases, mild topical corticosteroids, possibly alternating with emollients, may be used. Combination of mild steroid and antifungals is often prescribed, but should be carefully applied in folds and for the shortest possible duration. There are concerns of systemic absorption with topical steroids, leading to adrenal suppression in infants (Turpeinen et al), while no systemic absorption for topical ketoconazole was found when it was used to treat infantile SD (Taieb et al). Topical agents containing salicylic acid or selenium sulphide should be avoided in neonates because of the dangers posed by their percutaneous absorption. In 'bipolar' ISD, careful hygiene of the fold should be prescribed, taking into account that a vigorous cleansing or a strong detergent can worsen the situation. In the napkin area, particular attention should be paid to more frequent napkin changes and to skin protection with zinc oxide-based pastes.

Adult SD (Table 10.2): As the disease runs a remitting relapsing course, careful treatment selection is essential. Maintenance treatment is required in those with frequent recurrences and relapses soon after stopping medications. The treatment is largely topical and antifungals form the first line in management. The following section discussed topical and systemic agents used and tabulates the first and second line of management.

Topical Therapy

Azoles

Azole class of antifungal agents is the most effective in growth inhibition of *Malassezia* species associated with the development of seborrheic dermatitis. Among the azoles, ketoconazole applied in various vehicles showed superior effects, and hence it is the first-line treatment. Ketoconazole is available in different over-the-counter topical preparations, such as shampoos, creams and gels. Ketoconazole shampoo 2% is effective in treating scalp seborrheic dermatitis, used twice weekly. Intermittent use of ketoconazole 2% shampoo (once weekly) has been shown to have a significant prophylactic effect. Ketoconazole 2% cream significantly improves SD of the face and chest used twice daily. It also has slight anti-inflammatory properties, and it is principally well tolerated in all available formulations. Bifonazole 1% cream, used once daily, is usually effective in the treatment of seborrheic dermatitis of the scalp and face. A combination ointment containing

1% bifonazole and 40% urea helps reduce the symptoms of scalp seborrheic dermatitis. Miconazole can also be effectively used in the treatment of seborrheic dermatitis as a monotherapy or in combination with hydrocortisone.

Ciclopirox

Ciclopirox olamine is a synthetic antifungal agent with a high affinity for trivalent metal cations. Ciclopirox has both antifungal and anti-inflammatory properties. Ciclopirox is available as 1% and 1.5% shampoos, alone or in combination with zinc pyrithione.

Zinc Pyrithione

Zinc pyrithione is a common active ingredient in most of the over-the-counter anti-dandruff shampoos and has antifungal effects. Its antifungal effect is thought to derive from its ability to disrupt membrane transport by blocking the proton pump that energizes the transport mechanism. Zinc pyrithione is available in concentrations of 1% and 2% in shampoos. It is effective when used alone or in combination with ketoconazole.

Selenium Sulfide

Selenium sulfide is a cytostatic agent with an antimitotic action resulting in a reduction in the turnover of epidermal cells. It also has antibacterial and mild antifungal activity, which may contribute to its effectiveness. Selenium sulfide 2.5% lotion is available for scalp use and short contact use on skin.

Corticosteroids

In severe cases of seborrheic dermatitis, low to mild potency topical corticosteroids are effective in fast clearing of visible signs and associated symptoms. Most commonly used are hydrocortisone and beclomethasone dipropionate which can be used alone or in combination with antifungal agents. However, frequent and prolonged use of topical corticosteroids is not recommended because

Table 10.2: Treatment of adult seborrheic dermatitis

Site	First line	Second line
Scalp and beard region	**Ketoconazole** 2% shampoo or selenium sulfide 2.5% shampoo: 2 times/week for a month, then 1–2 times/week for maintenance (Tolerance of ketoconazole is superior to selenium sulfide) **Ciclopirox olamine** 1.5% shampoo: 2–3 times a week × 4 weeks; followed by 1/week maintenance	• **Coal tar/salicylic** acid based shampoos (1–2 times/week) • **1% Zinc pyrithione** shampoos (2–3 times/week) • **Topical steroid** lotion for short term (1–2 weeks) • Ketoconazole stay on preparations • **Molecular replacement** therapy
Face and body	Ketoconazole 2% cream Bifonazole 1% cream Miconazole 2% cream Sertaconazole 2% cream Clotrimazole 1% cream (For four weeks, then weekly or less frequently)	• Mild topical steroid (hydrocortisone/desonide) for a short period of time • Topical calcineurin inhibitors (tacrolimus and pimecrolimus) for control of disease • Twice weekly tacrolimus 0.1% ointment may be considered for prevention of recurrence • Ketoconazole shampoo as body wash • Metronidazole gel
	Otitis externa Steroid drops compounded with an antifungal **Blepharitis:** Gentle cleansing with a cotton bud. Use of steroid eye drops is a simple remedy though off label	

Systemic agents:

Itraconazole: 200 mg/day for 1 week for clearance; then 200 mg/day for 2 days/month up to 11 months Or 200 mg every 2 weeks for maintenence.

Terbinafine: Continuous regimen: 250 mg/day for 4–6 weeks OR Intermittent regimen: 250 mg/day for 12 days per month for 3 months.

Fluconazole: 50 mg/day for 2 weeks or 200–300 mg weekly for 2–4 weeks.

Ketoconazole: 200 mg OD for 4 weeks.

Isotretinoin: 0.1–0.5 mg/kg/day OD/alternate day/3 days a week.

Prednisolone: Low evidence; 0.5 mg/kg/day for 15 days with gradual tapering produced benefit (in combination with topical ketoconazole).

In case of secondary infection an antibiotic course may be administered.

of their well-known side effects. Hence, antifungal agents are the first choice in the treatment of seborrheic dermatitis. Topical corticosteroids are useful in short term mainly to control erythema and itching and provide symptomatic relief.

Calcineurin Inhibitors

Topical calcineurin inhibitors decrease cutaneous inflammation by inhibiting T lymphocyte-driven cytokine production. Pimecrolimus 1% cream and tacrolimus 0.03% and 0.1% ointment twice daily therapy is effective and well tolerated in the treatment of seborrheic dermatitis. Twice weekly application of tacrolimus 0.1% ointment has also been shown to prevent recurrences after initial control (Kim et al, 2013).

Metronidazole

Metronidazole has anti-inflammatory activity via inhibition of free radical species. 1% metronidazole gel is an effective treatment for facial seborrheic dermatitis.

Coal Tar

Coal tar has keratoplastic effect (decreasing scaling), anti-proliferative, anti-inflammatory properties, antifungal action, and causes inhibition of sebum secretion. A combination of 4% coal tar and 2% ketoconazole is commonly used in the presence of thicker scaling.

Molecular Replacement Therapy (Bhattacharyya A)

Fatty acids in the form of phospholipids are important components of the lipid bilayer of the cell membrane of all cells. But interestingly, all fatty acids and their derivatives are not perceived as the same by *Malassezia*. Select a few can naturally insert themselves into the lipid bilayer of the fungal membranes and physically disturb the membrane, resulting in increased fluidity of the membrane. Such elevations in membrane fluidity can cause a generalized disorganization of the cell membrane that lead to conformational changes in membrane proteins, release of intracellular components, cytoplasmic disorder and eventual cell disintegration in quick succession. A product utilizing this has recently been launched in the Indian market, although scientific data regarding it are yet lacking.

For mild seborrheic dermatitis of the scalp, over-the-counter dandruff shampoos containing selenium sulfide, zinc pyrithione, or coal tar can control symptoms at a fraction of the cost of other treatments. For long-term control, antifungal shampoos containing ketoconazole 2% or ciclopirox 1% can be used until remission is achieved. Once-weekly use of these medicated shampoos can prevent relapse. There is no degradation in their effectiveness over time. The shampoos should remain on the hair for at least five minutes to guarantee adequate exposure to the scalp. Topical steroids in shampoo or lotion form are used in more severe cases, and they reduce acute symptoms more quickly and maintain control longer after discontinuing use, compared with ketoconazole alone. Recently many stay on preparations of ketoconazole have been launched for scalp SD. However, their efficacy over appropriate use of shampoo preparations is not yet established. For skin involvement too, topical antifungals form the mainstay of use. Topical steroids should be sparingly used for shortest possible durations. Maintenance can be considered for frequently relapsing cases.

Systemic Therapy

Oral therapies may be beneficial when multiple anatomic sites are involved, for patients who are unresponsive to traditional topical therapies and/or for those with severe SD. There is a lack of consistency between studies on oral treatment for SD preventing direct comparison between the different drugs.

Oral itraconazole has an affinity for highly keratinized areas of the body and persists in the skin for long durations allowing a single administration over a week time, hence enhances the chance of better adherence to the regime. Itraconazole has been used in the dose of 200 mg/day for the first week of the month followed by pulse maintenance theray as 200 mg every two weeks or on the first two days every month. The maintenance treatment has been continued for variable periods ranging from

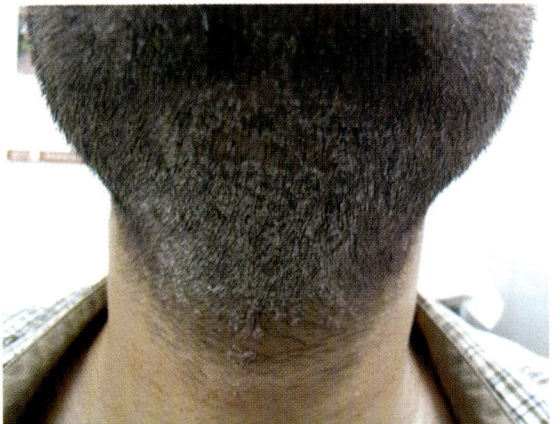 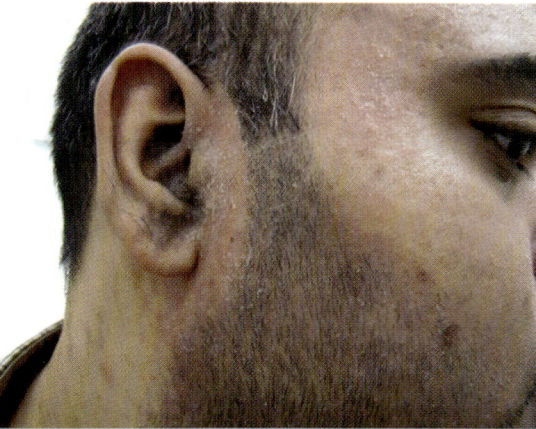

Fig. 10.14a: A case of severe SD in an adult male

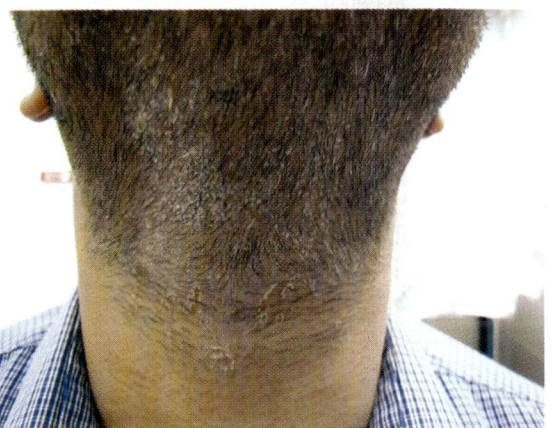 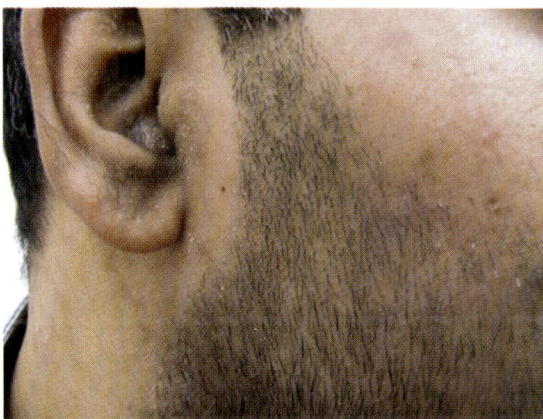

Fig. 10.14b: Oral ketoconazole (after LFT) was administered with tar 5% lotion alternating with flucort 0.01% w/v lotion. The latter being not under active promotion is a cheap option. Maintenance regimen intended is tacrolimus 0.1%

2–11 months. Terbinafine has been prescribed at 250 mg/day either as a continuous (4–6 weeks) or as an intermittent regimen (12 days per month) for 3 months. Fluconazole has been used daily (50 mg/day for 2 weeks) or weekly (200–300 mg) for 2–4 weeks. Ketoconazole dosing regimen is 200 mg daily for 4 weeks. However, ketoconazole therapy is associated with more relapses compared to other treatments.

Isotretinoin has been used in refractory cases, in varying dosing ranging from 0.1 to 0.5 mg/kg/day and dosing intervals from once daily to alternate day or 3 days a week. Isotretinoin, even in small doses, given for

6 months has been shown to reduce sebaceous gland size by 51% and sebum production by 64% (Giessler et al, 2003). The benefit in seborrheic dermatitis may be due to this effect only or may also be related to its recently detailed anti-inflammatory properties.

In most severe case a combination therapy is needed (Figs 10.14a and b).

Bibliography

1. Alexopoulos A, Kakourou T, Orfanou I, Xaidara A, Chrousos G. Retrospective analysis of the relationship between infantile seborrheic dermatitis and atopic dermatitis. Pediatr Dermatol 2014;31:125–30.

2. Baghestani S, Zare S, Mahboobi AA. Skin disease patterns in Hormozgan, Iran. Int J Dermatol 2005; 44: 641–645.

3. Banerjee S, Gangopadhyay DN, Jana S, Chanda M. Seasonal variation in pediatric dermatoses. Indian J Dermatol 2010;55:44–6.

4. Barba A, Piubello W, Vantini I, et al. Skin lesions in chronic alcoholic pancreatitis. Dermatologica 1982;164:322–326.

5. Bhattacharyya A, Jain N, Prasad S, Jain S, Yadav V, Ghosh S, Sengupta S. Evaluation of therapeutic potential of VB-001, a leave-on formulation, for the treatment of moderate adherent dandruff. BMC Dermatol 2017 May 3;17(1):5.

6. Binder RL, Jonelis FJ. Seborrheic dermatitis in neuroleptic induced parkinsonism. Arch Dermatol 1983;119:473–475.

7. Borda LJ, Wikramanayake TC. Seborrheic Dermatitis and Dandruff: A Comprehensive Review. J Clin Investig Dermatol 2015 Dec;3(2).

8. Cheong WK, Yeung CK, Torsekar RG, Suh DH, Ungpakorn R, Widaty S. Treatment of Seborrhoeic Dermatitis in Asia: A Consensus Guide. Skin Appendage Disord 2016 May;1(4):187–96.

9. Clark GW, Pope SM, JabooriKA. Diagnosis and treatment of seborrheic dermatitis. Am Fam Physician 2015 Feb 1;91(3):185–90.

10. Clift DC, Dodd JH, Kirby JD, et al. Seborrheic dermatitis and malignancy. An investigation of the skin flora. Acta Derm Venereol 1988;68:48–52.

11. Cohen S. Should we treat infantile seborrhoeic dermatitis with topical antifungals or topical steroids? Arch Dis Child 2004;89:288–9.

12. Cribier B, Samain F, Vetter D, et al. Systematic cutaneous examination in hepatitis C virus infected patients. Acta Derm Venereol 1992;72:454–455.

13. David E, Tanuos H, Sullivan T, Yan A, Kircik LH. A double-blind, placebo-controlled pilot study to estimate the efficacy and tolerability of a nonsteroidal cream for the treatment of cradle cap (seborrheic dermatitis). J Drugs Dermatol 2013; 12:448–52.

14. de Souza Leão Kamamoto C, Sanudo A, Hassun KM, Bagatin E. Low-dose oral isotretinoin for moderate to severe seborrhea and seborrheic dermatitis: a randomized comparative trial. Int J Dermatol 2017 Jan;56(1):80–8.

15. Ercis M, Balci S, Atakan N. Dermatological manifestations of 71 Down syndrome children admitted to a clinical genetics unit. Clin Genet 1996;50:317–320.

16. Fraitag S, Bodemer C. Neonatal erythroderma. Curr Opin Pediatr 2010; 22:438–44.

17. Gaitanis G, Magiatis P, Stathopoulou K, et al. AhR ligands, malassezin, and indolo 3, 2-b carbazole are selectively produced by Malassezia furfur strains isolated from seborrheic dermatitis. J Invest Dermatol 2008; 128:1620–5.

18. Goh CL, Akarapanth R. Epidemiology of skin disease among children in a referral skin clinic in Singapore. Pediatr Dermatol 1994;11:125–128.

19. Gross-Tsur V, Gross-Kieselstein E, Amir N. Cardio-faciocutaneous syndrome: neurological manifestations. Clin Genet 1990;38:382–386.

20. Gupta AK, Richardson M, Paquet M. Systematic review of oral treatments for seborrheic dermatitis. J Eur Acad Dermatol Venereol 2014 Jan;28(1):16–26.

21. Hald M, Arendrup MC, Svejgaard EL, Lindskov R, Foged EK, Saunte DM; Danish Society of Dermatology. Evidence-based Danish guidelines for the treatment of Malassezia-related skin diseases. Acta Derm Venereol 2015;95:12–9.

22. Hay RJ. Malassezia, dandruff and seborrhoeic dermatitis: an overview. Br J Dermatol 2011;165 Suppl 2:2–8.

23. Henderson CA, Taylor J, Cunliffe WJ. Sebum excretion rates in mothers and neonates. Br J Dermatol 2000;142:110–111.

24. Manapajon A, Kanokvalai K, Sukhum J. Clinical characteristics and quality of life of seborrheic dermatitis patients in a tropical country. Indian J Dermatology 2015; 60:519.

25. Marren P, Burge S. Seborrhoeic dermatitis of the scalp-a manifestation of Hailey-Hailey disease in a predisposed individual. Br J Dermatol 1992; 126:294–296.

26. Mathes BM, Douglass MC. Seborrheic dermatitis in patients with acquired immunodeficiency syndrome. J Am Acad Dermatol 1985;13: 947–951.

27. Naldi L, ReboraA.Clinical practice. Seborrheic dermatitis. N Engl J Med 2009;360:387–96.

28. Nanda A, Al-Hasawi F, Alsaleh QA. A prospective survey of pediatric dermatology clinic patients in Kuwait: an analysis of 10,000 cases. Pediatr Dermatol 1999; 16: 6–11.

29. Ostlere LS, Taylor CR, Harris DW, et al. Skin surface lipids in HIV positive patients with and

without seborrheic dermatitis. Int J Dermatol 1996; 35:276–9.

30. Palamaras I, Kyriakis KP, Stavrianeas NG. Seborrheic dermatitis: lifetime detection rates. J Eur Acad Dermatol Venereol 2012;26:524–6.

31. Pillai J, Okade R. A clinical spectrum of scalp dermatoses in adults presenting to a tertiary referral care centre. Int J Biol Med Res 2014;5:4434–4439.

32. Plunkett A, Merlin K, Gill D, Zuo Y, Jolley D, Marks R. The frequency of common nonmalignant skin conditions in adults in central Victoria, Australia. Int J Dermatol 1999; 38: 901–908.

33. Rademaker M. Low-Dose Isotretinoin for Seborrhoeic Dermatitis. J Cutan Med Surg 2017 Mar/Apr;21(2):170–171.

34. Ratzer MA. The incidence of skin diseases in the West of Scotland. Br J Dermatol 1969;81:456–461.

35. Sardana K, Mahajan S, Sarkar R, et al. The spectrum of skin disease among Indian children. Pediatr Dermatol 2009;26:6–13.

36. Shuster S. The aetiology of dandruff and the mode of action of therapeutic agents. Br J Dermatol 1984; 111:235–42.

37. Szepietowski JC, Reich A, Wesolowska-Szepietowska E, Baran E. National Quality of Life in Dermatology Group. Quality of life in patients suffering from seborrheic dermatitis: influence of age, gender and education level. Mycoses. 2009;52:357–63.

38. Taieb A, Legrain V, Palmier C, et al. Topical ketoconazole for infantile seborrhoeic dermatitis. Dermatologica 1990;181:26–32.

39. Tamer E, Ilhan MN, Polat M, Lenk N, Alli N. Prevalence of skin diseases among pediatric patients in Turkey. J Dermatol 2008; 35: 413–418.

40. Turpeinen M, Salo OP, Leisti S. Effect of percutaneous absorption of hydrocortisone on adrenocortical responsiveness in infants with severe skin disease. Br J Dermatol 1986;115:475–484.

41. Veraldi S, Menter A, Innocenti M. Treatment of mild to moderate seborrhoeic dermatitis with MAS064D (Sebclair), a novel topical medical device: results of a pilot, randomized, double-blind, controlled trial. J Eur Acad Dermatol Venereol 2008;22:290–6.

11

Infective Dermatitis

Aastha Gupta

DEFINITION

Infective eczema or microbial eczema is a distinctive pattern of eczema caused by microbial invasion as the primary event followed by secondary eczematization, which as a rule, clears when the causative pathogens are eradicated. It is important to distinguish this entity from infected eczema, where a secondary bacterial or viral infection complicates eczema due to some other cause.

PATHOPHYSIOLOGY

Infective eczema is a controversial entity. Though the microbial flora of an eczematous lesion differs quantitatively from that of normal skin, it is difficult to differentiate between microbial colonization and infection. Moreover, the mere presence of organisms in an eczematous lesion does not establish that they are modifying the lesion.

The pathogenesis of infected eczema is unclear. It is believed that bacterial super-antigens such as staphylococcal protein A and enterotoxin B can promote a cytotoxic reaction in the skin and can act as immune stimulants and can aggravate and perpetuate eczematous dermatitis. Also, studies show that cultured staphylococci applied topically on human skin can provoke an eczematous delayed hyper-sensitivity reaction.

PATHOLOGY

The histological features of infective eczema are that of a subacute or chronic eczema, with hyperkeratosis, patchy parakeratosis, acantho-sis and spongiosis in the epidermis and dermis showing polymorphonuclear and lymphocytic cell infiltration invading the epidermis to a variable extent.

CLINICAL FEATURES

Infective eczema usually presents as an area of advancing erythema with vesicles seen around an infected discharging wound, usually clearing with antibiotic treatment alone (Fig. 11.1). It is frequently seen in patients with venous leg ulcers, mimicking contact dermatitis due to topical medicaments.

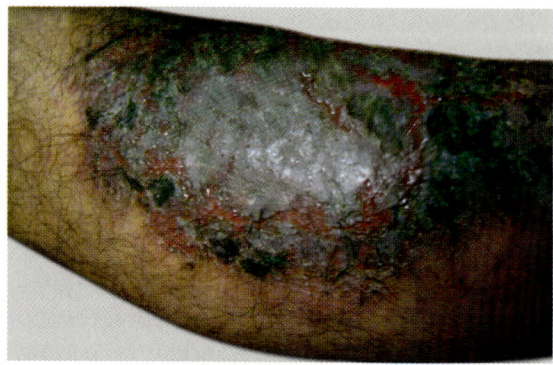

Fig. 11.1: Infected eczema in a patient with lichen simplex chronicus

Meyerson phenomenon, i.e. eczema developing around lesions of molluscum contagiosum, is another example. The eczema usually develops a few days after the appearance of the molluscum lesions, even if they have not been traumatized, and generally clears when the lesions subside. Infective dermatitis may also complicate tinea pedis and infestations like pediculosis, scabies and chronic threadworm infestation, though in such cases it is unclear whether the eczematization is due to the repeated scratching, secondary infection or the infestation per se.

Clinical Variants

Infective dermatitis of the forefeet is a distinctive type of infective eczema affecting the interdigital spaces of the medial toes particularly in patients with poor personal hygiene, hyperhidrosis and heavy footwear. Staphylococci or streptococci are commonly isolated from these cases, and the lesions improve dramatically with antibiotic therapy.

Infective dermatitis of children associated with human T cell leukemia virus 1 (HTLV-1) infection is a type of infective eczema that was initially used to describe the severe exudative and crusted eczema involving the scalp, axillae and groins, eyelids, perinasal and retroauricular areas in Jamaican children. A generalized fine papular rash was also present in a few cases and most patients complained of chronic nasal discharge. Cultures from the nasal cavity and/or skin were positive for *Staphylococcus aureus* or hemolytic streptococci and the eruption responded to antibiotic therapy, but relapsed on its cessation.

It was later found out that these children were infected with HTLV-1. Human T cell lymphotropic virus type 1 (HTLV-1), also referred to as human T cell leukemia virus type 1, infects T cells, B cells and monocytes. It is transmitted via sexual intercourse, needle sharing, blood transfusions and breastfeeding. HTLV-1 induces spontaneous T cell proliferation and increased secretion of interleukin

Table 11.1: Criteria for the diagnosis of infective dermatitis

Major

- Eczema of the scalp, axillae and groin, ears, paranasal skin, eyelid margins and/ or neck
- Chronic watery nasal discharge and/or crusting of the anterior nares
- Chronic relapsing dermatitis which responds quickly to antibiotics but relapses promptly after withdrawal
- Onset during early childhood
- Seropositivity for HTLV-1

Minor

- Positive cultures for *Staphylococcus aureus* and/ or β-hemolytic streptococci from the skin or anterior nares
- Generalized fine papular rash
- Anemia, elevated erythrocyte sedimentation rate
- Hyperimmunoglobulinemia
- Elevated CD4+ and CD8+ T cell counts; elevated CD4/CD8 ratio

(IL)-2, interferon-γ, TNF-α, IL-5 and IL-10. Infected individuals are usually asymptomatic and show increased susceptibility to a variety of infections and scabies and helminthic infestations. 2% of the perinatally infected children develop infective dermatitis in which a few cases persist till adulthood. Complications include corneal opacities and progression to other HTLV-1-associated disorders (adult T cell leukemia/ lymphoma and tropical spastic paraparesis). Diagnosis is established by major and minor criteria.

Table 11.1 shows criteria for the diagnosis of infective dermatitis.

To establish the diagnosis, four major criteria are required, with mandatory inclusion of human T cell lymphotropic/leukemia virus type 1 (HTLV-1) seropositivity.

For the first major criteria, the involvement of at least two body regions is required.

DIFFERENTIAL DIAGNOSIS

Infective dermatitis needs to be differentiated from infected eczema though the differentiation is quite difficult at times. Lesions of infected eczema show profuse exudation and crusting with an underlying erythemaous and raw surface. The margins are characteristically sharply defined and an encircling collarette may be seen. There are usually small pustules in the advancing edge along with fissuring when the flexures are involved.

Infective dermatitis of children associated with human T cell leukemia virus 1 (HTLV-1) infection should be differentiated from atopic dermatitis. Positive serology for HTLV-1 infection, and presence of more exuberant and obviously infected lesions with mild pruritus are clues for the diagnosis of infective dermatitis. Also, crusting of the nasal vestibule and blepharoconjunctivitis are more prominent in children with infective dermatitis. Other differential diagnoses include seborrheic dermatitis and impetigo.

MANAGEMENT

The management of infective dermatitis necessitates treating the primary infective etiology as the eczema generally settles as the infection subsides. Topical antibacterial agents are effective in mild forms of the disease, though systemic antibiotics may be needed in severe cases. For the forefeet variant of infective eczema and in acute exudative lesions, potassium permanganate soaks are helpful initially, in combination with systemic antibiotics. For the HTLV-1 associated infective eczema, oral antibiotics are generally required along with topical treatments including intranasal antibiotics, corticosteroids, and bleach baths. It is important to eliminate the predisposing factors for infection whenever possible, to prevent recurrences.

Bibliography

1. Goncalves DU, Gnedes AC, Proietti AB et al, Interdisciplinary HTLV 1/2 Research Group. Dermatologic lesions in asymptomatic blood donors seropositive for human T cell lymphotropic venus type-1. Am J Trop Med Hyg 2003; 68.562–5.

2. Griffiths C, Barker J, Bleiker T, Chalmers R, Creamer D. Rook's Textbook of Dermatology. 9th ed. Chichester. John Wiley & Sons; 2016. Chapter 39. Eczematous Disorders; p. 21–2.

12

Asteatotic Eczema

Kabir Sardana

This pruritic dermatitis is most commonly located in the lower extremities of elderly individuals, but may present in other parts of the body as well.

CLINICAL FEATURES

The affected areas appear dry, with fine scales and cracks that can coalesce in a perpendicular fashion, resembling cracks in porcelain (Fig. 12.1) or cement. The term eczema craquelé is appropriately used to describe this pattern. Though seen on the lower limbs, this can also involve the trunk in severe cases. Scratching or treatment with drying lotions such as calamine aggravates the eczematous inflammation and leads to infection with accumulation of crusts and purulent material (Fig. 12.2).

It is most commonly associated with vigorous cleaning and rubbing, hot baths, and a history of xerosis. In India, it is also seen in areas where "hard water" is used for bathing purposes. Patients with an atopic diathesis are more likely to develop this distinctive pattern.

PATHOGENESIS

It is thought to occur more commonly in the elderly population in the setting of xerosis, secondary to a decrease in sebaceous and sweat gland activity, in addition to epidermal water

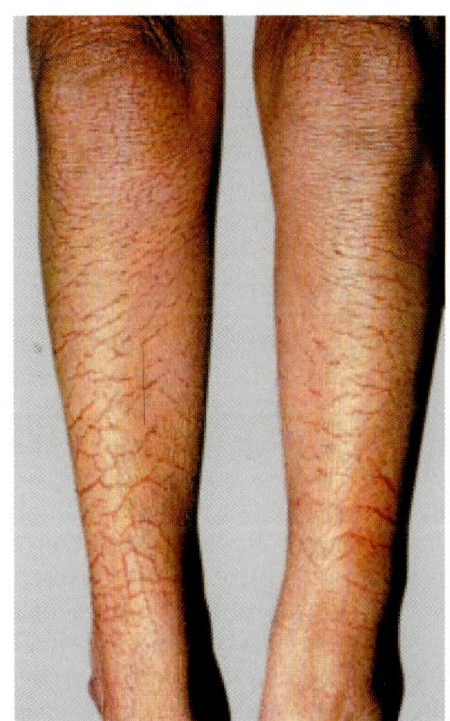

Fig. 12.1: Xerosis with cracked skin (eczema craquelé)

loss in the barrier. Frequent bathing with soap, especially during the winter, is a common factor in the elderly. The combination of hot water, harsh soaps and hard water leads to a increase in this condition. Fundamentally, asteatotic eczema represents a barrier defect. Spongiotic change is secondary. Some cases represent mild forms of nummular eczema.

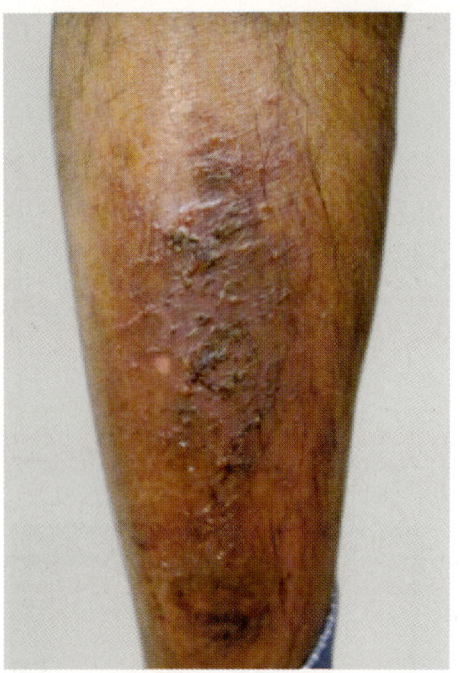

Fig. 12.2: Chronic scratching on a patch of asteatotic eczema with resultant subacute eczema

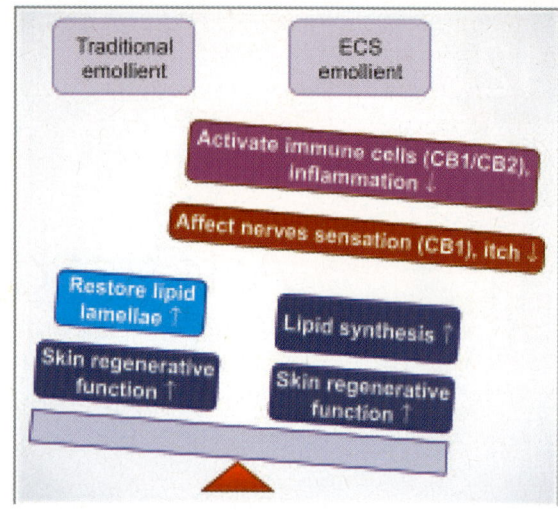

Fig. 12.3: Comparing the traditional emollient and PEA/AEA emollient

Note: Compared with the traditional emollient, the PEA/AEA emollient could simultaneously control both "passive" and "active" skin functions, including regeneration of skin and restoration of lipid lamellae, skin sensation, and immune competence.

Abbreviations: ECS, endocannabinoid system; CB, cannabinoid receptor; PEA, N-palmitoylethanolamine; AEA, N-acetylethanolamine.

The endocannabinoid system is believed to be actively involved in endogenous protective mechanisms in skin barrier function. Some endogenous lipids like N-palmitoylethanolamine (PEA) could markedly augment the effect of N-acetylethanolamine (AEA) at cannabinoid receptor type 1 and/or 2, as well as directly activate peroxisome proliferator-activated receptor alpha constitutively, and simultaneously control both "passive" and "active" skin functions, including regeneration of skin and restoration of lipid lamellae, skin sensation, and immune competence. Activation of cannabinoid receptor type 2 in the sebaceous glands by AEA could markedly enhance lipid synthesis. The literature indicates that the endocannabinoid system is a good treatment for uremic pruritus. Thus, this would help not only the dry skin, but by the action on endocannabinoids, play a role in decreasing the neural stimulation of itch (Fig. 12.3). PEA could downmodulate activation of skin mast cells and inhibit release of histamine, prostaglandin D_2, and tumor necrosis factor alpha.

Asteatotic eczema has been associated with drug therapy, bathing practices, nephrotic syndrome and is also listed as a paraneoplastic condition.

TREATMENT

Gentle cleaning with emollients and lukewarm water is recommended. In mild cases, the treatment is similar to cases of subacute eczema.

Though the conventional therapies revolve around the use of urea, lactic acid, or a lactate salt, a study found that the use of both endogenous lipids N-palmitoylethanolamine (PEA) and N-acetylethanolamine (AEA) were found to be superior to conventional emollients (Yuan C et al).

Topical corticosteroids can be considered, if there is an inflammatory component. In addition, 12% ammonium lactate lotion may help soften dry skin, but patients should be cautioned that it occasionally stings and irritates fissured areas. Urea-based ointments are useful as they increase hydration. The use of oral steroids should be avoided as the disease flares within 1 or 2 days once they are discontinued.

Bibliography

1. Chu CH, Chou CY, Lin FL. Generalized eczema craquelé (asteatotic dermatitis) associated with pemetrexed treatment. J Eur Acad Dermatol Venereol 2016 Oct;30(10):e81-e83.

2. Eczema in Sardana K, Mahajan S, Garg VK. Diagnosis and Management of Skin Disorders: An Evidence-Based Approach, 1/ e.: Lippincott Williams and Wilkins, 2012 (reprint 2015).

3. Fast Facts: Eczema and Contact Dermatitis by John Berth-Jones, Eunice Tan and Howard I Malbach Published 2004.

4. Koks N, Assen YJ, Libourel EJ, Eskes SA. [Asteatotic eczema as paraneoplastic syndrome.] Ned Tijdschr Geneeskd 2016;160(0):D391.

5. Thieme Clinical Companions Dermatology. Sterry, Dermatology© 2006 Thieme.

6. Yang CS, Lott JP, Bunick CG, Bolognia JL. Eczema craquelé associated with nephrotic syndrome. JAAD Case Rep 2016 Jun 4;2(3):241.

7. Yuan C, Wang XM, Guichard A, Tan YM, Qian CY, Yang LJ, Humbert. N-palmitoylethanolamine and N-acetylethanolamine are effective in asteatotic eczema: results of a randomized, double-blind, controlled study in 60 patients. Clin Interv Aging 2014 Jul 17;9:1163–9.

13

Discoid Eczema

Kabir Sardana, Shivani Bansal

Discoid eczema (also known as nummular dermatitis) is one of the many forms of dermatitis. It is also known as discoid dermatitis. The name comes from the Latin word nummus, which means coin. It is characterized by round or oval coin-shaped itchy lesions over the extensor surfaces of the extremities. It was first described in the mid-1800s by Marie-Guillaume-Alphonse Devergie and classically presents in younger- to middle-aged patients (Devergie M). It is to be distinguished from an irregular patchy form of eczema in which the lesions do not have recognizable, clear margins.

Hornstein's classification (Flowchart 13.1) reveals three basic eczema groups: Endogenous, exogenous, and dysregulative-microbial eczema with its subtype nummular eczema.

ETIOLOGY

The etiology of nummular eczema is multifactorial, involving **environmental**, **allergic**, **emotional, and nutritional factors**. It can occur in any season, but due to increased use of hot water, soaps, and detergents, it is most frequent in the **colder months** and was once termed "winter eczema" for this reason. It is associated with dryness of the skin, which may allow epidermal breach and permeation of allergens (Aoyama H). Severe, generalized nummular eczema has been reported in association with

Flowchart 13.1: Hornstein's classification of eczema

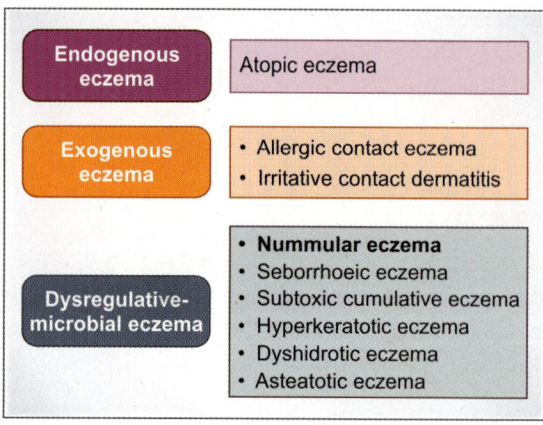

interferon and ribavirin therapy for hepatitis C and tumor necrosis factor inhibitors (Shen Y).

As in other forms of eczema, heavy colonization of the lesions by staphylococci may increase their severity, even in the absence of clinical evidence of infection (Wachs GN). Allergic sensitivity to staphylococci or micrococci may be responsible for secondary dissemination.

Emotional stress, liver dysfunction, or extensive alcohol consumption can have negative impact on the course of disease. A recent study reports elevated tryptase in children with nummular eczema in absence of mastocytosis or atopic eczema.

A summary of important factors is listed in Box 13.1.

Box 13.1: Common etiological factors implicated in the causation of discoid eczema	
Atopy and dry skin	Almost 50% cases may have atopy. Hard water in most parts of India may be an aggravating cause
Contact sensitization	Metals, fragrance, rubber, and preservatives
Hidden infections	Bacterial (dental infections, sinusitis, tonsillitis, bronchitis, prostatitis) and viral infections (hepatitis)
	Bacterial antigens (*Staphylococcus* spp.)
	Venous eczema
Drugs	Gold preparations, isotretinoin, antivirals (ribavirin, interferon, telaprevir)

CLINICAL FEATURES

Men usually get nummular eczema late in their life while women get it at a younger age.

Location is important to the diagnosis. Common affected areas are the distal limbs (lower extremities > upper extremities) and most commonly involves the dorsa of the hands, extensor surfaces of the forearms, upper arms, legs, thighs, and feet. The lesions start as solid plaques that enlarge and develop a peripheral papulovesicular border (Fig. 13.1).

There is often associated pruritus, but this varies greatly, with some patients complaining of almost constant itching and others noticing severe pruritus only at the time of initial outbreak of new lesions.

It may be convenient to recognize the following patterns:
1. Discoid eczema of the hands and forearms
2. Discoid eczema of the limbs and trunk
3. Dry discoid eczema.

Discoid eczema of the hands is a form of **irritant occupational dermatitis,** but may also occur in housewives or secretaries in whom the provoking factors are less clear. An atopic history appears to be more frequent in young women with discoid hand eczema than in other forms of the disease (Fig. 13.2).

The more usual form of discoid eczema affects the **limbs** and **trunk** (Figs 13.3 and 13.4).

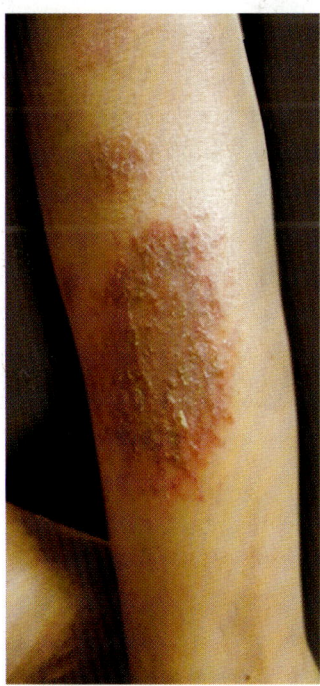

Fig. 13.1: A discoid patch of eczema (acute stage) with peripheral papulovesicles

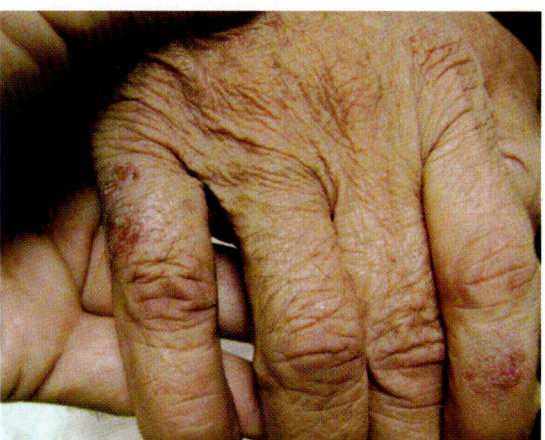

Fig. 13.2: Discoid eczema of the hands

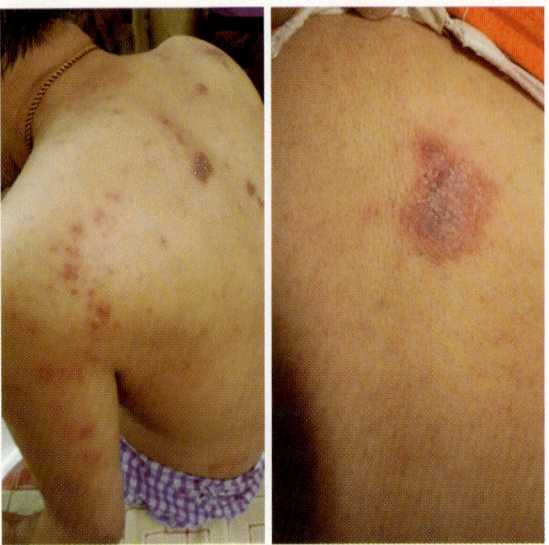

Fig. 13.3: Discoid eczema of limbs and trunk (subacute eczema stage)

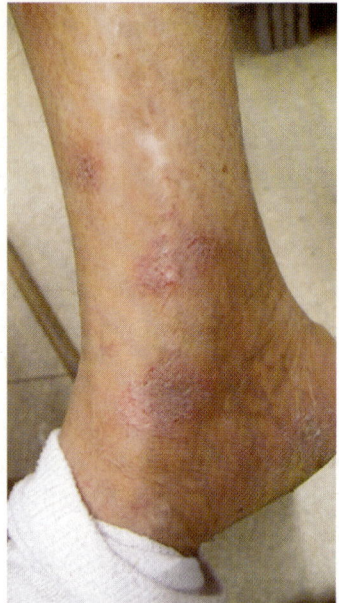

It appears to be particularly prevalent among managerial or professional classes. It is also seen in elderly people, often with a dry skin exacerbated by low humidity, central heating and car heating.

Dry discoid eczema is an uncommon variant, consisting of multiple, dry, scaly, round or oval discs on the arms or legs (Figs 13.4 and 13.5), but also with scattered microvesicles on an erythematous base on the palms and soles.

Course: Nummular dermatitis often waxes and wanes in winters. Cold or dry climates or swings in temperature may be exacerbating factors. It may improve with sun or humidity exposure or with moisturizer use. Occasionally, it may worsen with heat or humidity. New nummular dermatitis lesions often recur in the same locations as old lesions.

After a period between 10 days and several months, secondary lesions occur, often in a mirror-image configuration on the opposite side of the body. It is very characteristic of this disease that patches which have apparently become dormant may become active again, particularly if treatment is discontinued prematurely.

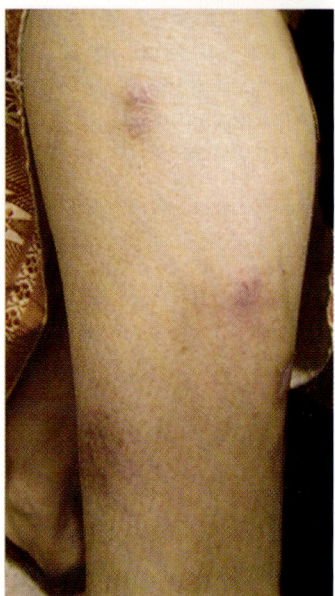

Figs 13.4 and 13.5: Dry discoid eczema of the limbs

Like most eczemas, nummular eczema will show the various phases of acute or subacute/chronic eczema.

DIAGNOSIS

A potassium hydroxide wet mount can be obtained to evaluate for dermatophyte infection, but typically no tests are ordered.

Table 13.1: Relevant investigations for discoid eczema	
Complete blood count ESR	*Leucocytosis and raised ESR:* Bacterial infections *Lymphopenia:* Viral Infections *Monocytosis:* Viral infection
Hepatitis serology	Hepatis A, B, C
HIV	AIDS
ASO titre	*Elevated:* Streptococcal infections
Anti-staphylolysin antibodies (ASTA)	*Elevated:* Staphylococcal infections
VDRL,TPHA	Syphilis
Total-IgE, RAST, prick test	Atopic dermatitis
Patch test	Contact dermatitis

Skin biopsy findings are non-specific. In the early stages, subacute dermatitis indistingui-shable from other forms of eczema with spongiotic vesicles, and a predominant lymphocytic infiltrate is found. Eosinophils may be observed in the papillary dermis. Chronic lesions demonstrate epidermal hyperplasia, hyperkeratosis, and a pronounced granular cell layer. The papillary dermis may be fibrotic, with a perivenular infiltrate of lymphocytes and monocytes.

Blood investigations may be performed to detect underlying infectious diseases, atopy or allergies (Table 13.1).

DIFFERENTIAL DIAGNOSIS

Diagnostically, this rash can be mistaken for tinea given the annular shape and sharp demarcation with raised peripheral border, but should be differentiated by location, appearance of crusting and scaling surface, lack of central clearing, and past history of eczema. Allergic contact dermatitis, irritant contact dermatitis and asteatotic eczema are the other differential diagnoses.

TREATMENT

Treatment is aimed at **rehydration** of the skin, **repair** of the epidermal lipid barrier, reduction of **inflammation**, treatment of any **infection** and witholding the inciting agent (often hot water showers and harsh soaps).

Steroids are the most commonly used therapy to reduce inflammation. In the early stages, a potent or very potent steroid may be needed. Oral, intramuscular, or parenteral steroids may be required in cases of severe, generalized eruptions.

Traditionally, a range of coaltar pastes or ointments were used in the less acute stages, and sometimes a combination of tar and dilute corticosteroid proved useful in long-term management.

Topical immune modulators (tacrolimus and pimecrolimus) also reduce inflammation. These are often initiated a few days after the topical steroid to decrease the risk of a burning sensation that may occur when applied to extremely irritated skin.

When eruptions are generalized and prolonged, phototherapy (generally UVB) may be helpful.

Oral antihistamines or sedatives may help reduce itching and improve sleep.

Oral antibiotics such as dicloxacillin, cefalexin, or erythromycin, should be used in cases of secondary infection. Swab cultures of the skin guide selection of antibiotics.

Phototherapy may be helpful. Broadband or narrow band UV B is most commonly used, although PUVA (Psoralen + UVA) may be used in severe cases.

The treatment is usually administered according to the stage of the disease (Table 13.2). An evidence-based overview is given in Table 13.3.

Table 13.2: Stage-wise treatment of discoid eczema

Acute discoid eczema	1. Systemic therapy with *steroids* (0.5–1.0 mg/kg prednisone) for about one week, in tapering dose 2. Systemic *antibiotic* therapy (penicillins, cephalosporins, lincosamides) 3. Glucocorticoid cream (O/W): Antibiotic combinations with wet dressings 4. In case of an underlying infection (tonsillitis, urethritis, bronchitis), specific antimicrobial therapy
Chronic discoid eczema	1. Glucocorticoid cream or ointment 2. Occlusive lipophilic ointment 3. Tars (3–5%) 4. Keratolytic ointments (urea 10% or salicylic acid 5%) 5. Ultraviolet B phototherapy

Table 13.3: An overview of therapeutic options for discoid eczema

	Topical	Systemic	Phototherapy	
First line	Topical corticosteroids ± antibacterial agents (fucidic acid-based preparations)* Emollients Tar-based preparations	Oral **antibiotics** Oral **antihistamines**	UVB and PUVA	
Second line		**Tacrolimus**	**Cyclosporine** **Steroids**	
Third line			**Azathioprine** **Methotrexate** **Mycophenolate** mofetil	

*Neomycin-based preparations can cause allergic contact dermatitis.

Bibliography

1. Aoyama H, Tanaka M, Hara M, Tabata N, Tagami H. Nummular eczema: An addition of senile xerosis and unique cutaneous reactivities to environmental aeroallergens. Dermatology 1999;199:135–9.

2. Devergie M. Traite Pratique des Maladies de la Peau. 2nd edn (French). Paris: V. Masson; 1857.

3. Shen Y, Pielop J, Hsu S. Generalized nummular eczema secondary to peginterferon Alfa-2b and ribavirin combination therapy for hepatitis C infection. Arch Dermatol 2005;141:102–3.

4. Wachs GN, Maibach H. Co-operative double blind trial of an antibiotic corticoid combination in impetiginized atopic dermatitis. Br J Dermatol 1976;95:323–8.

14

Pityriasis Alba

Kabir Sardana, Shivani Bansal

DEFINITION

It is derived from word **'pityriasis'** means scaly and **'alba'** which is a Latin word for white although patches are not totally depigmented. This is a pattern of dermatitis in which hypopigmentation is the most conspicuous feature. Although it is common worldwide, its incidence is markedly higher in darker skin phototypes. It is characterized by the presence of ill-defined, scaly, faintly erythematous patches. These lesions eventually subside, leaving hypopigmented areas that then slowly return to normal pigmentation. It is a common skin disorder in children and young adults.

ETIOLOGY

Pityriasis alba (PA) is found almost entirely in preadolescent children. In most instances, the lesions clear at puberty, however, persistence into adulthood has been reported (O'Farrell). No known cause of pityriasis alba has been reported. The condition is not contagious, and no infectious agent has been identified.

Leading theories as to the origin of the lesions in pityriasis alba involve atopy and post-inflammatory changes, with a large number of patients with pityriasis alba having a history of atopic disease, and atopic patients being more prone to develop the condition (Martin RF et al, Vinod S et al).

Nutritional deficiency, anemia and parasitic infestations were proposed as contributing factors (Bassaly et al). In addition, a positive correlation between some personal hygiene habits and PA has been recorded. Long, frequent baths, mechanical exfoliation, and other similar treatments may reduce the level of defensins and skin-protecting factors, contributing to the development of lesions.

CLINICAL FEATURES

It most frequently affects children aged 3 to 16 years. Both sexes are equally susceptible. Pityriasis alba lesions often occur on the face, with the cheek being a particularly common site. In 20% of affected children, the neck, arms and shoulders are involved as well. The legs and trunk are less commonly involved. There are three clinical variants of PA: **classic (CPA)**, **extensive (EPA)**, and **pigmenting (PPA)**. The first two variants occur in all skin phototypes. The pigmenting variant is typical of non-Caucasian populations from the Republic of South Africa, Middle East (Jadotte et al) and India.

Classic pityriasis alba: The individual lesion is a rounded, oval or irregular hypopigmented patch with indistinct margins. Lesions are often slightly erythematous and have fine scaling (Fig. 14.1). Initially, the erythema may

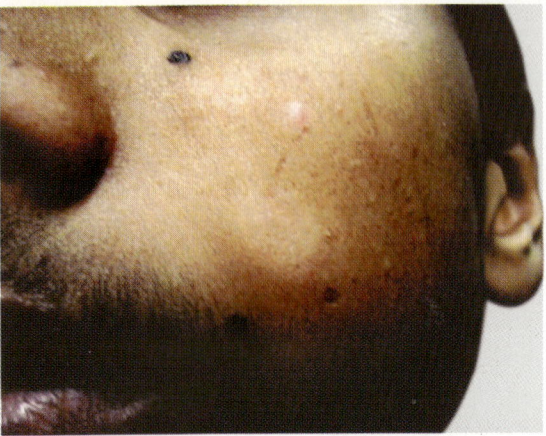

Fig. 14.1: An initial stage of pityriasis alba with fine scaling and an underlying area of hypopigmentation

be conspicuous and there may even be minimal serous crusting. Later, the erythema subsides completely, and at the stage at which the lesions are commonly seen by a physician, they show only persistent fine scaling and hypopigmentation. It is this that commonly induces the patient to seek advice. The hypopigmentation is most conspicuous in pigmented skin, and in lighter skins may become more evident after sun exposure (Fig. 14.2).

Lesions may progress through the following three clinical stages:
- Papular (scaling) erythematous
- Papular (scaling) hypochromic
- Smooth hypochromic

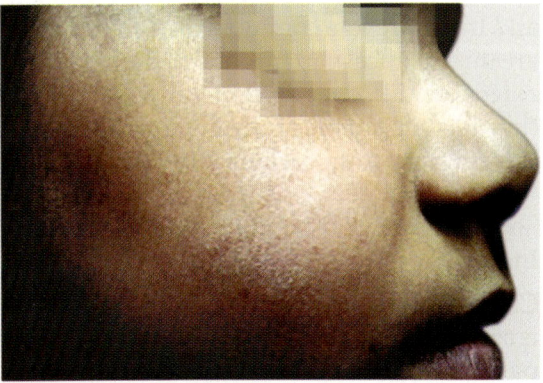

Fig. 14.2: Uniform scaling which eventually heal to leave behind an area of pigmentary loss

Uncommon variants of pityriasis alba are as follows:

- *Pigmented pityriasis alba:* Typical lesion has a central zone of bluish hyperpigmentation surrounded by a hypopigmented, slightly scaly halo of variable width; the lesions are usually confined to the face and are often associated with dermatophyte infection. The pigmented area is attributed to melanin deposits in dermis. One-third of the patients have concurrent classic pityriasis alba.

- *Extensive pityriasis alba:* It is more commonly seen in adults. Differentiated from the classic form by the generalized involvement often involoving the inferior torso in symmetric fashion, the absence of a preceding inflammatory phase, and histologically, the absence of spongiosis.

  Debate exists as to the validity of the term extensive pityriasis alba, which some believe to be a confusing misnomer applied to a pathoetiologically different entity. Some authors believe that extensive pityriasis alba overlaps with another condition, described as "progressive and extensive hypomelanosis" in persons of mixed racial background and also reported as "progressive and confluent hypomelanosis of the melanodermic metis" or "creole dyschromia". The alternate name of "progressive extensive hypomelanosis" has been proposed (Di Lernia V).

- *Follicular pityriasis alba:* A "follicular" variety of pityriasis alba consists of follicular hyperkeratosis within or around the hypopigmented macules, resembling keratosis pilaris; the hypopigmentation helps in the diagnosis of this condition. Others feel that this is similar to pityriasis alba with follicular eczema.

In patients of "skin of color", various follicular morphologies have been described and follicular pityriasis alba can be seen even without AD (Fig. 14.3a and b).

DIAGNOSIS

The age incidence, the fine scaling and the distribution of the lesions usually suggest the diagnosis. A workup, as follows, may be undertaken to exclude other causes of hypopigmentation:

- **Wood's light examination:** It may help in determining the presence of vitiligo, which will glow more brightly and have edges with sharper demarcation.
- **Skin biopsy:** The histological changes are acanthosis and mild spongiosis, with moderate hyperkeratosis and patchy parakeratosis. There may be follicular plugging, spongiosis and sebaceous gland atrophy, and irregular pigmentation by melanin of the basal layer of epidermis. Irregular pigmentation in the late stage has been recorded in all patients and is thus considered to be characteristic of PA.

DIFFERENTIAL DIAGNOSIS

- Post-inflammatory hypopigmentation
- Nevus anemicus
- Nevus depigmentosus
- Tuberous sclerosis
- Vitiligo
- Tinea versicolor
- Mycosis fungoides

MANAGEMENT

Pityriasis alba is generally self-limited, and the prognosis is good, with eventual complete repigmentation. No long-term residual effects are expected. Treatment consists primarily of good general skin care and education of a young patient's parents about the benign nature of this self-limited disorder. Supportive measures such as decrease sun exposure, use of sunscreens and reduction of frequency and temperature of baths should be recommended. Therapy may also include the following:

- **Low-potency topical steroids (e.g. hydro-cortisone):** They may help in stage 1 and stage 2 of pityriasis alba and may accelerate repigmentation of existing lesions. However, their use should be limited to avoid long-term skin atrophy and steroid changes.
- **Emollient cream:** Used to reduce the scaling of lesions, especially on the face.
- **Psoralen plus ultraviolet light A (PUVA) photochemotherapy:** It may be used to help with repigmentation in extensive cases; recurrence rate is high after treatment is stopped.
- **Tacrolimus ointment 0.1% and pimecro-limus cream 1%:** It has been reported to be beneficial in the treatment of pityriasis alba (Rigopoulos et al, Fujita et al). It is effective when applied to hypopigmented areas in the third stage of disease as it has an activating effect on tyrosinase and causes enhancement of melanin biosynthesis.

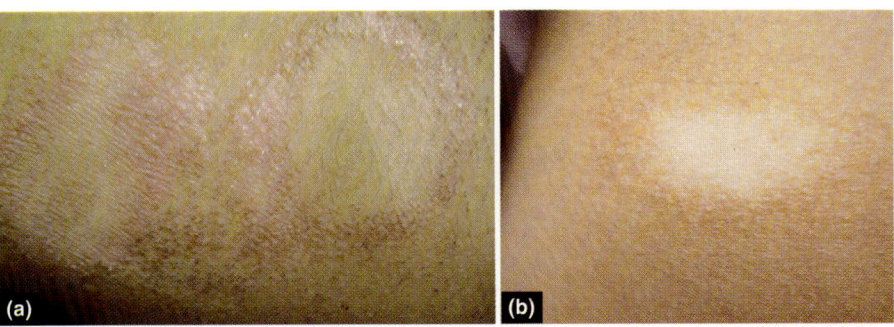

Fig. 14.3a and b: Follicular pityriasis alba, note the follicular papules that surround a central area of hypopigmentation. Though described in AD, they are commonly seen in patients of "skin of color" and some believe that are similar to follicular eczema

- **Tar:** We often use 3–5% tar preparations which is safe and is an efficient way of treating both the inflammatory phase of pityriasis alba and also helps to pigment the lesion.
- **Laser therapy:** Treatment with a 308-nm excimer laser twice a week has been shown to be effective against pityriasis alba (Al-Mutairi et al).

Bibliography

1. Al-Mutairi N, Hadad AA. Efficacy of 308 nm xenon chloride excimer laser in pityriasis alba. Dermatol Surg 2012 Apr. 38(4):604–9.

2. Bassaly M, Miale A. Studies on pityriasis alba—a common facial skin lesion in Egyptian children. Arch Dermatol 1963;88: 88–91.

3. Di Lernia V, Ricci C. On atopic and idiopatic extensive pityriasis alba. Pediatr Dermatol 2007 Sep-Oct. 24(5):578–9.

4. Fujita WH, McCormick CL, Parneix-Spake A. An exploratory study to evaluate the efficacy of pimecrolimus cream 1% for the treatment of pityriasis alba. Int J Dermatol 2007 Jul 46(7):700–5.

5. Jadotte YT, Janniger CK. Pityriasis alba revisited: perspectives on an enigmatic disorder of childhood. Cutis 2011;87:66–72.

6. Martin RF, Lugo-Somolinos A, Sanchez JL. Clinicopathologic study on pityriasis alba. Bol Asoc Med P R 1990 Oct. 82(10):463–5.

7. O'Farrell NM. Pityriasis alba. Arch Dermatol 1956;73: 376–377.

8. Rigopoulos D, Gregoriou S, Charissi C, Kontochristopoulos G, Kalogeromitros D, Georgala S. Tacrolimus ointment 0.1% in pityriasis alba: an open-label, randomized, placebo-controlled study. Br J Dermatol 2006 July; 155(1): 152–5.

9. Sardana K. Follicular disorders of the face. Clin Dermatol 2014 Nov-Dec;32(6):839–72.

10. Sardana K, Arora P, Mishra D. Follicular eczema: a commonly misdiagnosed dermatosis. Indian Pediatr 2012 Jul;49(7):599. Pub Med PMID: 22885452.

11. Vinod S, Singh G, Dash K, Grover S. Clinico-epidemiological study of pityriasis alba. Indian J Dermatol Venereol Leprol 2002 Nov-Dec. 68(6):338–40.

15

Hand Eczema

Konchok Dorjay, Kabir Sardana, Ananta Khurana, Pooja Arora Mrig

INTRODUCTION

Hands are an important part of our body as they help us in our daily activities and also have aesthetic importance. They can become a cause of serious disability when afflicted with chronic disease and can lead to significant psychosocial impairment.

"Hand dermatitis/eczema" is predominant involvement of the hands with eczema. If the hands are involved as a part of extensive disorder, then it is called hand involvement. Hand eczema is a common and distressing condition. A high incidence of hand eczema is associated with female sex, contact allergy, atopic dermatitis and wet work. It often affects people who work in cleaning, catering, hairdressing, healthcare and mechanical jobs where they may come into contact with chemicals or other irritants. It causes domestic, psychological, social and occupational undesirable outcomes leading to negative impact on quality of life.

CLASSIFICATION

No single classification of hand dermatitis is completely satisfactory. But, hand eczema can be classified on the basis of etiology, morphology and stages of disease (Tables 15.1 to 15.3).

During the normal practice, it is very common to observe mixed forms where development of HE involves multiple factors that may be present at the same or at different times. Thus the classification of hand eczema is challenging and it can be carried out

Table 15.1: Etiological classification of hand eczema
Exogenous
1. Contact irritants: • Chemical (e.g. soaps, detergents, solvents)   • Physical (e.g. friction, minor trauma, cold dry air)
2. Contact allergens: • Delayed hypersensitivity (type IV) (e.g. chromium, rubber)   • Immediate hypersensitivity (type I) (e.g. seafood)
3. Ingested allergens (e.g. drugs, possibly nickel, chromium)
4. Infection (e.g. following bacterial infection of hand wounds)
5. Secondary dissemination (e.g. dermatophytide reaction to tinea pedis)
Endogenous
1. Idiopathic (e.g. discoid, hyperkeratotic palmar eczema)
2. Immunological or metabolic defect (e.g. atopic)
3. Psychosomatic: Stress aggravates, but may not be causative
4. Dyshidrosis: Increased sweating aggravates, but may not be causative

Table 15.2: Morphological classification of hand eczema

1. Recurrent vesicular/dyshidrotic hand eczema or pompholyx
2. Hyperkeratotic/tylotic hand eczema
3. Nummular hand eczema
4. Wear and tear/asteatotic/housewives' dermatitis/ dermatitis palmaris sicca.
5. Chronic fingertip eczema/pulpitis
6. Ring eczema
7. Recurrent focal palmar peeling
8. Apron eczema
9. Chronic acral dermatitis
10. Interdigital (webspace) eczema
11. Gut/slaughterhouse eczema
12. Patchy/papulosquamous eczema

Table 15.3: Classification of hand eczema based on the stages of disease

Stages of disease	Clinical features
Acute	Erythema, edema, vesiculation, exudation, bullae formation
Subacute	Erythema, papules and crusting
Chronic	Lichenification (thickening of skin, accentuated skin markings, hyperpigmentation)

according to etiological and morphological criteria as well as the affected location as reported in Tables 15.1 to 15.3.

Though we will be listing and detailing the various forms of HE, it must be appreciated that we can distinguish **four** main types of HE: Irritant (subtoxic-cumulative) HE, allergic HE, atopic HE, and other forms of HE. The last category includes various entities but the discrete one are pompholyx and discoid eczema. **Chronic hand eczema** (CHE) is not a uniform disease. It can be described as persistent HE (with own etiology and clinical manifestation) over 3 months or returns twice or more within 12 months. An overview of the main features of this crucial and often missed entity is listed in Box 15.1.

Though the section that follows lists numerous types of morphologies, it must be appreciated that the 4 main types can encompass most of the entities.

ETIOLOGY

Hand eczema has multifactorial etiology. Both exogenous (extrinsic) and endogenous (intrinsic) factors may be involved in the pathogenesis of hand eczema. There are a few predictive factors for hand eczema of which a history of childhood eczema was the most important predictive factor for hand eczema. Other factors are listed in Box 15.2.

Endogenous Causes

Atopic diathesis is the commonest endogenous cause of hand eczema. Twin studies suggest hereditary factors play a role in the development

Box 15.1: Snapshot of chronic hand eczema (CHE)	
Etiopathogenesis	• It can be the result of the IHD, AHD, AE, or other forms becoming chronic (*see* below)
	• The hyperkeratotic-rhagadiform, vesicular, and mixed pattern HE are the most common manifestation
Site	• Palmar and dorsum site
	• Tendency to recur at the same site
Morphology	• Irregularly bordered, symmetrical, hyperkeratotic, lichenified lesions with painful rhagades
	• Absence or mild pruritus
	• Absence of vesicular eruptions is characteristic

Box 15.2: Predictive factors for hand eczema

- History of childhood eczema
- Female gender
- Occupational exposure
- History of asthma and/or hay fever
- Service occupation (e.g. professional cleaners)

Meding B, Swanbeck G: Contact Dermatitis 23:154, 1990.

of hand eczema. In genetically predisposed individuals, environmental exposure to allergens and irritants results in development of chronic hand eczema. Filaggrin mutations increase the risk and persistence of hand eczema in subjects with atopic dermatitis.

Atopic Hand Eczema (AHE)

Patients often have a history of asthma, hay fever or childhood eczema. The following factors predict the occurrence of hand eczema in adults with a history of atopic dermatitis:
1. Hand dermatitis before age 15
2. Persistent eczema on the body
3. Dry or itchy skin in adult life
4. Widespread atopic dermatitis in childhood

Many people with atopic dermatitis develop hand eczema independently of exposure to irritants, but such exposure causes additional irritant contact dermatitis. Hands are the most frequent site to be involved in adults with atopic dermatitis. The clinical features that point to an atopic etiology are listed in Box 15.3

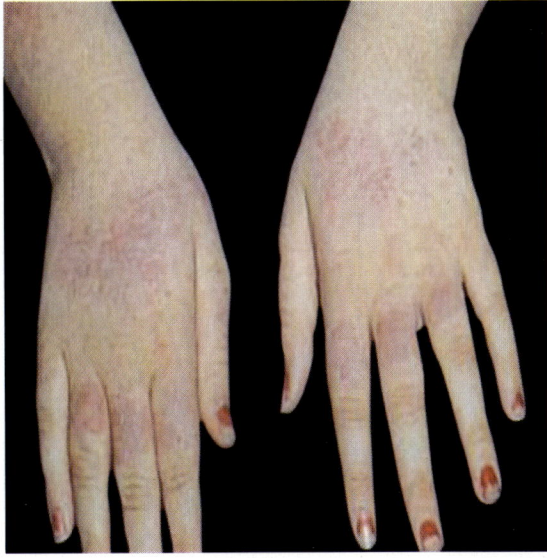

Fig.15.1: Atopic hand eczema involving dorsum of hand

and include involvement of dorsal hand surfaces (Fig. 15.1) and the volar wrist (Simpson et al). Out of all types of hand eczema, atopic hand eczema has the worst prognosis (Meding et al).

Exogenous Causes

Irritant Contact Dermatitis (ICD) (Syn: Irritant (Subtoxic-Cumulative) Hand Dermatitis (IHD)

Contact irritants are the commonest exogenous cause of hand eczema. In ICD, eczema occurs without prior sensitization. Exposure to

Box 15.3: Snapshot of atopic hand eczema	
Etiopathogenesis	• Frequently unrelated to occupation but it is worthy to remember that irritant or occupational factors can trigger skin manifestation
Site	• Often involves the **back** of the hands (especially the **dorsal** site of the fingers)
	• Involvement of the nails can be present
	• Hand eczema can be the only site of AD involvement, or the hand can be a site of an AD spreader involvement (as flexor surfaces, face, neck)
	• Involvement of the **wrist** and of the "**snuff box**"
Morphology	• Vesicles (dyshidrosiform morphology) in palmar and interdigital areas
	• Poorly bordered lichenified patches
	• Scaling and rhagades in the lichenified patches
	• Rarely discoid morphology

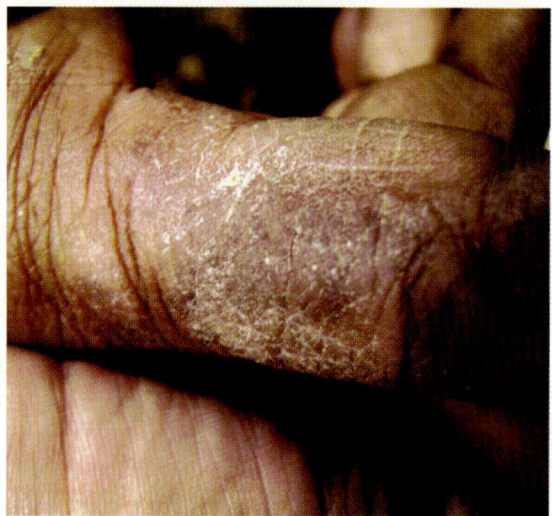

Fig.15.2a: A chronic patch of eczema on the finger

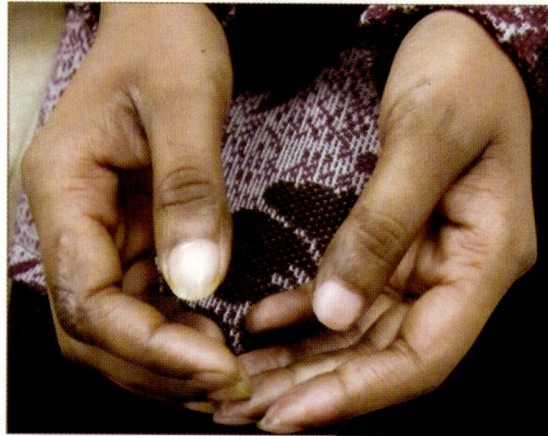

Fig. 15.2b: IHD involving the dorsum of thumb and extending to the inner aspects of fingers

Allergic Contact Dermatitis (Allergic Hand Eczema)

irritants impair the barrier functions of the skin. ICD of the hands is frequently seen in female, cleaners, hospital workers, hairdressers, painters and laborers. Most of the patients have a history of exposure to "wet" work. Common irritants are detergents, solvents, alkalis, abrasives. ICD can be acute (single external exposure to irritant for short duration) or chronic (repeated exposure to irritants over a prolonged period) (Fig. 15.2a and b). An overview is given in Box 15.4.

It is a delayed type hypersensitivity reaction to an allergen or chemical in which prior sensitization occurs. Allergic contact dermatitis (ACD) occurs 1 to 2 days after contact and is initially localized to the site of exposure. Vegetables, detergents, soaps, topical drugs, metals, industrial agents, and nuts are the major allergens found in Indian series. The chemicals responsible are nickel (tools, jewellery), chromate (leather, cement), rubber additives (in gloves), and preservatives (in creams).

Box 15.4: Snapshot of irritant (subtoxic-cumulative) hand dermatitis (IHD)	
Etiopathogenesis	• Repeated subirritant doses • Common cause in India is "hard" water • If the etiology is an irritant within the work environment, an improvement during the weekend (and healing possible with extended periods away from work) is classic
Site	• Back of the hands, fingers, exposed areas of the forearms, and, later, the inner surfaces of the hands (Fig.15.2b) are the most commonly involved areas
Morphology	• *Acute:* Skin is raw, dry, and scaly. • *Subacute/chronic:* Redness, infiltration, and lichenification • Lastly, painful rhagades development and hyperkeratotic plaques interspersed with rhagades (hyperkeratotic-rhagadiform eczema) • Lesions present relatively well-defined borders and are not so itchy (as in allergic contact dermatitis)

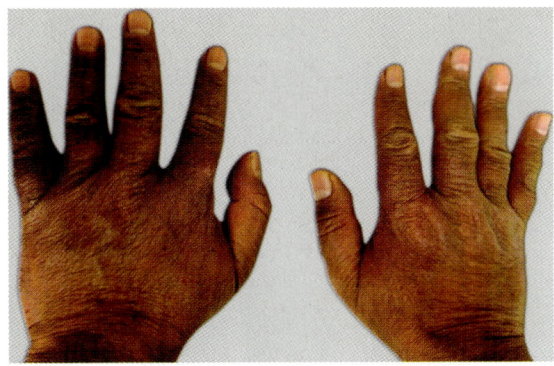
Fig. 15.3: ACD to gloves in a health care worker

Figure 15.3 depicts a patient with allergic contact dermatitis to gloves. Oral ingestion of allergen (e.g nickel) can also provoke hand eczema, though rare (Jensen et al). A list of common allergens implicated is given in Box 15.5 and an overview is given in Box 15.6 with marked involvement of the dorsum of the hands.

Pompholyx/Recurrent Vesicular Dyshidrotic Hand Eczema

In this variant of hand eczema, deep-seated "sago-like" clear vesicles appear on palms and sides of fingers (cheiropompholyx). Lesions can also occur on plantar aspect of feet (podopompholyx). There is no associated erythema. Pompholyx accounts for 5–20% of all cases of hand eczema (Figs 15.4 and 15.5). The condition is extremely itchy. A prickling sensation precedes the attacks. Resolution occurs in 2–3 weeks with desquamation. Summer exacerbation may be seen. Pompholyx has multifactorial etiology, most important of which is atopy. Other factors are sweat gland dysfunction, exposure to irritants (soluble oils), allergens (nickel, chromium, cobalt, dichromates, perfumes, fragrances). Oral contraceptive pills (OCP), aspirin intake and smoking increase the risk of pompholyx. Differential diagnosis includes pustular psoriasis and erythema multiforme.

Also see Chapter 17.

Discoid Eczema

It is characterized by round to oval plaques of eczema that have a well-demarcated edge. Various factors involved in its pathogenesis

Box 15.5: A list of common allergens and the common objects implicated	
Nickel	Door knobs, handles on kitchen utensils, scissors, knitting needles, industrial equipment, hairdressing equipment, metallic mobile phones
Potassium dichromate	Cement, leather articles (gloves), industrial machines, oils
Rubbers	Gloves, industrial equipment (hoses, belts, cables)
Fragrances	Cosmetics, soaps, lubricants, topical medications
Formaldehyde	Wash and wear fabrics, paper, cosmetics, embalming fluids
Lanolin	Topical lubricants and medications, cosmetics

Box 15.6: Snapshot of allergic hand eczema	
Etiopathogenesis	• It is the result of delayed contact hypersensitivity (type IV hypersensitivity) to one or more allergens in a sensitized individual (verification with patch test is mandatory) • Protein contact dermatitis is also reported (rarely) • Like IHD a break from work improves the condition
Site	• Corresponds to contact site • Spread of the dermatitis around the site of the exposure
Morphology	• *Acute:* Skin is raw, dry, and scaly • *Subacute/chronic:* Redness, infiltration, and lichenification • Lesions present relatively ill-defined borders and are itchy

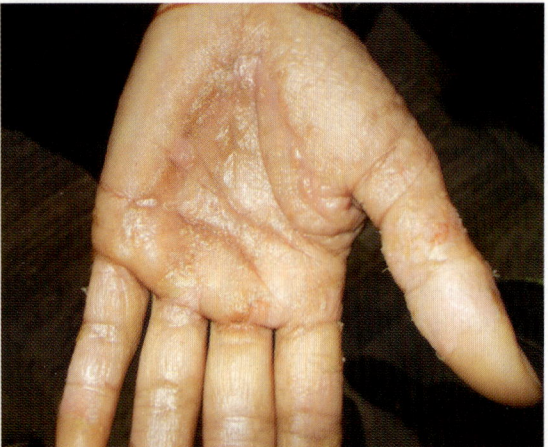

Fig. 15.4: Pompholyx on palm

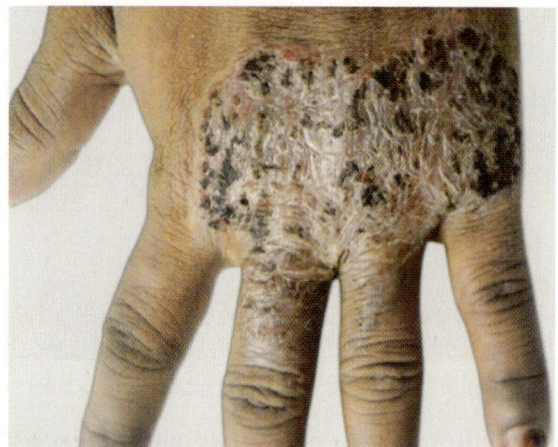

Fig. 15.6: Single well-defined discoid eczema on dorsum

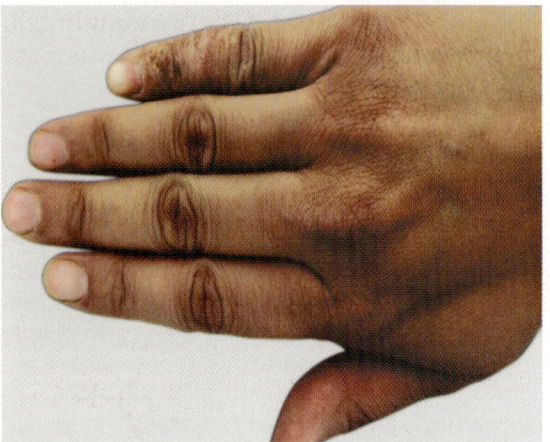

Fig. 15.5: The fifth digit depicts an area of pompholyx in the healing stage

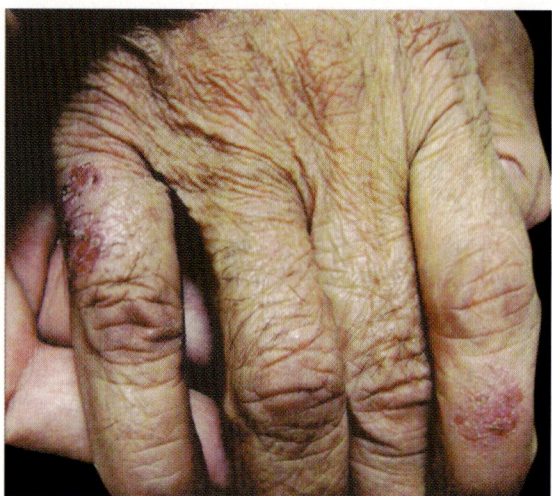

Fig.15.7: Discoid eczema on dorsum of hand of fingers

are atopy, infection, trauma, allergic sensitivity and emotional stress. Discoid eczema of the hands generally affect the dorsal aspect of hands or the back or sides of fingers (Figs 15.6 and 15.7). Single plaque is seen initially followed by appearance of secondary lesions on fingers or forearms. Secondary infection with *S. aureus* may occur.

Protein Contact Eczema

It is a type I hypersensitivity reaction mediated by IgE (allergen specific) in a sensitized individual. It is clinically characterized by chronic or recurrent dermatitis usually of the fingertips. Urticarial or vesicular lesions occur within minutes of contact with incriminated proteins (e.g. fruits, vegetables, spices, grains). Repeated exposure causes eczema. It is usually seen in cooks, caterers, food handlers, housewives).

Hybrid Hand Eczema

It combines aspects of ICD, ACD and atopic dermatitis.

Unclassified

In patients with chronic hand eczema, it is difficult to characterize the cause.

Hyperkeratotic (Tylotic) Hand Eczema

It is characterized by well-defined hyperkeratotic plaques on the palms and palmar surfaces of the fingers. Simultaneous involvement of plantar aspect of feet may be seen. It is common in middle-aged men. An Indian study (Minocha et al) has revealed contact sensitivity (to vegetables, detergents, metals, rubber) in patch test done in patients with hyperkeratotic hand eczema (Minocha et al). The condition is resistant to treatment. Figures 15.8 and 15.9 show a patient with hyperkeratotic hand eczema. Psoriasis is a close differential diagnosis. However, the latter has well demarcated lesions that are non-itchy (*see* Chapter 16).

Wear and Tear/Asteatotic/Housewives' Dermatitis

Various factors are involved in its pathogenesis. These are exposure to irritants, asteotosis, or friction. It is seen in occupations that involve wet work and exposure to detergents. Hence common in housewives and cleaners. The palmar skin of bilateral hands becomes dry, cracked and criss-crossed. Exudation and pruritus are not seen (Figs 15.10 and 15.11).

Fingertip Eczema/Pulpitis

Eczema develops on the palmar surface of the tips of fingers. Skin becomes dry, cracked and fissured (Figs 15.12 and 15.13). The condition can be due to irritant or allergic contact dermatitis.

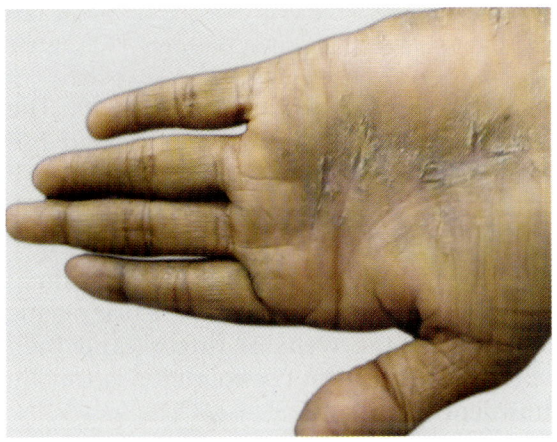

Fig. 15.8: Tylotic eczema on palm

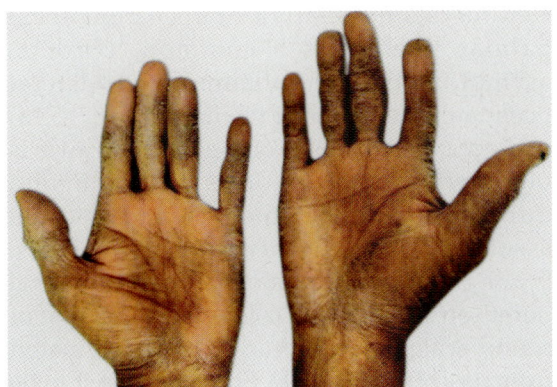

Fig. 15.9: Symmetrical chronic eczematous patches on the palms with tylotic eczema

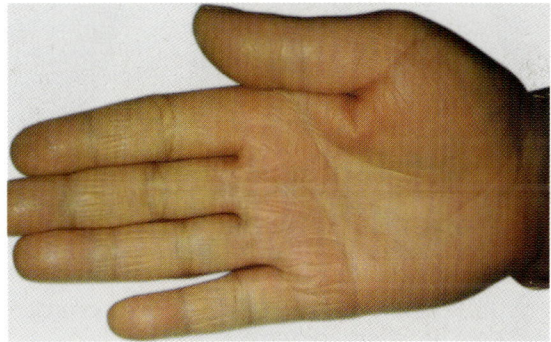

Fig. 15.10: Wear and tear dermatitis on palm

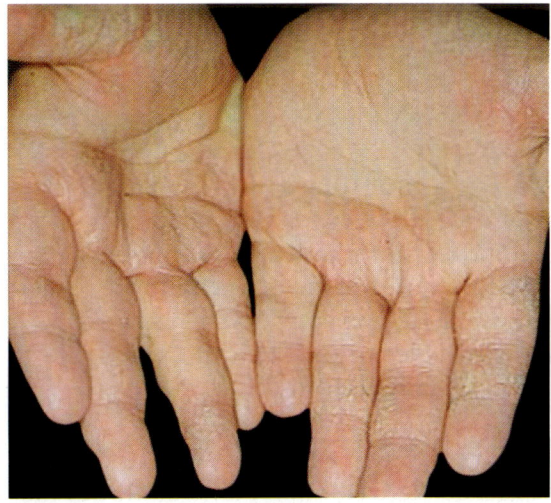

Fig. 15.11: Wear and tear dermatitis on bilateral palm

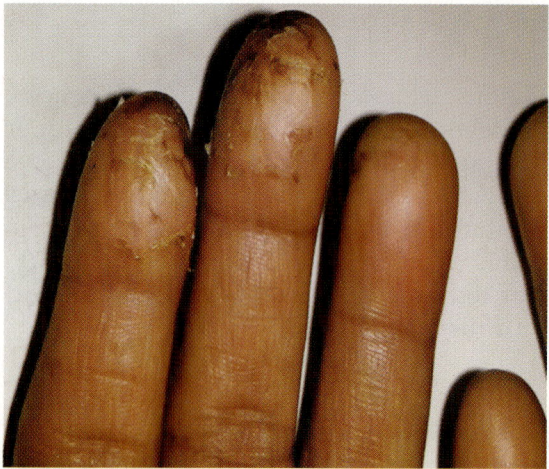

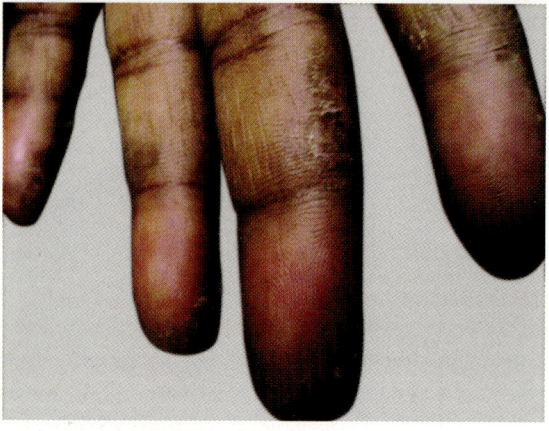

Figs 15.12 and 15.13: Fissuring with desquamation in a case of fingertip eczema

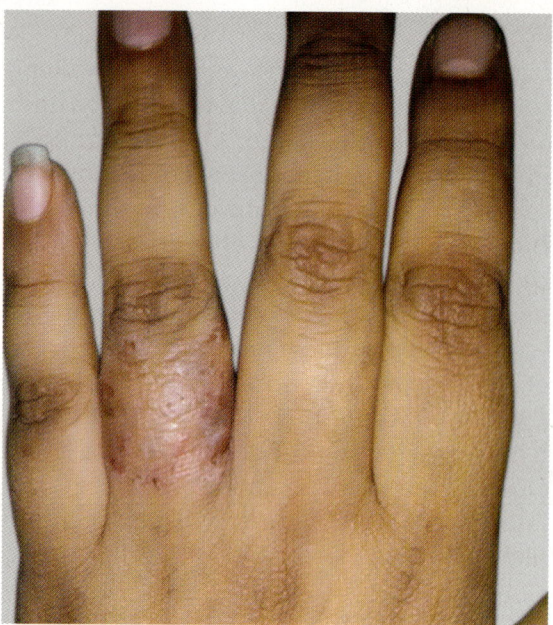

Fig. 15.14: Ring eczema

usually seen in middle-aged patients. The condition is associated with elevated IgE levels.

Gut/Slaughterhouse Eczema

It is seen in people who deal with animal carcasses in slaughterhouses. Vesicular plaque starts from the webs of fingers and then spreads to the sides. The condition is usually transient.

Ring Eczema

A patch of eczema develops under a ring and can spread to the adjacent skin. It occurs due to accumulation of soaps and detergents under the ring (Fig.15.14).

Apron Eczema

It involves the proximal palmar aspect of two adjacent fingers. It can extend onto the palmar skin over the metacarpophalangeal joints. It is usually seen in women. It can be due to irritant or allergic contact dermatitis.

Chronic Acral Dermatitis

It is characterized by hyperkeratotic papulo-vesicular eczema of hands and feet. It is

Recurrent Focal Palmar Peeling

Keratolysis exfoliativa or recurrent focal palmar peeling is a common, chronic, asymptomatic, non-inflammatory bilateral peeling of the palms of the hands (Fig. 15.15) and occasionally soles of the feet; its cause is unknown. The eruption is most common during the summer months and is often associated with sweaty palms and soles. Scaling starts simultaneously from several points on the palms or soles with 2 or 3 mm of round scales that appear to have originated from a ruptured vesicle. Some believe it to be associated with dyshidrosis and is believed to be a mild case of pompholyx.

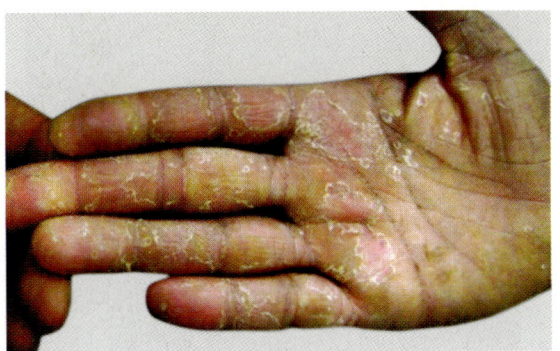

Fig. 15.15: Focal and annular patch of scaling on the palms in a case of keratolysis exfoliativa

DIFFERENTIAL DIAGNOSIS

Hand eczema may be confused with other dermatological conditions (Table 15.4).

MANAGEMENT

The management of HE shall be discussed under following headings.
1. Assessment of severity
2. Diagnostic (history and investigations); identifying etiological factors
3. Preventive and protective measures
4. Treatment

Assessment of Severity

Various scoring indices have been developed to assess the severity of hand eczema but are hardly used in clinical practice. The hand eczema severity index (HECSI) was developed as a clinical grading tool but is mainly used for research. The Dyshidrotic Eczema Area and Severity Index is a scoring system developed for the assessment of dyshidrotic eczema.

Diagnosis (History and Investigations)

History and Clinical Examination

1. A carefully taken history is the first step in diagnosing hand eczema. One should elicit history pertaining to mode of onset, frequency and duration of symptoms and any seasonal exacerbation. Details about exposure at workplace, history of contact with chemicals, oils, and wet work should be sought out. Exposure to allergens during household work as well as during leisure activities should be inquired. Personal or family history of atopy should be ruled out. Patient should be asked about treatment taken and any exposure to medication.
2. The localization of the lesions (e.g. palmar, dorsal, interdigital, wrist, involvement of the feet, and eczematous lesions at other body localizations) should be checked.
3. The morphology of the lesions (dry scaly skin, hyperkeratosis, fissures, vesicles, blister, etc.) should carefully examined.

Table 15.4: Differential diagnosis of hand eczema			
Location	Redness and scaling	Vesicles	Pustules
Dorsum of hand	• Atopic dermatitis • Irritant contact dermatitis • Lichen simplex chronicus • Nummular eczema • Psoriasis • Tinea	• Id reaction • Scabies (web spaces) • Tinea	• Bacterial infection • Psoriasis
Palmar surface	• Finger tip eczema • Hyperkeratotic eczema • Recurrent focal palmar peeling • Psoriasis • Tinea	• Allergic contact dermatitis • Pompholyx	• Bacterial infection • Pompholyx • Psoriasis

4. Time-course of flare up and remissions of lesions (seasonal variations, remission over weekends or holidays, the time duration of a flare up after re-exposure at the workplace, etc.) must be asked.

5. Exposure assessment of possible irritants and allergens at workplace, household, or leisure must be identified.

Investigation

A detailed investigation is useful apart from patch testing (Table 15.5).

Patch testing (Figs 15.16 and 15.17): Patch testing at present is the only scientific method to detect the cause of contact dermatitis. In various Indian studies, positive patch test ranges from 30 to 82% of patients with hands eczema. The vegetables, potassium dichromate and nickel are more common sensitizer found in most of the Indian studies. The most commonly used allergens are Indian standard

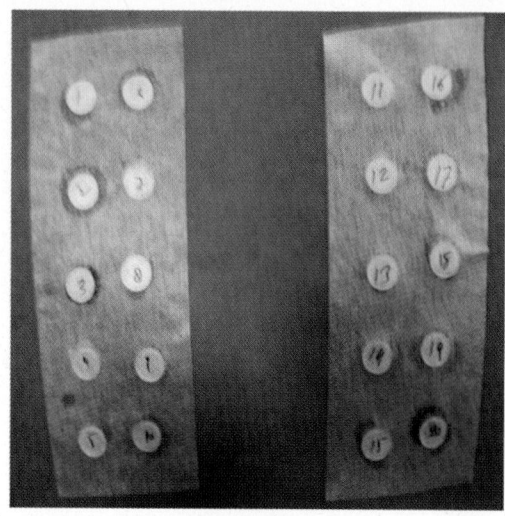

Fig. 15.16: Allergens applied on the back

series approved by CODFI. The Indian standard series is useful but insufficient. Hence, testing with vegetables and other suspected product are suggested along with standard series.

Table 15.5: Diagnostic work-up for a patient with hand eczema	
Investigations	
1. KOH mount	Done from active border of the lesion to rule out tinea
2. Gram stain	To rule out secondary bacterial infections in cases with oozing and purulent discharge
3. Absolute eosinophil count and IgE	To rule out atopic diathesis
4. Skin biopsy	In doubtful cases to differentiate form conditions like psoriasis
5. Patch testing	In cases of suspected ACD or cases failing to respond to treatment, chronic hand and foot eczema
6. 24 hours patch testing	With detergent and soap solutions (8% v/v) for patient in whom detergents are a cause of hand eczema (e.g. housewives, cleaners)
7. Prick test	In cases of suspected protein contact dermatitis or contact urticaria caused by latex or fish proteins
8. RAST	Radioallergosorbent test for specific IgE
9. RPA (RNase protection assay) test	This measures small quantities of RNA obtained from tape stripping of human skin and is very sensitive. The RPA test discriminates between irritant and allergic patch test reactions
10. Chemical spot test	For nickel (dimethylgloxime), chromate (diphenylcarbazide test), cobalt (cobalt cotton stick test), formaldehydes (lutidine test)

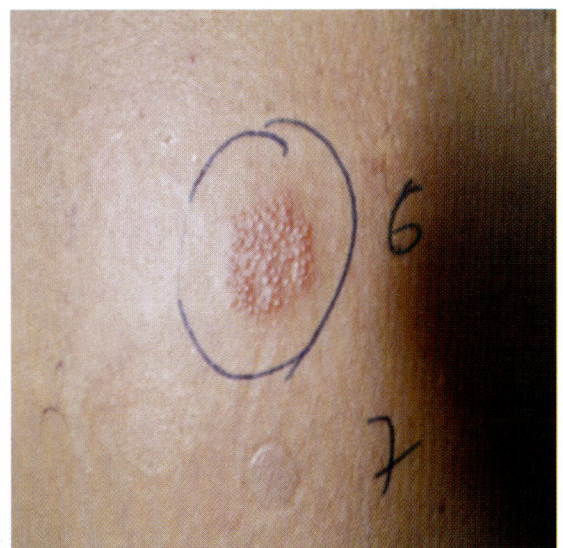

Fig. 15.17: Strong positive reaction (++) to potassium dichromate

Prick testing: Prick test should be done with standardized allergens and/or fresh food stuffs. Histamine as positive control and saline as negative control should be used. The maximum wheal diameter is measured in mm.

Skin Protection (Box 15.7)

Prevention

1. Appropriate changes in lifestyle should be carried out to minimize exposure to irritants and allergens. Patients in high-risk occupations, like cleaners, hairdressers, healthcare workers, foodhandlers, should be identified and educated appropriately. Patients should be informed about high-risk factors like wet work and low humidity. Wet hands for more than 2 hours daily, frequent hand washing >20 times/day and wearing tight fitting gloves for more than 2 hours per day are considered as wet hand according to German standard giving rise to irritant hand eczema.
2. Various protective measures can be adopted at the workplace and at home. Barrier creams can be used before and during work. These contain aluminium chlorhydrate,

Box 15.7: Skin protection program

1. Rinse your hands with lukewarm water, rinse and dry your hands thoroughly after washing.
2. Use protective gloves when starting wet work tasks.
3. Protective gloves should be used when necessary but for as short a time as possible.
4. Protective gloves should be intact and clean and dry inside.
5. When protective gloves are used for more than 10 min, cotton gloves should be worn underneath.
6. Do not wear rings at work.
7. Disinfectants should be used according to the recommendations for the work place.
8. Apply moisturizers on your hand during the working day and after your work select a lipid rich moisturizer free from fragrances and with preservatives having the lowest allergen potential.
9. Moisturizers should be applied all over the hands including finger webs, finger tips and back of the hands.
10. Take care also when doing house work, use protective gloves for dishwashing and warm gloves when going outside in winter.
11. Avoid contact with certain food items: tomatoes, peeling of oranges, citrus fruits, and such like. Avoid juice from fish, meat, and certain vegetables. The patient's own experience will show what must be avoided.
12. Avoid hair dying and potent allergens (i.e. p-phenylenediamine, acrylic compounds, nickel, etc.).

zinc oxide, talcum and have to be applied on intact skin. They decrease penetration of irritants. Alcohol-based hand rubs (containing emollients) and mild skin cleansers can be used for cleaning hands after work (instead of soaps and detergents). Gloves can be used to avoid exposure to irritants and allergens. In case of rubber allergy, recently a variety of gloves for medical use, including gloves with antigen removed, hypoallergenic gloves, powder-free gloves, and urethane gloves, have become commercially available.

3. Emollients and moisturizers should be used liberally after work. They moisturise the

skin and prevent drying. They provide protection from irritants and help restore the skin barrier. However, urea-containing moisturisers should be avoided as they increase skin permeability and might enhance penetration of a few irritants (Wohlrab et al). Emollients and moisturisers are the mainstay of prevention and treatment of chronic hand eczema.

TREATMENT (Table 15.6)

Although there are different therapeutic strategies for each group of HE, all patients should be educated and should adhere to skin protection measures (see above) and lifestyle changes to minimize exposure to allergens or irritants.

Allergen avoidance may also be beneficial, but not all contact allergies are clinically relevant. A good overview is given in Fig. 15.18 but most clinicians use their own combination therapies. The treatment of hand eczema must take into account the following features in order to perform the correct management and therapy:

- Disease etiology (atopic, allergic, irritant, vesicular)
- Acuteness (acute vs. chronic eczema)
- Morphology (redness, scaling, lichenification, blistering, hyperkeratosis, rhagades, pruritus, etc.)
- Location (dorsal aspects of hands, interdigital spaces, palms)

In the acute stage, it is important to soothe the irritated skin with wet compresses or soaks (saline, aluminium acetate, potassium permanganate solution may be used), and not

Table 15.6: A summary of the treatment options in hand eczema

Skin protection program	Topical	Systemic
1. Education 2. Avoidance and substitution 3. Protection 4. Prevention 5. Lifestyle changes	1. Moisturizers 2. Keratolytics (salicylic acid 20%, urea 5–10%) 3. Corticosteroids (1*) 4. Calcineurin inhibitors (tacrolimus, pimecrolimus) (2*) 5. Retinoids (bexarotene) 6. Coal tar, ichthyol 7. Dithranol 8. Vitamin D$_3$ derivatives (calcipotriol and maxacalcitol 9. Calcipotriol/betamethasone ointment combination 10. Botulinum toxin 11. Iontophoresis 12. Potassium dichromate, aluminium acetate	1. Corticosteroids 2. Retinoids-acitretin (3*), alitretinoin (1*) 3. Cyclosporine (2*) 4. Methotrexate 5. Azathioprine 6. Mycophenolate mofetil 7. Ranitidine 8. Interferon 9. Intravenous immunoglobulins 10. Infliximab 11. H1 anti-histamines
Physical therapy	Others	
1. Phototherapy (UVA, UVB, PUVA) (2*) 2. Ionizing radiation: X-rays, radiotherapy, Grenz rays.	1. Low nickel diet and short course of oral disulfiram therapy disodium cromoglycate [HE-04] 2. Iron therapy with low nickel diet 3. Low nickel diet with disodium chromoglycate 4. Oxybutynin 5. Others—triethylenetetramine, topical antibiotics	

Level of evidence*

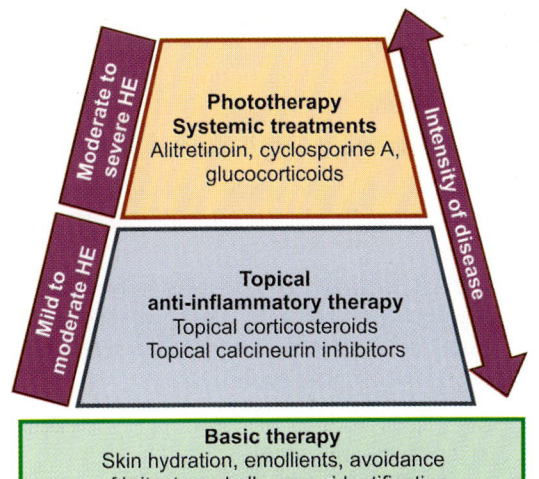

Fig. 15.18: Overview of therapy of hand eczema according to the severity (English et al)

use occlusive ointments. In the sub-acute stage, creams may be introduced and in the chronic stage, ointments. Topical treatment with emollients and topical corticosteroids in addition to skin protection measures form the mainstay of therapy to control an acute flare of hand eczema.

Generally, mild hand eczema should be treated with anti-inflammatory drugs [topical corticosteroids (TCS)] together with a proper skin protection measures. This therapy, if performed quickly, is effective in controlling the symptoms in lots of these patients.

The short- and long-term management aims to prevent new relapses and to avoid the condition becoming chronic (which happens in a considerable number of cases despite basic therapy and potent TCS). It is important to note that a complete functional regeneration of the epidermal barrier requires several weeks or months after healing.

Chronic hand eczema is very difficult to treat and manage. They should be referred immediately and the treatment should not be delayed. A successful management requires treatments that restore the skin barrier and control the inflammation.

Topical Therapy

The specific and proper use of topical corticosteroids (TCS) remains the first-line anti-inflammatory treatment of HE. Though they are effective, skin atrophy may contribute to further weakening of the skin barrier and further inflammation.

The choice of the potency of corticosteroids and the duration of treatment depend on the morphology, location, and severity of hand eczema.

It is commonly suggested to use immediately a potent to very potent steroid (according to the severity of the disease and the age of the patient) once or twice a day, followed by a less potent preparation for a few days.

In mild to severe forms of HE, TCS have to be combined with the basic therapy. It is worthy to remember that the hand barrier is not restored at all after the end of the treatment. Thus a continued use of a nonsteroidal topical therapy (emollient) is necessary together with a basic education.

An overview of morphology specific topical therapy is given in Table 15.7.

1. *Moisturizers:* They help to restore the skin barrier that is affected by eczema. They should be applied frequently and liberally. Ointments may be preferred over creams. The latter contain preservatives that can be sensitizing and emulsifiers that can act as irritants. White petrolatum is the moisturiser of choice as it is both an emollient and a barrier cream.

2. *Keratolytics:* These can be used in cases of chronic hand eczema especially the hyperkeratotoic type. Keratolytics include salicylic acid (up to 20%) and urea (5–10%). Urea increases the water binding capacity of skin. However, it might enhance the penetration of a few chemicals as mentioned previously.

3. *Topical steroids:* Topical steroids and moisturizers are the mainstay of treatment of hand eczema. Potent topical steroids can be used initially for one

Table 15.7: Morphology specific topical therapy (Diepgen et al)	
Vesicular ("dyshidrosiform")	• Astringent solutions (i.e. potassium permanganate 0.025%), zinc oxide barrier cream • If hyperhidrosis, possible used aluminum chloride hexahydrate
Weeping/superinfection	• Moisturizing (containing glycerol, urea 5–10%, coal tar, etc.) • Astringent solution • Disinfectant and antibacterial (chlorhexidine, polyhexanide, povidone iodine, hydrogen peroxide, silver sulfadiazine) • Treat immediately the superinfection (when it is clinically manifest) with pharmacological treatment
Hyperkeratosis	• Keratolytic agents (salicylic acid-based ointments, ointments containing sodium chloride or urea)
Rhagades/fissures	Hydrocolloid dressings (rhagades)
Subacute eczematous reaction/ lichenification	Moisturizing (containing glycerol, urea 5–10%, coal tar, etc.)
Dry, scaling	Moisturizing (containing glycerol, urea 5–10%, coaltar, etc.)

month followed by maintenance therapy three times per week (Drake et al). Potent steroids are more effective than moderately potent steroids (Moller et al). They also reduce the risk of recurrences. However, long-term use can cause side effects like skin atrophy (causing further weakening of skin barrier), tachyphylaxis and adrenal suppression. Calcineurin inhibitors can be added along with a moderately-potent topical steroid to reduce the side effects. Worsening of eczema suggests contact allergy to steroid cream or other ingredients and patch test should be done in such cases. Some authors advocate the "soak and smear" technique where mid- to high-potency steroids are applied after thorough hydration of the hands with an emollient.

4. *Intradermal injection of steroid:* Intradermal injection of triamcinolone acetonide (10 mg/ml) for recalcitrant localized patches of hand eczema has been recommended.

5. *Topical calcineurin inhibitors (tacrolimus/ pimecrolimus):* These are immunomodulators and act as steroid sparing agents.

These are not licenced for the treatment of hand eczema, however, trials have shown favorable results. These can also be combined with moderate potent steroids for maintenance therapy. Side effects include mild burning sensation that is transient and sensitivity to light.

6. *Topical retinoids:* Topical bexarotene gel has shown good efficacy in a randomised trial in patients with chronic severe hand eczema (Hanifin et al). It can cause side effects like irritation of skin, burning sensation and flare of dermatitis.

7. *Topical coal tar:* It can be used in patients with subacute andchronic eczema. It has anti-inflammatory, anti-proliferative and antipruritic effects.

8. *Vitamin D derivatives:* A recent study showed good results with topical vitamin D_3 derivatives (calcipotriol 50 μg/g and maxacalcitol 25 μg/g) in recalcitrant hyperkeratotic palmoplantar eczema and suggested them as safe and effective alternate forms of treatment in the same.

9. *Botulinum toxin:* It can be used as an adjunctive therapy for vesicular eczema associated with hyperhidrosis. Significant drop in DASI score has been seen.

10. *Iontophoresis:* Iontophoresis is the transfer of ions through the skin induced by direct current. In a randomized half-side study of 20 patients with mild-to-moderate dyshidrotic eczema, patients received steroid free topical therapy of both hands and daily unilateral tap water iontophoresis. Significant improvement in eczema, as assessed by DASI scores, was noted only in iontophoresis treated hands.

Systemic Therapy

This is largely reserved for chronic hand eczema. The ideal drug would be alitretinoin but in its absence as is the case in India, an useful option remains cyclosporine. It is approved for atopic dermatitis (of hands), and it can be used in severe, treatment-refractory HE, as a second-line treatment in patients unresponsive to alitretinoin or where the use of alitretinoin is not possible or is contraindicated.

1. **Oral corticosteroids:** These can be used for the management of acute flares. However, side effects preclude use of oral steroids for long term. Dexamethasone or methylprednisolone pulse therapy is a feasible option in severe extensive dermatitis.

2. **Oral retinoids:** There is a little evidence supporting the use of oral retinoids in hand eczema. One study reported 50% improvement with oral acitretin 40 mg daily in patients with hyperkeratotic hand eczema (Pederson et al). Hence, combined therapy may be used. Alitretinoin (9-cis-retinoic acid) is an endogenous physical retinoid that is structurally similar to isotretinoin. It is the only evidence-based treatment option for patients with severe chronic hand eczema who are unresponsive to topical steroids. Randomized controlled trials (RCTs) have shown good response with alitretinoin 10–30 mg once daily for up to 24 weeks (Ruzicka et al). Also side effects are less compared to other retinoids. Common side effects with alitretinoin are headache, mucosal and cutaneous dryness, reduction in TSH levels and hypertriglyceridemia. When using alitretinoin, it is important to counsel the female patients regarding contraception during treatment and one month after stopping treatment.

3. **Cyclosporine:** Cyclosporine is the most frequently used especially in patients with history of atopic eczema. It is given in a dose of 2.5–3 mg/kg/day and gradually tapered over a few months. Serum electrolytes, creatinine and blood pressure should be monitored during treatment.

4. **Azathioprine:** Azathioprine is used in a dose of 2 mg/kg/day. Patients with atopic dermatitis respond well to azathioprine.

5. **Methotrexate:** Methotrexate, in a dose of 5–20 mg once weekly, has been found to be effective in hand eczema (Shaffrali et al). It should be remembered that all immunosuppressive agents pose a risk of serious side effects (hematological toxicity, hepatic dysfunction, opportunistic infections, etc.) and should only be used in unresponsive patients.

6. **Mycophenolate mofetil:** Mycophenolate mofetil is a relatively new immunomodulating agent that inhibits the synthesis of guanosine nucleotides. A case report described a patient with a four-year history of recurrent dyshidrotic eczema resistant to corticosteroids, iontophoresis, and phototherapy who responded to 1.5 g of mycophenolate mofetil administered twice daily. Complete clearing was achieved in four weeks and the dose was tapered gradually over 12 months without recurrence.

7. **Ranitidine:** Ranitidine works better than placebo in double blind placebo-controlled trial in atopic hand eczema.

8. Other, occasionally used therapies (off-label) such as interferon, intravenous

immunoglobulins and infliximab. The use of systemic antihistamines may be appropriate in some patients for the symptomatic relief of itching and redness, but they have not been shown to alter the overall course of hand eczema.

Physical Therapy

1. **Phototherapy:** It is widely used for hand eczema. PUVA, broadband UVB and UVA1 all are used in the treatment. A study has shown that PUVA is more efficacious than UVB in chronic eczema of hands. However, a few side effects, e.g. nausea (due to oral methoxsalen), edema and pain, can occur. Long-term side effects include increased risk of skin cancer.

    This treatment can also be useful in combination with other topical or systemic therapies. It can be a therapeutic option in moderate to severe forms, as well as in HE unresponsive to TCS, including also very potent TCS.

2. **Radiotherapy:** Grenz rays and superficial X-rays both have been used in the treatment of hand eczema. Superficial X-rays penetrate deeper and hence are more effective. But Grenz rays are safer.

Others

1. **Low nickel diet and short course of oral disulfiram therapy:** A study done by Sharma AD have shown low nickel diet and short course of oral disulfiram therapy can be considered as a good and safe option for the control of chronic, recurring hand eczema in nickel-sensitive individuals.

2. **Iron therapy:** It was observed that adequate iron intake reduces nickel absorption from intestine. Iron is absorbed in preference to nickel by divalent metal transporter (DMT) because of high affinity.

3. **Disodium cromoglycate:** Some reports have shown that oral disodium cromoglycate is effective in patients whose nickel allergy is confirmed and worsened by dietary intake of nickel.

4. **Oxybutynin:** There is remarkable improvement of relapsing dyshidrotic eczema after treatment of co-existant hyperhidrosis with oxybutynin.

Bibliography

1. Diepgen TL, Elsner P, Schliemann S, Fartasch M, Köllner A, Skudlik C, John SM, Worm M, Deutsche Dermatologische Gesellschaft. Guideline on the management of hand eczema ICD-10 Code: L20. L23. L24. L25. L30. J Dtsch Dermatol Ges 2009;7 Suppl 3:S1–16.

2. Drake LA, Dinehart SM, Farmer ER, et al. Guidelines of care for the use of topical glicocorticosteroids. J Am Acad Dermatol 1996; 35:615–9.

3. English J, Aldridge R, Gawkrodger DJ, Kownacki S, Statham B, White JM, Williams J. Consensus statement on the management of chronic hand eczema. Clin Exp Dermatol 2009;34(7):761–9.

4. Hanifin JM, Stevens V, Sheth P, et al. Novel treatment of chronic severe hand dermatitis with bexarotene gel. Br J Dermatol 2004; 150(3):545–53.

5. Jensen CS, Menne T, Johansen JD. Systemic contact dermatitis after oral exposure to nickel: a review with a modified meta-analysis. Contact Dermatitis 2006; 54:79–86.

6. Meding B, Swanbeck G. Epidemiology of different types of hand eczema in an industrial city. Acta Derm Venereol 1989; 69: 227–33.

7. Meding B, Swanbeck G. Contact Dermatitis 1990;23:154.

8. Minocha YC, Dogra A, Sood VK. Contact sensitivity in palmar hyperkeratotic dermatitis. Indian J Dermatol Venerol Leprol 1983;59: 60–3.

9. Moller H, Svartholm H, Dahl G. Intermittent maintenance therapy in chronic hand eczema with clobetasol propionate and fluprednilen acetate. Curr Med Res Opin 1983;8:640–4.

10. Ruzicka T, Lynde CW, Jemec GB, Diepgen T, Berth-Jones J, Coenraads PJ, et al. Efficacy and safety of oral alitretinoin (9-cis retinoic acid) in patients with severe chronic hand eczema refractory to topical corticosteroids: Results of a randomized, double-blind, placebo-controlled, multicentre trial. Br J Dermatol 2008;158:808–17.

11. Shaffrali FC, Colver GB, Messenger AG, Gawkrodger DJ. Experience with low-dose

methotrexate for the treatment of eczema in the elderly. J Am Acad Dermatol 2003;48:417–9.

12. Simpson EL, Thompson MM, Hanifin JM. Prevalence and morphology of hand eczema in patients with atopic dermatitis. Dermatitis 2006; 17:123–27.

13. Thestrup-Pederson K, Andersen KE, Menne T, Veien NK. Treatment of hyperkeratotic dermatitis of the palms (eczema keratoticum) with oral acitretin. A single-blind placebo-controlled study. Acta Derm Venereol 2001;81:353–5.

14. Wohlrab W. The influence of urea on the penetration kinetics of topically applied corticosteroids. Acta Derm Venereol (Stockh) 1984;64:233-8.

15. Vocks E, Plötz SG, Ring J. The Dyshidrotic Eczema Area and Severity Index - A Score Developed for the Assessment of Dyshidrotic Eczema. Dermatology 1999;198:265–269.

16. Thyssen JP, Carlsen BC, Menne T et al. Filaggrin null mutations increase the risk and persistence of hand eczema in subjects with atopic dermatitis: results from a general population study. Br J Dermatol 2010; 163: 115–20.

17. Yang M, Chang JM. Successful treatment of refractory chronic hand eczema with calcipotriol/betamethasone ointment: A report of three cases. Experimental and therapeutic medicine. 2015;10: 1943–1946.

18. Epstein E. Hand dermatitis: Practical management and current concepts. J Am Acad Dermatol 1984;10:395–424.

19. Veien NK, Kaaber K, Larsen PO, Nielsen AO, Thestrup-Pedersen K. Ranitidine treatment of hand eczema in patients with atopic dermatitis: A double blind placebo controlled trial. J Am Acad Dermatol 1995;32:1056–7.

20. Sehgal VN, Srivastava G, Dogra S. Tacrolimus in dermatology: Pharmacokinetics, mechanism of action, drug interactions dosages and side-effects-Part 1. Skinmed 2008;7:27–30.

21. Reitamo S, Granlund H. Cyclosporine A in the treatment of chronic dermatitis of the hands. Br J Dermatol 1994;130:75–8.

22. Hanifin JM, Stevens V, Sheth P, Breneman D. Novel treatment of chronic severe hand dermatitis with bexarotene gel. Br J Dermatol 2004;150:545–53.

23. Egawa K. Topical vitamin D3 derivatives in treating hyperkeratotic palmoplantar eczema: A report of 5 patients. J Dermatol 2005;32:381–6.

24. Lakshmi C, Srinivas CR. Hand eczema: An update. Indian J Dermatol Venereol Leprol 2012;78:569–82.

25. Sehgal VN, Aggarwal AK, Srivastava G, Sharma AD. Hand dermatitis: Current treatment options. Indian J Dermatol Venereol Leprol 2008;74:433–5.

26. Pickenaker A, Luger TA, Schwarz T. Dyshidrotic eczema treated with mycophenolate mofetil. Arch Dermatol 1998;134:378–9.

27. Markantoni V, Kouris A, Armyra K, Vavouli C and Kontochristopoulos G. Remarkable improvement of relapsing dyshidrotic eczema after treatment of coexistant hyperhidrosis with oxybutynin. Dermatol Ther 2014;27: 365–368.

28. Georgieva FG. Hand eczema and its impact on wellbeing and quality of life of patients. J of IMAB 2017 Jan-Mar;23(1)

29. Sharma AD. Disulfiram and low nickel diet in the management of hand eczema: A clinical study. Indian J Dermatol Venereol Leprol 2006;72:113–8.

30. Diepgen TL, Agner T, Aberer W, Berth-Jones J, Cambazard F, Elsner P, McFadden J and Coenraads PJ Management of chronic hand eczema. Contact Dermatitis 2007; 57: 203–210.

16

Hyperkeratotic Eczema of the Palms

Kabir Sardana, Ananta Khurana

Hyperkeratotic eczema of the palms (also called hyperkeratotic hand eczema) is a relatively frustrating recalcitrant form of hand dermatitis which more often than not gets labeled as psoriasis and has then different connotations for the clinician and the patient.

CLINICAL FEATURES

Morphology: Although the nomenclature and the clinical and pathological presentations of the variants of hand eczema often overlap and render the diagnostic classification imprecise, this condition presents as chronic, scaly, slightly erythematous, hyperkeratotic, fissure-prone plaques on the palms (Fig. 16.1a). Typically, plaques are discrete, with relatively sharp margins (Fig. 16.1b). They have a multifocal and symmetrical distribution (Fig. 16.1c). Sometimes the plaques coalesce together to cover most of the palmar surface. They typically occur on the central palms (Fig. 16.1a). The border of the palms and the volar surfaces of the fingers may also be involved (Fig. 16.2). The eruption tends to spare dorsal hand and fingertips. Plantar involvement is seen in some cases.

Symptoms: The eruption may be asymptomatic but in nearly half of the patients, it is itchy. When fissures are present, it may be painful.

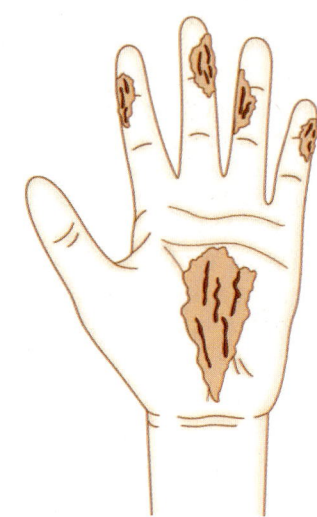

Fig. 16.1a: A depiction of the sites of involvement in hyperkeratotic eczema including the **palms** and **volar** aspects of fingers

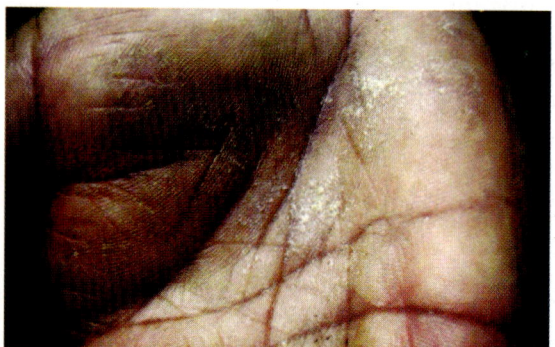

Fig. 16.1b: A hyperkeratotic plaque in the center of the palm

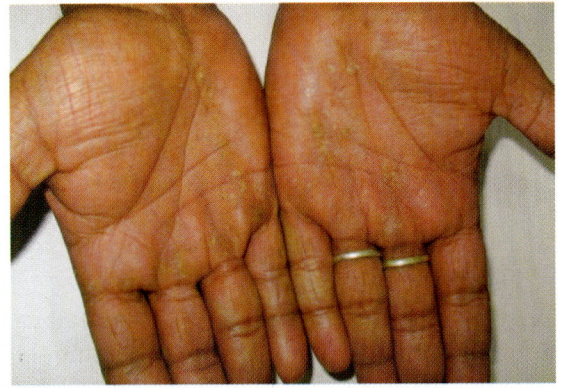
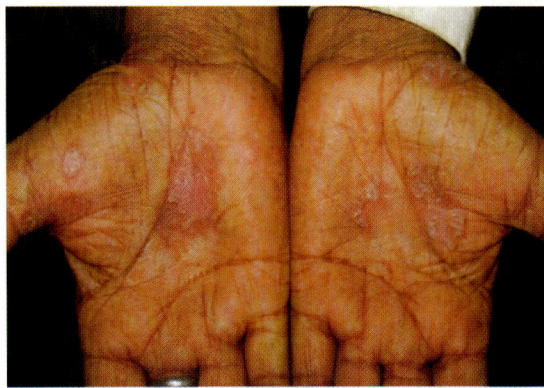

Fig. 16.1c: Multifocal and symmetrical involvement of the palms

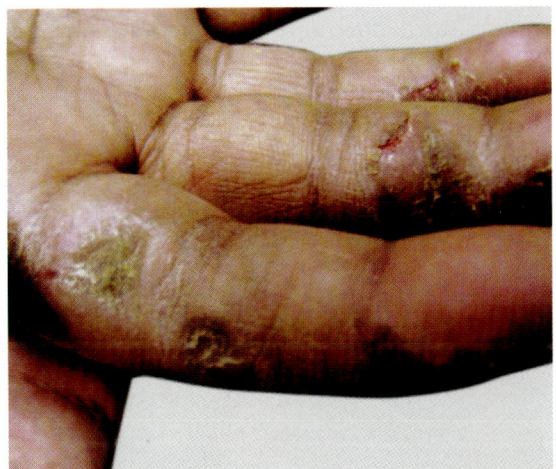

Fig. 16.2: Fissured, thick plaques on the volar aspects of the fingers

EPIDEMIOLOGY

Hyperkeratotic eczema of the palms constitutes 2–13% of hand eczema. Its prevalence varies in different populations. Compared to other types of hand eczema, the hyperkeratotic type typically affects older age groups. It is most prevalent in people 40–60 years of age. This entity is more common in men than women.

Some seasonal variability in severity of symptoms has been reported. In one study, 30% of the patients with hyperkeratotic hand dermatitis experienced some degree of exacerbation in summers and 70% in winters (Chopra A).

ETIOLOGY

Hyperkeratotic eczema of the palms is considered an endogenous dermatitis. The etiology is unknown. The patients usually have no relevant irritant exposure or contact sensitization, patch tests are usually negative, and the incidence of atopy is not greater than in the general population. The prevalence of psoriasis in close relatives does not differ from what can be found in the general population.

Although some authors consider hyperkeratotic hand dermatitis as an entity independent of mechanical irritation, some use the term "frictional hand dermatitis" to describe a subset of hyperkeratotic hand dermatitis that is precipitated by repeated mechanical trauma and friction to the hands (Hersle K). Frictional hand dermatitis is usually seen in manual workers and is more prominent on the dominant hand, where the mechanical stress is more severe. Once removed from the repeated mechanical trauma, the eruption improves after a few days to months, depending on the severity of the dermatitis. At least in some cases, what we call frictional hand dermatitis may actually be a form of chronic irritant contact dermatitis or may be palmar psoriasis with Koebner phenomenon.

There is a debate about whether hyperkeratotic eczema is merely a variant of psoriasis as the histologic features of palmoplantar psoriasis and eczema overlap with each other (see below).

HISTOLOGY

The characteristic histologic features of hyperkeratotic hand eczema include spongiosis and psoriasiform hyperplasia of the epidermis, although the elongation of the rete ridges is usually not as regular as in typical cases of psoriasis. Overlying compact orthokeratosis with small foci of parakeratosis is typical. The dilated blood vessels in the upper dermis are surrounded by a moderately dense mononuclear cell infiltrate. Lymphocyte exocytosis may be prominent in the epidermis, but there are usually no neutrophils (Weedon D). Histopathological findings cannot differentiate hyperkeratotic eczema of the palms from other types of chronic hand dermatitis.

Many features of eczematous palmar dermatitis overlap with those of plaque-type palmar psoriasis. Both dermatoses of this skin area share similar histologic features (Posada C). Some histologic features that have been suggested to be helpful in differentiating *psoriasis* from *eczematous dermatitis* include:

a. The absence of granular layer
b. Regular epidermal hyperplasia
c. Thinned suprapapillary plate
d. Tortuous capillaries in the papillary dermis
e. Lack of spongiosis

In 2007, Aydin et al conducted a study comparing histologic findings of palmoplantar psoriasis with those of palmoplantar eczema. The patients with eczema were not limited to hyperkeratotic type. Diagnostic criteria for distinguishing these two were not described, except for the presence of psoriatic lesions in other body areas in patients with psoriasis. Interestingly, in this study, spongiosis and vesiculation were more common in patients clinically classified as having palmoplantar psoriasis than in patients with dermatitis. One study demonstrated that a significant difference exists in the thickness of the granular layer between psoriasis and hand eczema, which might be helpful in differentiating between

these two conditions. There was no difference between psoriasis and hyperkeratotic hand eczema (Park JY). In our opinion and experience, these two entities are different as we have seen patients with no evidence of psoriasis anywhere else in the body , with a non-diagnostic biopsy (Figs 16.3 and 16.4).

Dermoscopy

Dermoscopic features of hand eczema have recently been described. The most commonly reported feature is focally distributed yellow scales followed by brownish orange dots (Fig. 16.5) on a yellowish/less erythematous background and yellowish orange crusts

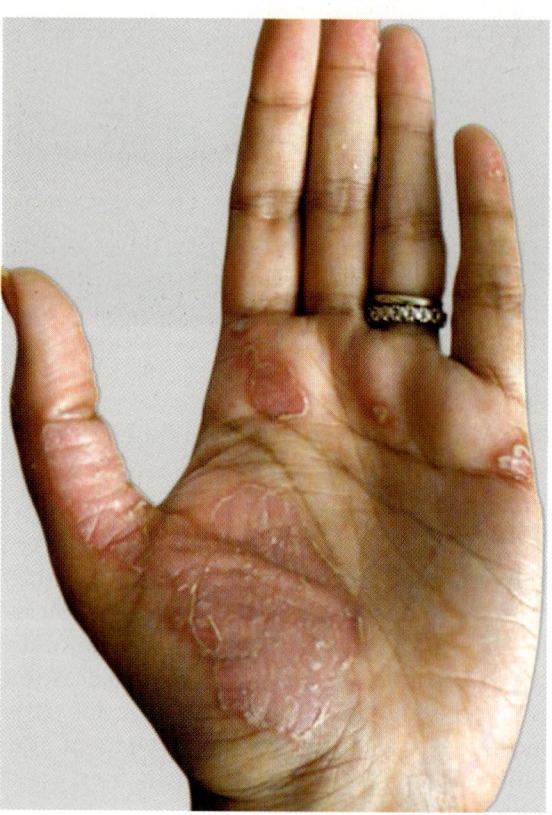

Fig. 16.3: This patient was diagnosed as psoriasis and offered biologicals as the patient could not tolerate methotrexate. In our experience, merely having hyperkeratotic psoriasiform plaques on the palms does not make it psoriasis. A repeat evaluation of biopsy at two centers could not confirm a diagnosis of psoriasis

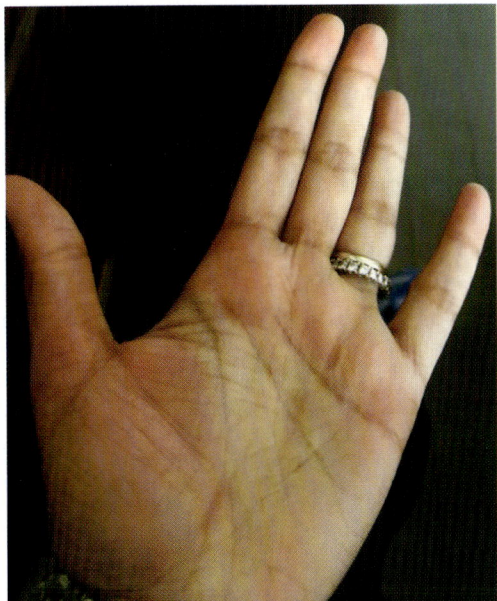

Fig. 16.4: Topical emollients with a calcipotriol steroid combination achieved heartening results

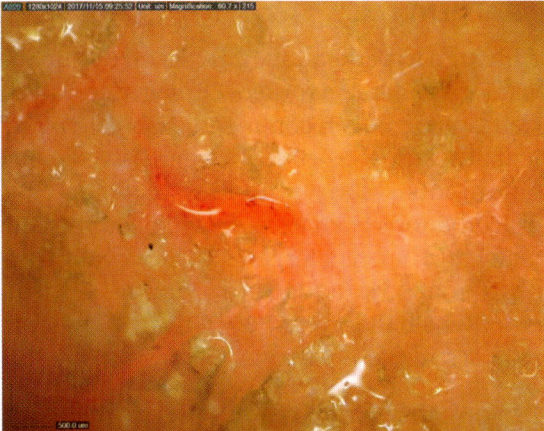

Fig. 16.5: Dermoscopy of hand eczema showing focal vascular pattern and brownish red dots

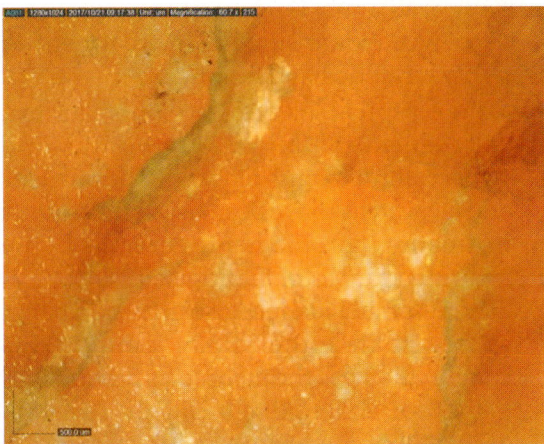

Fig. 16.6: Diffuse yellow background with dirty white scales and crusts

(Fig. 16.6). Less common features include focally distributed dotted vessels, patchily distributed white scales and sparse yellowish-orange crusts. This is similar to dermoscopy of eczema elsewhere on the body.

DIFFERENTIAL DIAGNOSIS

Other types of hand dermatitis, such as contact dermatitis or atopic dermatitis, may be hyperkeratotic in chronic stages. Distribution of lesions and sharp margins of plaques in hyperkeratotic eczema are clinically useful findings.

Acrokeratosis paraneoplastica (Bazex syndrome) may be difficult to distinguish from hyperkeratotic eczema of the palms and palmoplantar psoriasis clinically and histologically.

Distribution of lesions is usually a clue to the diagnosis. The lesions appear around the tips of the fingers and nail folds, dorsal hand and foot, the nose, and the conchae of the ears.

The term "keratoderma climactericum" is used to describe a condition that is sometimes similar to hyperkeratotic hand eczema clinically and pathologically, occurring on the soles in females over the age of 45 years. Pressure areas, such as the heel and the forefoot, are involved first. Keratoderma climactericum is generally a clinical diagnosis, based on the age and sex of the patient and on typical clinical findings, including initial involvement of the feet.

Palmoplantar keratoderma is seen in a variety of genetic disorders and syndromes. Reiter's syndrome (keratoderma blennorrhagica), cutaneous T cell lymphoma, palmoplantar pustulosis, lichen planus, pityriasis rubra pilaris, lupus erythematosus, Darier's disease, syphilis, and tinea manuum should be considered in differential diagnosis of hyperkeratotic hand dermatitis.

TREATMENT

Although hyperkeratotic (HK) hand dermatitis is not considered a form of contact dermatitis, traditionally, the recommendation is to avoid irritants and to encourage aggressive use of emollients. Many patients suffer disease exacerbations from excessive exposure to hot water and harsh detergents. Use of cool water, mild soaps, adequate protection, and an emollient hand cream is critical to prevent relapses in these patients.

Topical Agents

a. Topical **corticosteroids** are usually first-line treatment for hyperkeratotic hand dermatitis.
b. Topical **vitamin D₃** derivatives have been used with some success in treatment of hyperkeratotic hand eczema.
c. **Other** topical treatments such as tar, calcineurin inhibitors (tacrolimus and pimecrolimus), and retinoids (bexarotene and tazarotene) have been used successfully in treating chronic hand eczema. Using tazarotene in combination with a topical corticosteroid like clobetasol may be a better choice than either drug alone. This combination has the theoretical advantages of the topical steroid reducing the irritation of the vitamin A analog and the vitamin A analog potentially reducing the risk of atrophy associated with the topical corticosteroid.
d. In patients with significant hyperkeratosis, topical lactic acid 5–12% or urea 10–40% preparations may be added to the above treatment. These will reduce the scale and enhance the penetration of the active agents.

Phototherapy

Various forms of phototherapy have been used though PUVA is a better option and safer, if used topically in the so-called "paint PUVA" protocol. Though there are reports of the use of NB-UVB, its penetration is less than UVA and is thus would not be as effective as PUVA, though some trials report an equipotent effect.

A study compared the efficacy of cream PUVA therapy with monochromatic excimer light therapy. Ten patients with psoriasis of the palms and soles were randomly assigned to receive cream PUVA on one side and 308 nm UVB on the contralateral side for 5 weeks. At the end of the treatment period, the test groups showed similar psoriasis area and severity index (PASI) score reduction (308 nm UVB, 64%; cream PUVA, 65%) (Neumann NJ).

Systemic Agents

Acitretin is considered an effective treatment for hyperkeratotic hand eczema and is especially useful for thinning out thick hyperkeratotic areas and making the lesions more susceptible to other treatments such as topical agents and phototherapy. A dose of 30 mg daily is good enough for a predictable response. A controlled study of comparative efficacy of oral acitretin, 25–50 mg/day, and topical betamethasone/salicylic acid ointment for chronic hyperkeratotic palmoplantar dermatitis showed that acitretin was significantly better than ointment after 30 days, and improvement persisted 5 months after suspension of treatment. Lesions improved more rapidly with acitretin, with minimal side effects. Patients were more satisfied with acitretin (Capella GL).

In severe refractory cases, cyclosporine A 3–5 mg/kg, mycophenolate mofetil 2 gm/day, or methotrexate 10–25 mg once weekly, may be considered.

Alitretinoin (not available in India) may also be a highly effective therapeutic for refractory disease of the hyperkeratotic presentation of hand dermatitis.

Bibliography

1. Aydin O, Engin B, O ğ uz O, Ilvan S, Demirkesen C. Non-pustular palmoplantar psoriasis: is histologic differentiation from eczematous dermatitis possible? J Cutan Pathol 2008;35(2):169–73.

2. Chopra A, Maninder, Gill SS. Hyperkeratosis of palms and soles: clinical study. Indian J Dermatol Venereol Leprol 1997;63(2):85–8.

3. Diepgen TL, Andersen KE, Brandao FM, Bruze M, Bruynzeel DP, Frosch P, et al. Hand eczema classification: a cross-sectional, multicentre study of the aetiology and morphology of hand eczema. Br J Dermatol 2009;160(2):353–8.

4. Errichetti E, Stinco G.Dermoscopy in differential diagnosis of palmar psoriasis and chronic hand eczema. J Dermatol 2016 Apr;43(4):423–5.

5. Hersle K, Mobacken H. Hyperkeratotic dermatitis of the palms. Br J Dermatol 1982;107(2):195–201.

6. Neumann NJ, Mahnke N, Korpusik D, Stege H, Ruzicka T. Treatment of palmoplantar psoriasis with monochromatic excimer light (308-nm) versus cream PUVA. Acta Derm Venereol 2006; 86(1):22–4.

7. Park JY, Cho EB, Park EJ, Park HR, Kim KH, Kim KJ. The histopathological differentiation between palmar psoriasis and hand eczema: A retrospective review of 96 cases. J Am Acad Dermatol 2017 Jul;77(1):130–135.

8. Pettey AA, Balkrishnan R, Rapp SR, Fleischer AB, Feldman SR. Patients with palmoplantar psoriasis have more physical disability and discomfort than patients with other forms of psoriasis: implications for clinical practice. J Am Acad Dermatol 2003; 49(2): 271–5.

9. Posada C, García-Doval I, de la Torre C, Cruces MJ. Value of palmar and plantar biopsies of hyperkeratotic and vesicular pustular lesions: a cross-sectional study. Actas Dermosifiliogr 2010; 101(1):103–5.

10. Steven R. Feldman and Arash Taheri. Hyperkeratotic eczema of the palms. A. Alikhan et al. (eds.), Textbook of Hand Eczema, © Springer: Verlag Berlin Heidelberg 2014.

11. Veien NK, Hattel T, Laurberg G. Hand eczema: causes, course, and prognosis I. Contact Dermatitis 2008;58(6):330–4.

12. Weedon D. Skin pathology. 2nd ed.New York: Churchill Livingstone; 2002.

17

Acute and Recurrent Vesicular Hand Eczema (Syn: Pompholyx)

Kabir Sardana

Acute and recurrent vesicular hand eczema is defined as the infrequent or repeated eruption of vesicles on the palms, palmar aspects of the fingers, and/or sides of the fingers (Fig. 17.1a) that cannot be explained by contact with external contactants.

Acute and vesicular hand dermatitis should be preferred over pompholyx and dyshidrosis as we still do not know what causes this intriguing clinical manifestation.

CLINICAL TYPES

In 2007, Storrs et al proposed a new classification of dyshydrosis—acute and recurrent vesicular hand dermatitis.

The term acute and recurrent vesicular hand eczema has been chosen, because there appear to be two clinical types of this dermatitis. One type is explosive, with eruptions of severe vesiculation (Fig. 17.1b) or even bullous lesions. This type is rare and is representative of the initial descriptions of the dermatosis made in the late nineteenth century. Most of the cases described over the past 30 years are of a less severe type, with repeated eruptions of tiny, severely pruritic vesicles (Fig. 17.1c and d).

Doshi and Kimbal classified vesicular palmoplantar eczema into four categories based on clinical features—pompholyx, vesiculobullous eczema, hyperkeratotic hand

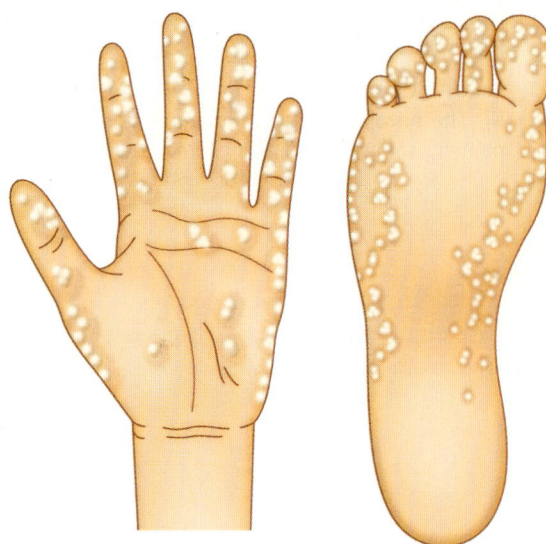

Fig. 17.1a: Pompholyx. A depiction of multiple "sago grain" like vesicles on the sides of fingers

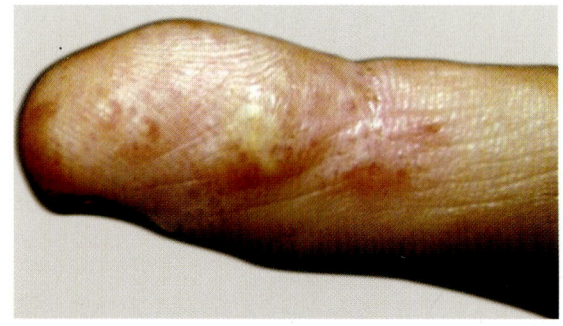

Fig. 17.1b: Large vesicles coalescing into a bulla in a case of vesicular hand eczema

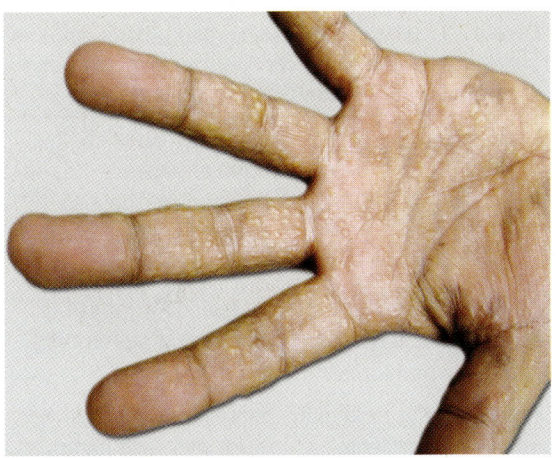

Fig. 17.1c: Multiple "sago grain" like vesicles on the palms

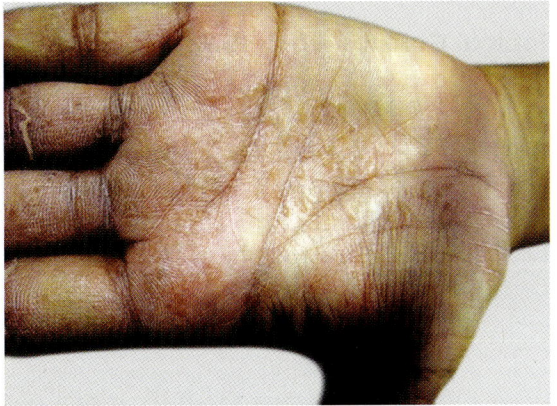

Fig. 17.1d: A patient with a history of recurrent vesicles on the palmar aspect of hand

dermatitis, and "Id" vesicular reactions. Cheiropompholyx and podopompholyx respectively refer to involvement of only the hands or only the feet. Vesiculobullous hand eczema is characterized by vesicles and/or bullae on the lateral aspects of the fingers. The Id eruption is usually due to an infective process.

EPIDEMIOLOGY

Most cases are sporadic. It has been seen worldwide but appears to be less common in Asia. There is no gender preference and while it is more frequent in adults, it can also occur in children. Familial dyshidrosis was first described in 1969 [Curth] and occurs through autosomal dominant transmission. A genetic study on 23 fourth generation individuals from a Chinese family with familial dyshidrosis found that the gene for this familial form maps to chromosome 18q22.1–18q22.3 between the markers D18S465 and D18S1362 (Chen JJ).

ETIOLOGY

A variety of causes have been described with varying levels of evidence and they constitute a useful list to run through before hurriedly labeling the patient as an idiopathic disorder (Table 17.1). A study by Guillet MH found that the common causes were mycosis (10.0%); allergic contact pompholyx (67.5%), with cosmetic and hygiene products as the main factor (31.7%), followed by metals (16.7%); and internal reactivation from drug, food, or haptenic (nickel) origin (6.7%). The remaining 15.0% of patients were classified as idiopathic patients, but all were atopic.

Uncommon causes include intravenous immunoglobulin infusions, mycofenolate mofetil, certain cosmetics containing balsam of Peru, perfumes, certain rubbers particularly those containing paraphenylenediamine, as well as many exogenous irritants such as

Table 17.1: Possible causes of acute and recurrent vesicular hand eczema
• Atopy
• Dermatophytid
• Drug reactions
• Systemic contact dermatitis
• Allergic contact dermatitis (*garlic, compositae plants, balsam of Peru*)
• Metals (*dental metals, orthodontic treatment, Ni, chromium*)
• Ingested metals (*Ni, chromium*)
• Food (*Tuna, coffee, tomato, pineapple, American cheese, milk, egg, wheat, lamb, chocolate, and chicken.*)

irritant cosmetics and prolonged wearing of gloves.

MANAGEMENT

The most important aspect of the management of acute and recurrent vesicular hand eczema is the determination of the cause of the eruptions where the list (Table 17.1) can be a useful initial exercise.

The history should include information about external and possible systemic exposures. Vesicular eruptions have been described as occurring less than 1 h after exposure to proteins in persons with protein contact dermatitis. Oral challenge with nickel has caused vesicular palmar eruptions after 1–3 days in nickel-sensitive patients. A history of exposures up to **3 days** before the eruption of vesicular hand eczema is, therefore, an essential element in the diagnosis of this condition. The history should include information regarding dermatophytosis of the feet, particularly that caused by *T. mentagrophytes*. Patients with recurrent vesicular hand eczema should ideally be patch tested with a standard tray, including the metals nickel, cobalt, and chromium, as well as balsam of Peru and perfume ingredients. When protein contact dermatitis is suspected, prick testing and prick-prick testing should be carried out with suspected food items.

If a diet trial is initiated, it should last from 1 to 3 months. If improvement is not apparent, the diet trial should be discontinued. If improvement is seen, the diet should be moderated to make life easier for the patient.

A basic investigative option is given in Box 17.1.

Given the extreme complexity of "dyshidrosis" syndrome and the highly variable course of the condition in a given individual, the treatment of this disorder has never been studied by a scientifically coherent approach. As double-blind studies are scarce and have a number of biases, treatment should be dictated by "experience" and common sense and is listed in Table 17.2.

Box 17.1: Recommended investigations prior to initiating treatment in patients with pompholyx: identification of factors that trigger flares

Patch tests	Document any allergic contact eczema (cosmetics, metals, perfumes, other contact allergens)
Detection of concomitant palmar or plantar hyperhidrosis	Questioning (possibly with iodine starch test)
History-taking to identify other environmental triggers	Smoking, alcohol, stress, work with "wet hands" and/or in a hot or humid environment

Topical Corticosteroids (TCS)

TCS are applied in the evening; creams are preferred to ointments. During acute flares, superpotent corticosteroids (such as clobetasol propionate and betamethasone dipropionate) are recommended. During the erythematosquamous regressive phase, mid-strength corticosteroids are used.

Calcineurin Inhibitors

0.1% topical tacrolimus (2 applications per day) was as effective on dyshidrotic palmar lesions as 0.1% mometasone furoate ointment.

Topical pimecrolimus can also be used though it is less effective and costlier.

Topical Retinoids

1% bexarotene gel (Targretin Gel®) can be tried and has been found to be as effective as TCS.

Systemic Treatments

Systemic Corticosteroids

Systemic corticosteroid therapy is rarely indicated in dyshidrosis. There are no convincing published data to support it and it obviously involves adverse effects. Despite an absence of controlled studies, it has been used in extremely acute flares.

	Topical	Systemic	Other
Table 17.2: Management of pompholyx based on best available evidence			
First line	**Dermocorticoids** (mometasone furoate cream; clobetasol propionate)	**Oral antihistamines** **Oral steroids**	**UVA-1** **PUVA therapy**
Second line	**Calcineurin inhibitors** 0.1% tacrolimus	**Alitretinoin**	
Third line	**1% bexarotene gel**	**Immunosuppressive agents** *Azathioprine:* 100–150 *Methotrexate:* 15–25 mg weekly *MMF:* 2 g *Cyclosporine:* 2.5 mg/kg/day *Etanercept:* 25 mg twice weekly for 6 weeks	**Iontophoresis** **Botulinum toxin** **Radiotherapy**
Emergency measure		**Prednisolone 40 mg OD × 5 d**	

If secondary infection of the lesions occurs with resultant lymphangitis and lymphadeno-pathy, systemic antibiotics can rapidly treat this complication.

Immunosuppressive Therapy

This is not a preferred option. Azathioprine 100–150 mg daily, low-dose methotrexate 15–25 mg weekly and mycophenolate mofetil 2 g daily have been used in recalcitrant cases of dyshidrosis. Cyclosporine is another option in a dose of 2.5 mg/kg/day but recurrence is common after discontinuing treatment.

Retinoids

Alitretinoin (9-cis-retinoic acid) was used at different doses in a 12-week European randomized, double-blind, placebo-controlled study in 319 patients with chronic hand eczema refractory to standard therapy, including 70 patients with dyshidrosis. Significant improvement was seen in 53% of patients, but there was no significant difference between alitretinoin and placebo in the dyshidrosis group (Ruzicka et al).

In conclusion, while oral alitretinoin is effective in chronic hand dermatitis, it appears to have only moderate efficacy in pompholyx.

Biologicals

A patient with palmar dyshidrosis refractory to standard therapy was treated with etanercept 25 mg twice a week. Complete remission was achieved after six weeks of treatment. Etanercept was then maintained for four months during which time the condition recurred despite a doubling of the dose (Ogden S).

OTHER TREATMENTS

Botulinum Toxin

Botulinum toxin has potent antihidrotic activity and can be used as hyperhidrosis is an aggravating factor. In a study of 6 patients, intradermal injections of 100 U of botulinum toxin in one palm, as an adjuvant to topical corticosteroids, produced significant improvement in the DASI score compared with corticosteroids alone (Wollina U). In another study involving intradermal injections of 162 U of botulinum toxin in one palm compared with the other untreated palm, 7 of the 10 patients showed improvement in dyshidrosis (reduction of pruritus and vesiculation) (Swartling C, et al).

Phototherapy

PUVA therapy is effective, but localized treatment on affected hands or hands/feet may cause generalized photosensitization.

Bath-PUVA with an 8-methoxypsoralen (8-MOP) bath before UVA exposure is effective against palmoplantar eczema and dyshidrosis. Smokers with dyshidrosis are less responsive to bath-PUVA than non-smokers.

Topical PUVA therapy with application of 8-MOP cream was not statistically different from UVA alone in a randomized, double-blind study of 12 patients with dyshidrosis (Grattan CE).

Local UVB (TL-01) therapy was compared with local PUVA (with 8-MOP) in a prospective study of 15 patients, 3 of whom had chronic dyshidrosis. Local UVB was as effective as local PUVA (although the group with dyshidrosis was not studied separately) (Sezer E).

UVA-1 irradiation was determined to be effective in dyshidrosis in a non-controlled study in patients with hand dyshidrosis and was more effective than placebo in a randomized, controlled, double-blind, placebo-controlled study when administered 5 times per week (40 joules/cm^2) [Polderman MC].

Iontophoresis

By controlling excessive palmoplantar sweating, tap water iontophoresis appears to be an interesting adjuvant to topical corticosteroids, as shown in a study of 20 patients with dyshidrosis. It significantly improves pruritus and the duration of remission, as compared with corticosteroids alone (Wollina U).

Bibliography

1. Chen JJ, Liang YH, Zhou FS, et al. The gene for a rare autosomal dominant form of pompholyx maps to chromosome 18q22. 1-18q22.3. J Invest Dermatol 2006, 126: 300–4.

2. Curth HO. Familial pompholyx. Arch Dermatol, 1969, 100: 520.

3. Doshi DN, Kimbal AB. Vesicular palmoplantar eczema. In Fitzpatrick's Dermatology in General Medicine, vol. 1, Seventh edition. McGraw-Hill Medical, 2007, 162–7.

4. Grattan CE, Carmichael AJ, Shuttleworth GJ, Foulds IS. Comparison of topical PUVA with UVA for chronic vesicular hand eczema. Acta Dermatol Venereol 1991, 71: 118–22.

5. Guillet MH, Wierzbicka E, Guillet S, Dagregorio G, Guillet G. A 3-year causative study of pompholyx in 120 patients. Arch Dermatol 2007; 143(12):1504–8.

6. Ogden S, Clayton TH, Goodfield MJ. Recalcitrant hand pompholyx: variable response to etanercept. Clin Exp Dermatol, 2006, 31: 145–6.

7. Polderman MC, Govaert JC, Le Cessie S, Pavel S. A double-blind placebo-controlled trial of UVA-1 in the treatment of dyshidrotic eczema. Clin Exp Dermato 2003, 28: 584–7.

8. Ruzicka T, Larsen FG, Galewicz D, et al. Oral alitretinoin (9-cis-retinoic acid) therapy for chronic hand dermatitis in patients refractory to standard therapy: results of a randomized, double-blind, placebo-controlled, multicenter trial. Arch Dermatol 2004, 140: 1453–59.

9. Sezer E, Etikan I. Local narrowband UVB phototherapy vs. local PUVA in the treatment of chronic hand eczema. Photodermatol Photoimmunol Photomed 2007, 23: 10–4.

10. Storrs F. Acute and recurrent vesicular hand dermatitis not pompholyx or dyshidrosis. Arch Dermatol 2007;143(12):1578–80.

11. Swartling C, Naver H, Lindberg M, Anveden I. Treatment of dyshidrotic hand dermatitis with intradermal botulinum toxin. J Am Acad Dermatol 2002, 47: 667–1.

12. Wollina U, Karamfilov T. Adjuvant botulinum toxin A in dyshidrotic hand eczema: a controlled prospective pilot study with left-right comparison. J Eur Acad Dermatol Venereol 2002, 16: 40–2.

13. Wollina U, Uhlemann C, Elstermann D et al. Therapy of hyperhidrosis with tap water iontophoresis. Positive effect on healing time and lack of recurrence in hand-foot eczema. Hautarzt 1998, 49: 109–13.

14. Wollina U. Pompholyx. A review of clinical features, differential diagnosis, and management. Am J Clin Dermatol. 2010;11(5):306–14.

18

Juvenile Plantar Dermatosis

Aastha Gupta

Synonyms: Chapped fissured feet (sweaty sock dermatitis, peridigital dermatitis, juvenile plantar dermatosis, dermatitis plantaris sicca, atopic winter feet).

CLINICAL FEATURES

This is seen initially with scaling, erythema, fissuring, and loss of the epidermal ridge pattern. The tendency to severe chapping declines with age and disappears around the age of puberty. Though most books use the term juvenile plantar dermatoses and some associate it with a atopic tendency, this may not be the case always. The mean age of onset is 7.3 years; the mean age of remission is 14.3 years. Onset is in early fall or when the weather becomes cold and heavy socks and impermeable shoes or boots are worn. An artificial intertrigo is created when moist socks are kept in contact with the soles. Friction and enhanced sweating play a contributory role. Humid environment leads to increased hydration of the horny layer, making it much less resistant to wear and tear, resulting in its shedding off due to friction. The skin in pressure areas, toes, and metatarsal regions becomes dry, brittle, and scaly, glazed and then fissured. The chapping extends onto the sides of the toes. Eventually, the entire sole may be involved; sometimes the hands are also affected. The lesions are characteristically symmetrical and soreness is often present in the affected areas. The dorsa of the feet, toe clefts and the instep are typically spared (Fig. 18.1).

The eruption lasts throughout the winter, clears without treatment in the late spring, and predictably recurs. A common differential is atopic dermatitis of the feet in children which occurs on the dorsal toes and usually not on the plantar surface, and is itchy.

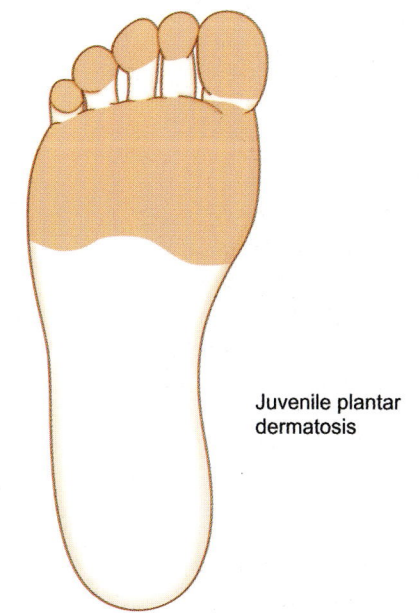

Juvenile plantar dermatosis

Fig. 18.1: An artist's depiction of the distribution of juvenile plantar dermatoses

The diagnosis is primarily clinical. Histopathological examination may be helpful in difficult cases showing features of subacute or chronic spongiotic dermatitis. Eccrine duct inflammation is seen in some cases.

DIFFERENTIAL DIAGNOSIS

The differential diagnosis includes psoriasis, tinea pedis, and allergic contact dermatitis.

Psoriasis: The erythema in psoriasis is more prominent and the scales in chapped fissured feet are adherent, and removal of the scales causes bleeding.

Fungal infections: Tinea of the feet in children is rare. Feet with the rare case of familial *Trichophyton rubrum* are pale brown and have a fine scale. Fissuring is minimal, and there is little seasonal variation. Interdigital spaces are spared in chapped fissured feet.

Allergic contact dermatitis to shoes usually affects the dorsal surface and spares the soles, webs, and sides of the feet. The eruption is bright red and scaly rather than pale red and chapped.

TREATMENT

Topical steroids and lubrication provide some relief. Group II or III topical steroids are applied twice each day, preferably, with plastic wrap occlusion at bedtime. Lubricating creams and/or keratolytics are beneficial. Emollients should be applied several times each day, especially directly after removing moist socks to seal in moisture. The feet should not be allowed to remain moist inside shoes. Preventive measures include changing into light leather shoes and changing cotton socks one or two times each day.

Bibliography

1. Eczema, in. Sardana k, Mahajan S, Garg VK. Diagnosis and Management of Skin Disorders: An Evidence-Based Approach, 1/e.: Lippincott Williams and Wilkins, 2012 (reprint 2015).
2. Fast Facts: Eczema and Contact Dermatitis By John Berth-Jones, Eunice Tan and Howard I Malbach Published 2004.
3. Griffiths C, Barker J, Bleiker T, Chalmers R, Creamer D. Rook's Textbook of Dermatology. 9th ed. Chichester. John Wiley & Sons; 2016. Chapter 39. Eczematous Disorders; p. 21–2
4. Thieme Clinical Companions Dermatology. Sterry, Dermatology© 2006 Thieme.

19

Venous Eczema

Kabir Sardana, Shivani Bansal

Stasis dermatitis (also known as "gravitational eczema," "stasis eczema," and "varicose eczema") refers to a common form of eczema/dermatitis that affects one or both lower legs, in association with venous insufficiency. Insufficient venous return results in increased pressure in the capillaries with the result that both fluid and cells may "leak" out of the capillaries. This results in red cells breaking down, with iron-containing hemosiderin possibly contributing to the pathology of this entity.

ETIOLOGY

Stasis dermatitis occurs as a direct consequence of venous insufficiency. Disturbed function of the one-way valvular system in the deep venous plexus of the legs results in a backflow of blood from the deep venous system to the superficial venous system, with accompanying venous hypertension. This loss of valvular function can result from an age-related decrease in valve competency. This distends the local capillary bed and widens the endothelial pores, thus allowing fibrinogen molecules to escape into the interstitial fluid, where they form a fibrin sheath around the capillaries. This layer of fibrin presumably forms a pericapillary barrier to the diffusion of oxygen and other nutrients which are essential for the normal vitality of the skin.

Cutaneous inflammation in venous hypertension may result from increased sequestration of white cells in the venules, with consequent release of proteolytic enzymes and free radicals which produce tissue damage (Fig. 19.1).

Alternatively, specific events, such as deep venous thrombosis, surgery (e.g. vein stripping, total knee arthroplasty, harvesting of saphenous veins for coronary bypass), or traumatic injury, can severely damage the function of the lower extremity venous system.

Some have speculated that stasis eczema is consequent to an allergic response to an epidermal protein antigen created through increased hydrostatic pressure, whereas others believe that the skin has been compromised and is more susceptible to irritation and trauma.

CLINICAL FEATURES

It is usually seen around the ankle and lower leg. It typically occurs in medial supramalleolar region where microangiopathy is more intense. The eczema may develop suddenly or insidiously. The patients are usually middle-aged or elderly and most often female. The skin appears thin, brown and tissue-like, with possible skin lesions (macule or patches), red spots, superficial skin irritation and/or

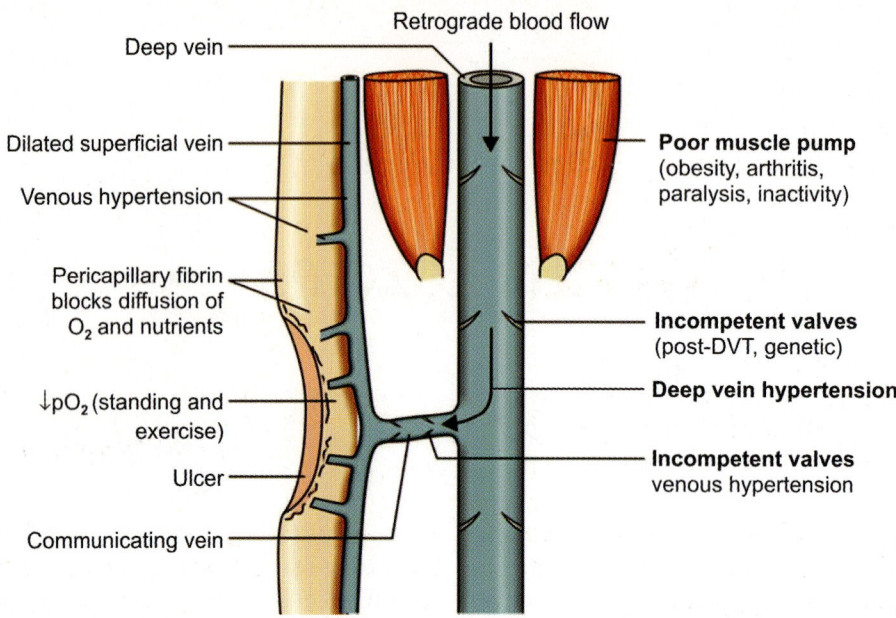

Fig. 19.1: An overview of the factors that determine leg ulcers and venous eczema

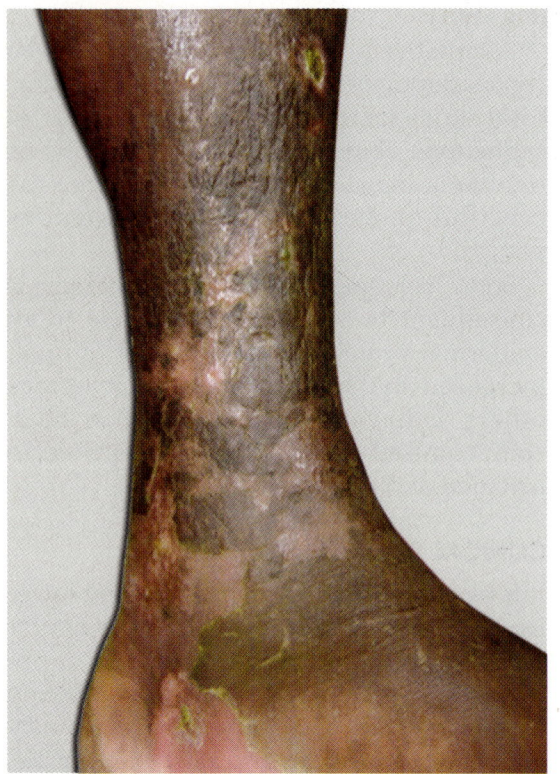

Fig. 19.2: A case of venous eczema with changes of subacute eczema seen on the medial aspect of the limb. Note early signs of lipodermatosclerosis

darkening and/or thickening of the skin at the ankles or legs (Fig. 19.2). The skin may be weakened and may ulcerate in areas. Legs, ankles, or other areas may become swollen. The patient complain of itching, soreness and pains in the legs.

Subacute Inflammation

Subacute inflammation usually begins in the winter months when the legs become dry and scaly. Brown staining of the skin (hemosiderin) may have appeared slowly for months. The pigment is iron remaining after disintegration of red blood cells that leaked out of veins because of increased hydrostatic pressure. Scratching induces first subacute and then chronic eczematous inflammation.

Acute Inflammation

A red, superficial itchy plaque may suddenly appear on the lower leg. This acute process may be eczematous inflammation, cellulitis, or both. Weeping and crusts appear and is associated with a vesicular eruption (Id reaction) on the palms, trunk and/or extremities.

Chronic Inflammation

Recurrent attacks of inflammation eventually compromise the poorly vascularized area, and the disease becomes chronic and recurrent. The typical presentation is a cyanotic red plaque over the medial malleolus. Fibrosis following chronic inflammation leads to permanent skin thickening. The skin surface in these irreversibly changed areas may have a bumpy, cobblestone appearance that results from fibrosis and venous and lymph stasis. The skin remains thickened and diffusely dark brown (post-inflammatory hyperpigmentation) during quiescent periods (Fig. 19.3).

COMPLICATIONS OF STASIS DERMATITIS

Cellulitis: The cracks and poor skin condition of this disorder predisposes for the entry of bacterial infection causing spreading cellulitis in the leg. Crusting or scaling is the most important sign in eczema and this is not seen in cellulitis, where the skin is smooth and shiny. Small blisters (vesicles) are common in eczema. These breakdown and the serous fluid released dries to form crusts (Fig. 19.2). Although blister formation is uncommon in cellulitis, if blisters do develop they are large and herald the onset of skin necrosis. If the skin condition deteriorates further and breaks down, a venous ulcer (also known as a stasis ulcer) may form.

Lipodermatosclerosis: Stasis dermatitis can lead to fat necrosis with the end stage being permanent sclerosis (lipodermatosclerosis) with inverted champagne bottle appearance (Figs 19.2 and 19.3). The eczema can also be accompanied with small patches of white, atrophic, telangiectatic scarring (atrophie blanche) (Fig. 19.4).

DIFFERENTIAL DIAGNOSIS

An approach to common causes of red leg is given in Fig. 19.5. Other differentials include:
• Atopic dermatitis
• Allergic contact dermatitis
• Discoid eczema

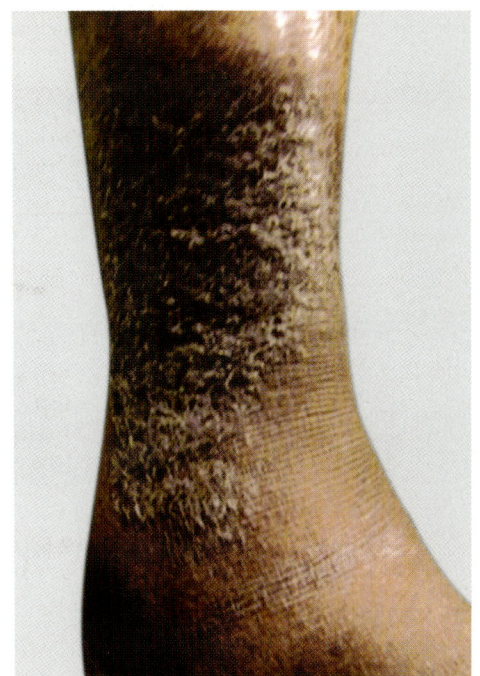

Fig. 19.3: A case of chronic venous eczema resulting in fibrosis, pigmentation and early signs of "inverted champagne" leg

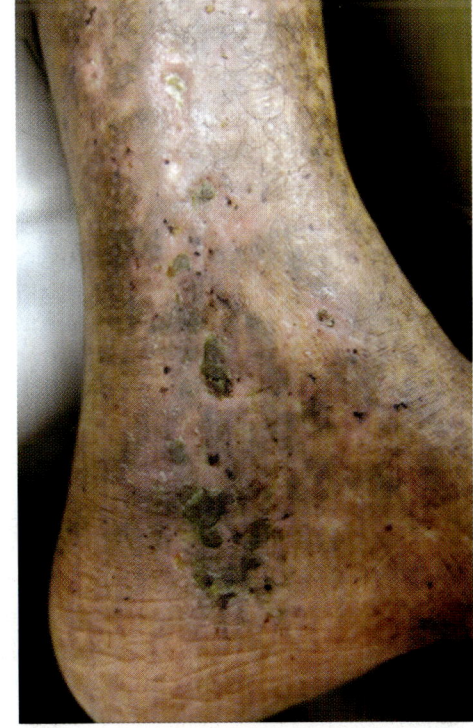

Fig. 19.4: Lipodermatosclerosis with atrophie blanche

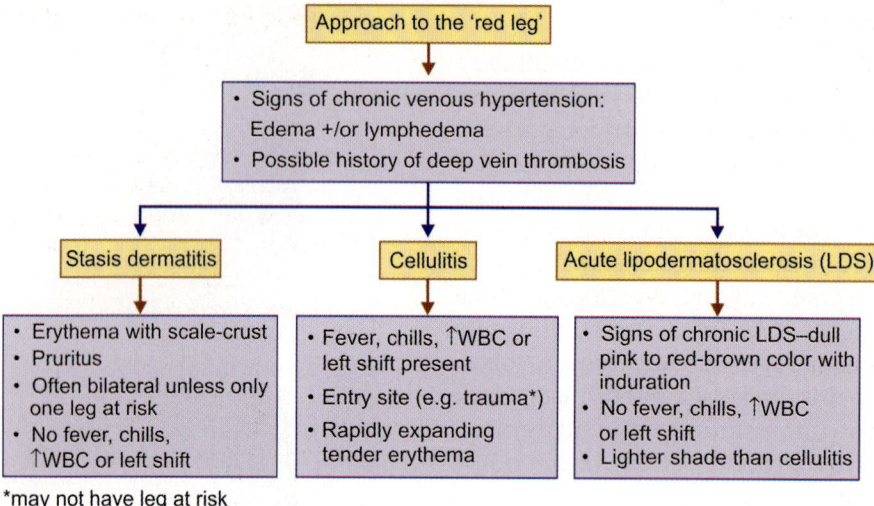

Fig. 19.5: Approch to the red leg

- Infective eczema
- Necrobiosis lipoidica
- Nummular dermatitis
- Pigmented purpuric dermatitis
- Pretibial myxedema

INVESTIGATION

Contact sensitization to active drugs or to their constituents is a continuously operating factor and is one of the factors responsible for the chronicity and deterioration in stasis dermatitis. Patch test should be used to identify the topical agents that may be responsible for perpetuation or aggravation of eczema, especially in patients who do not improve despite adequate treatment of other underlying cause(s). Additionally, it is imperative to consider unprescribed medications causing sudden exacerbation of existing dermatitis.

TREATMENT

General Measure

The underlying venous hypertension should be controlled. Obese patients should be urged to lose weight. Well-fitted support stockings or firm bandages can be helpful if worn regularly and care is taken to avoid the formation of a band at the top of the leg. The legs should be elevated as effectively as possible.

Wet Compresses

Moist exudative inflammation and moist ulcers respond to tepid wet compresses of Burow's solution or merely saline or water for 30 to 60 minutes several times a day. Wet dressings suppress inflammation while debriding the ulcer.

Topical Steroids

Mild topical steroids may be used to relieve irritation, but the use of potent steroids should be limited to short periods of a few days as they may cause cutaneous atrophy and increase the risk of ulceration.

Topical Tacrolimus

Topical tacrolimus has been reported to be effective.

Systemic Antibiotics

Bacterial infection must be treated where appropriate, but the risk of sensitization to topical antibiotics and antiseptics should be borne in mind, and systemic antibiotics may be preferable.

Venoprotective Agents

Aspirin (300 mg per day), pentoxifylline, calcium dobesilate, hesperidin diosmin and rutoside may improve healing of venous ulcer.

Venous disease is progressive and irreversible. Patient must be educated about the need for continual hemodynamic support. It is a mistake to place compression stocking on edematous limbs, if they are tender. One should use compression bandaging until all edema and inflammation has resolved. But compression stockings must be regularly used to reduce the edema and regularise various flow.

Bibliography

1. Eczema, in. Sardana K, Mahajan S, Garg VK. Diagnosis and Management of Skin Disorders: An Evidence-Based Approach, 1/ e. Lippincott Williams and Wilkins, 2012 (reprint 2015).
2. Fast Facts: Eczema and Contact Dermatitis by John Berth-Jones, Eunice Tan and Howard I Malbach Published 2004.
3. Thieme Clinical Companions Dermatology. Sterry, Dermatology© 2006, Thieme.

20

Lichen Simplex Chronicus

Kabir Sardana

This is a self-inflicted dermatosis which is seen in patients with high stress levels and some clinicians believe that the patients derive pleasure from itching and this is possibly a stress reliever.

It is typified by epidermal hypertrophy secondary to chronic, habitual rubbing or scratching of localized areas of skin.

CLINICAL FEATURES

It is perpetuated by constant scratching and rubbing. The lesions are seen on sites accessible by the dominant hand and are characterized by very thick oval plaques with a persistent course or with frequent recurrences (Figs 20.1 to 20.3). Occasionally they may be bilateral (Fig. 20.4). As most patients derive great pleasure in the relief that comes from frantically scratching the inflamed site, this habit forming dermatoses has frequent recurrences. The individual lesion is thickened like a bark of the tree with accentuation of skin lines (lichenification) (Fig. 20.1). The sites of involvement often conform to the reach of the dominant hand (Box 20.1, Figs 20.5 and 20.6).

Sometimes due to chronic scratching and use of potent topical steroids, a depigmentation is seen within the plaque (Fig. 20.7).

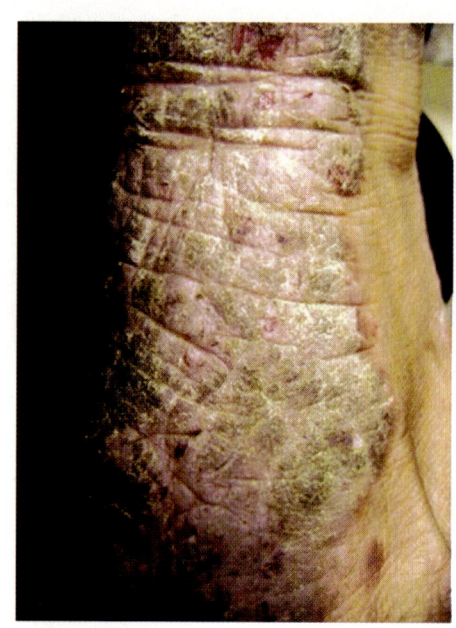

Fig. 20.1: A plaque of lichen simplex chronicus on the back of the foot. Note the thickened and lichenified skin

INVESTIGATIONS

Histologic features are similar to those of prurigo nodularis with compact hyperkeratosis, acanthosis with irregular elongation of rete ridges, hypergranulosis, and vertically oriented collagen bundles in the papillary dermis (Fig. 20.8).

An evidence-based tabulation of treatment options is given in Table 20.1.

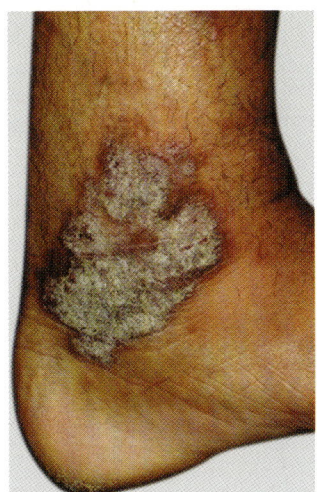

Fig. 20.2: Side of the ankle is a common site of this dermatosis and patients often use blunt objects to scratch these areas

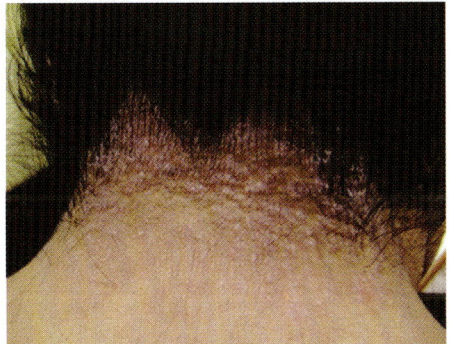

Fig. 20.3: Initial stage of lichen simplex nuchae on the neck in a female patient

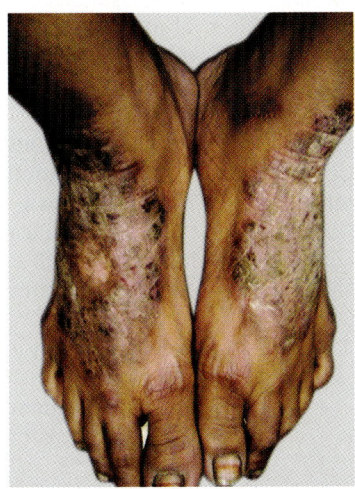

Fig. 20.4: Bilateral lichen simplex chronicus

Box 20.1: Sites of involvement of lichen simplex chronicus

- Outer lower portion of lower leg
- Genital: Scrotum, vulva, anal area, pubis
- Wrists and ankles (Figs 20.1 and 20.2)
- Upper eyelids
- Back (lichen simplex nuchae) and side of neck (Fig. 20.3)
- Orifice of the ear
- Extensor forearms near elbow
- Fold behind the ear
- Scalp (Picker's nodules)

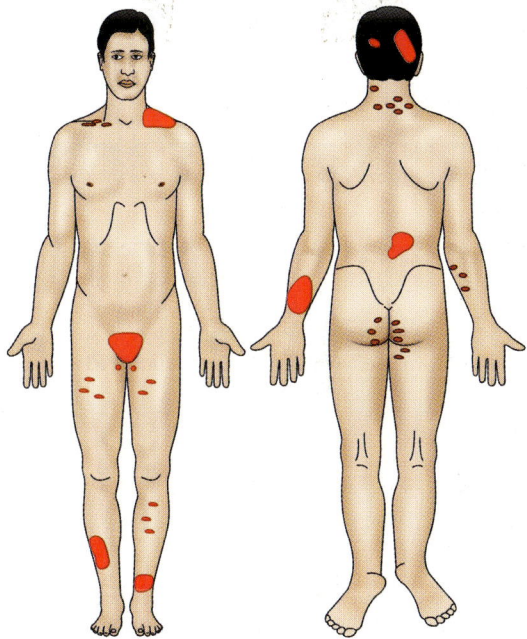

Fig. 20.5: Sites of involvement in lichen simplex chronicus

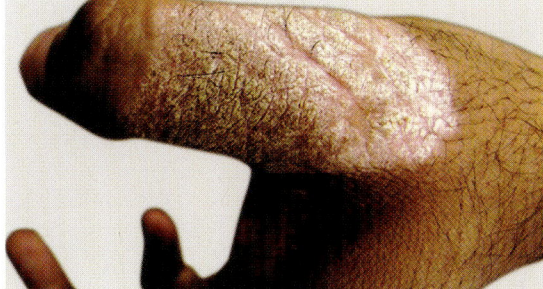

Fig. 20.6: An unusual site of lichen simplex chronicus, here the patient used to rub the finger on the side of the office table

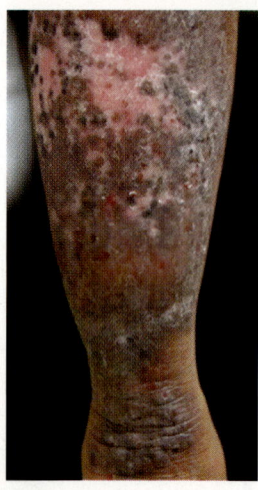

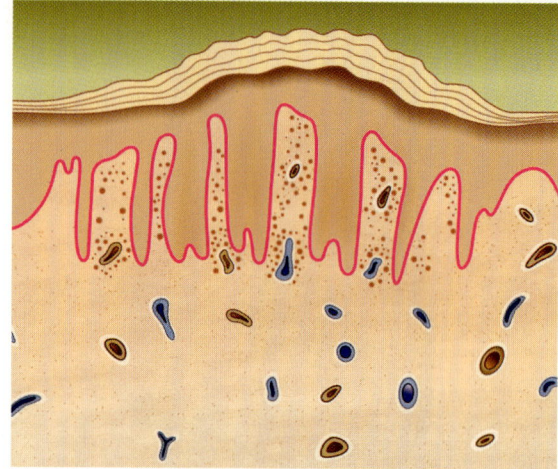

Fig. 20.7: A case of lichen simplex chronicus with loss of pigment due to scratching

Fig. 20.8: An artist's depiction of histology of lichen simplex chronicus

Table 20.1: Line of treatment of lichen simplex chronicus based on best available evidence			
	Topical	*Systemic*	*Other*
First line	• **Steroids (topical /IL)** (0.05% halobetasol, 0.05% clobetasol 17-propionate) • **Tar + Salicylic acid** • **Urea**	Higher doses of second-generation antihistamines **Doxepin** (30–75 mg)	
Second line	• **Doxepin*** • **Zinc, menthol and camphor**	• **Gabapentin** (300 mg/day increase by 300 mg/day every 3 days to a final dose of 900 mg/day) • **Pregabalin**	
Third line	• **Benzocaine, lidocaine, pramoxine** • **Tacrolimus and pimecrolimus** • **Capsaicin** (0.025–0.3%)	• **Nalmefene, naloxone and naltrexone** • **Cyclosporine** (100–150 mg) • **Thalidomide** (50–100 mg) • **Antidepressants** Paroxetine (12.5–25 mg) Mirtazapine (7.5–15 mg)	• **Transcutaneous electrical stimulation** • **Ketotifen** (1 mg BD) • **Acupuncture and electroacupuncture** • **Botulinum toxin** (20 units of botulinum toxin type A (100 U/mL) per 2 cm × 2 cm area) • **Aspirin** • **Psychotherapy** • **Hypnosis** • **Psychopharmacotherapy** • **Surgical excision**
Research drug		**Aprepitant**	

*Not available in India.

TREATMENT

The patient must be made to understand that the rash will not clear until even minor scratching and rubbing are stopped, but in most cases this is a habitual tendency and most patients cannot stop the tendency to scratch. Scratching frequently takes place during sleep, and the affected area may have to be covered to avoid this trauma.

The fundamentals of treatment are outlined in the introduction section on eczematous inflammation.

Clobetasol foams (not available in India) are very effective and can be used for lesions on the neck, legs, wrists, ankles, and vulva. Treatment of the anal area or the fold behind the ear does not require potent topical steroids as do other forms of lichen simplex chronicus. Lichen simplex nuchae (Fig. 20.3), because of its location, is difficult to treat. Inflammation that extends into the scalp may be treated with a group II steroid gel. Moist, secondarily infected areas respond to oral antibiotics and topical steroid solutions (e.g. clobetasol solution). A 2- to 3-week course of prednisone (20 mg twice daily) should be considered when an extensively inflamed scalp does not respond rapidly to topical treatment. Nodules may require monthly intralesional injections with triamcinolone acetonide (10 mg/ml).

Botulinum A toxin injected intradermally into lichenified lesions may block acetylcholine release and control pruritus.

Use of topical lidocaine 5% or capsaicin 8% patches, licensed for the treatment of postherpetic neuralgia, may be helpful in recalcitrant cases.

Bibliography

1. Eczema. In. Sardana K, Mahajan S, Garg VK. Diagnosis and Management of Skin Disorders: An Evidence-Based Approach, 1/ e. Lippincott Williams and Wilkins, 2012 (reprint 2015).

2. Fast Facts: Eczema and Contact Dermatitis by John Berth-Jones, Eunice Tan and Howard I Malbach Published 2004.

3. Thieme Clinical Companions Dermatology. Sterry, Dermatology© 2006 Thieme.

21

Exfoliative Erythroderma

Ananta Khurana

Erythroderma, first described by Hebra in 1868, is a reaction pattern, characterized by diffuse and confluent erythema with desquamation.

Exfoliative dermatitis is a synonymous term, though technically erythroderma is characterized by extensive and pronounced erythema with diffuse slight scaling, whereas exfoliative dermatitis presents a more conspicuous and marked scaling. The prerequisite to make the clinical diagnosis of erythroderma is ≥ 90% involvement of the skin surface.

CLINICAL FEATURES

A clinical classification distinguishes **three** different types of erythroderma:

1. Dry with large scales **(Wilson-Brocq)** (Figs 21.1 to 21.3)
2. Dry with small scales **(Hebra)**
3. Vesiculoedematous

The erythema has a variable intensity and scales may be dandruff-like or lamellar; large in acute forms and small in chronic cases.

Common signs in erythrodermic patients include pedal edema, facial edema, lymphadenopathy, ectropian, keratoderma of palms and soles and nail changes. Nails may be lost but are usually regrow unless a scarring process (e.g. lichen planus) is involved. Persons with long-standing erythroderma

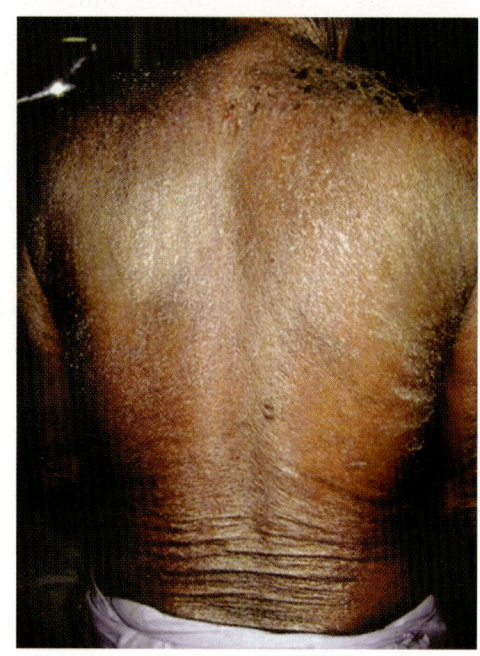

Fig. 21.1: Diffuse involvement of the skin with erythema and scaling

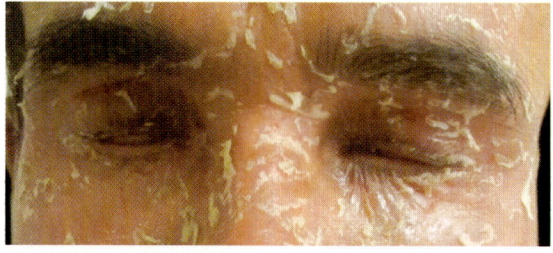

Fig. 21.2: Ectropion with erythroderma of 3 weeks duration

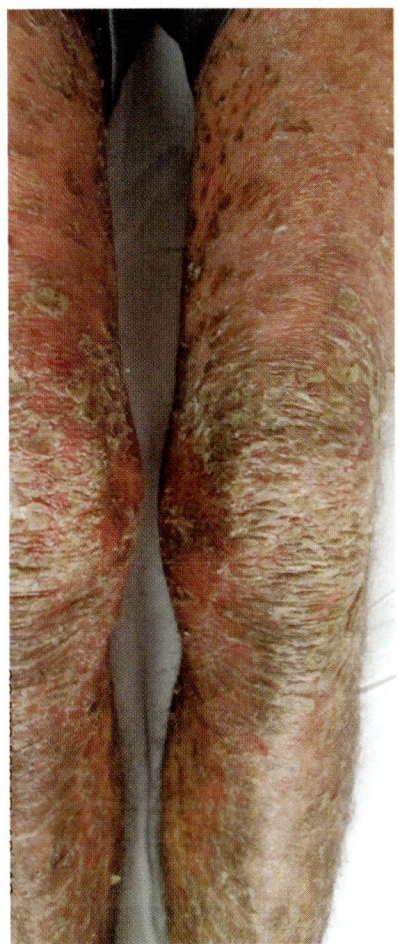

Fig. 21.3: Psoriatic erythroderma in a HIV positive male, with CD4 count of 218

may also present with cachexia (loss of weight, fatigue, weakness), diffuse alopecia, and ectropion (Fig. 21.2). Hepatomegaly occurs in approximately one-third of patients and is more commonly seen in drug-induced erythroderma. Splenomegaly may be associated with lymphoma, but it has rarely been reported otherwise.

The onset of symptoms is sudden and faster for drug-induced erythroderma and generally slower for a primary skin disease.

ETIOLOGY

Erythroderma results from a variety of specific dermatologic disorders (Table 21.1). Though the specific features of a disease are often lost when erythroderma develops, certain soft points may point to a particular diagnosis (Table 21.2).

The etiology may vary according to the **age** of the patient.

Adults

It is commonly idiopathic in 6–32% of cases, while it may be linked to an exacerbation of a pre-existing dermatosis in more than 50% of cases; therefore, patients should be carefully evaluated for an underlying skin disease.

The underlying causes frequently implicated include eczema (40% of cases), psoriasis (25%), lymphomas and leukemias (15%), drug intake, vitamin deficiency (10%), and, rarely, other dermatoses or skin infections and infestations (2%).

In adults, the **most common** causes of erythroderma include:

   a. Protracted pre-existing dermatoses,
   b. **Drug** intake,
   c. **Pre-lymphomatous** conditions, and
   d. **Occult malignancies**.

Drugs are a commonly overlooked cause. The most common causative drugs include calcium channel blockers, carbamazepine, phenytoin, and phenobarbital. Other medications include antibiotics, corticosteroids, diaminodiphenyl sulfone, NSAIDs, phenothiazines, antihypertensive drugs, cimetidine, lithium and gold, synthetic antimalarials, sulfonamides, peptic ulcer drugs, sulfasalazine, allopurinol, thalidomide, cytokines, trimethoprim, sodium clodronate, zidovudine, and codeine. Usually, drug-induced erythroderma is *sudden* and *rapid* and its resolution is fast, except in case of DRESS (drug rash with eosinophilia and systemic symptoms) due to antibiotics, anticonvulsants, and allopurinol. DRESS develops within 2–5 weeks after the start of treatment and may persist for weeks despite stopping the medication. Edema, fever, leukocytosis with marked eosinophilia, lymphadenopathy, organomegaly, and liver and renal dysfunction are characteristic of DRESS.

Table 21.1: Underlying causes of erythroderma
Dermatitis: Atopic dermatitis, chronic actinic dermatitis, seborrheic dermatitis, allergic contact dermatitis, irritant contact dermatitis, stasis dermatitis
Papulosquamous disorders: Psoriasis (Figs 21.2 to 21.4), pityriasis rubra pilaris (Fig. 21.5), Reiter syndrome, lichen planus
Connective tissue diseases: Systemic lupus erythematosus,dermatomyositis
Malignancy related: Leukemia, lymphoma (including Sezary syndrome), graft-versus-host disease, solid organ malignancy
Bullous diseases: Pemphigus foliaceus (Fig. 21.6), bullous pemphigoid
Infection related *HIV:* With seroconversion; seborrheic; lymphoma related; drug induced or unknown cause • Viral hepatitis • Staphylococcal scalded skin syndrome • Toxic shock syndrome • Dermatophytoses • Norwegian scabies
Drug reactions: Commonly antiepileptics (such as phenobarbitone, carbamazepine, and phenytoin), antibiotics (such as penicillin, sulphonamides and antituberculous drugs), gold, lithium salts and allopurinol
Idiopathic: (6–32% of cases in different series)
Rare: Sarcoidosis, Hailey-Hailey disease, toxic shock syndrome, pityriasis rosea, cutaneous graft-versus-host disease, angioimmunoblastic lymphadenopathy with dysproteinemia, Darier's disease, mastocytosis, Ofuji papuloerythroderma
Specific to pediatric age group • Immunodeficiencies (Omenn syndrome, Wiskott-Aldrich syndrome) • Ichthyotic disorders (Fig. 21.7) (congenital chthyosiform erythroderma, Netherton syndrome), metabolic diseases (holocarboxylase synthetase deficiency, biotinidase deficiency, essential fatty acid deficiency) • Infections (staphylococcal scalded skin syndrome (Fig. 21.8), congenital cutaneous candidiasis)

The suspicion of an underlying malignancy may arise when the development of erythroderma is insidious, the patient becomes progressively debilitated, no previous skin diseases are recognized, and the lesions resist standard therapies.

Children and Neonates

In children, atopic dermatitis is the most common cause. Other causes are listed in Table 21.1 but are dominated by ichthyoses. Uncommon causes include Netherton syndrome, primary immunodeficiency syndromes (PIDS), and metabolic diseases in neonates (aged less than 1 month of life). Psoriasis, Omenn syndrome, seborrheic dermatitis, and atopic dermatitis usually appear after the first month of life.

COMPLICATIONS

Erythroderma is a potentially fatal condition. Major complications are hemodynamic and metabolic disturbances. A high output cardiac failure may develop due to markedly increased blood flow through the skin. **hypothermia** may occur due to loss of thermal regulation. **Hypoalbuminemia** can develop leading to peripheral edema. Aberrations of the **immune response** with increased γ-globulins and CD4+ T lymphocytopenia in the absence of HIV infection have also been observed. **Infections** are common and

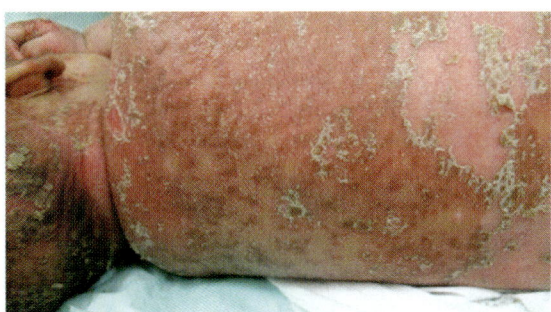

Fig. 21.4: Extensive pustular psoriasis leading to erythroderma in a 2-year-old child

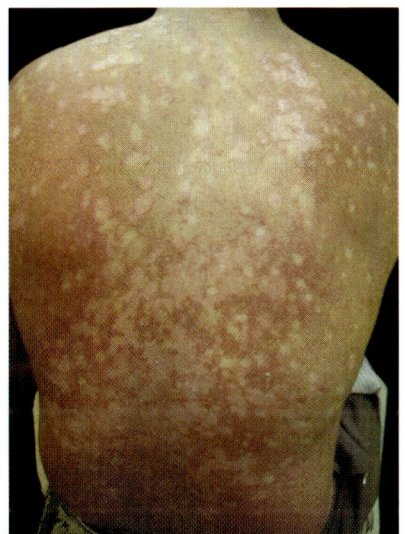

Fig. 21.5: Difffuse erythema with follicular keratotic lesions of PRP with "island of sparing"

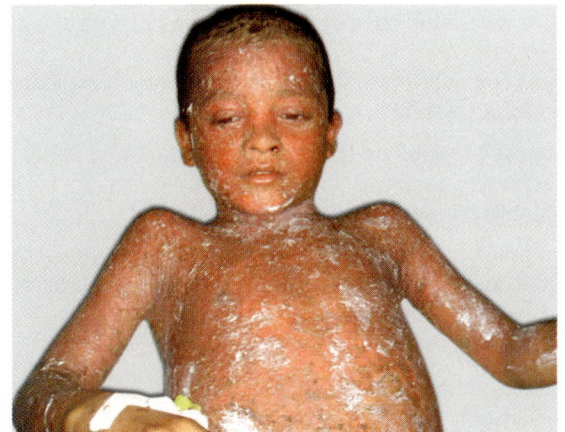

Fig. 21.6: Crusted plaques with erosions in a child of pemphigus foliaceus. The patient was being treated as a case of psoriasis by a general practitioner

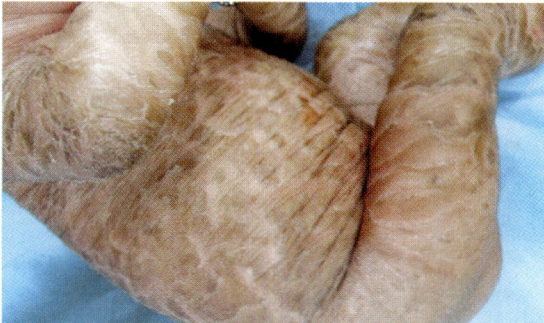

Fig. 21.7: Ichthyosiform erythroderma with large lamellar plate-like scales in a 3-week-old baby. The baby had a history of collodion membrane at birth

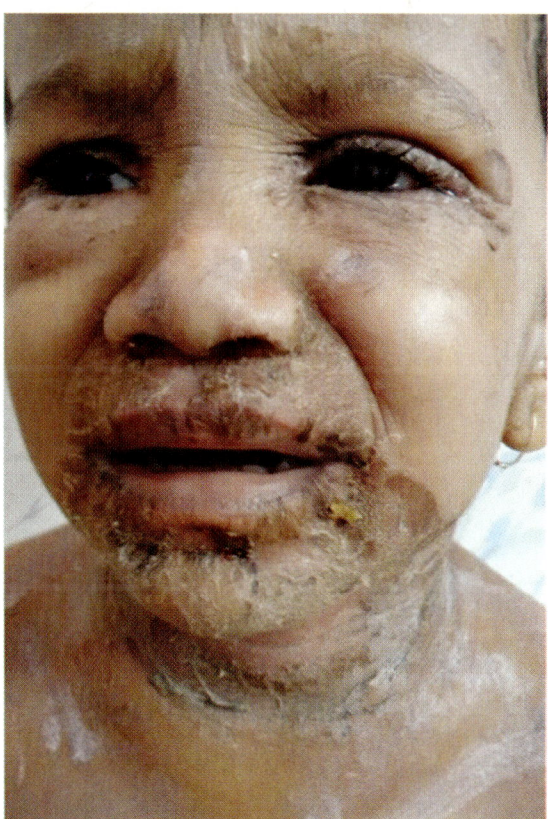

Fig. 21.8: A case of staphylococcal scalded skin syndrome with the classical "sad man facies" (Dr Gaurish Laad, Goa)

pneumonia remains the commonest cause of death. A list of complications are listed in Box 21.1.

Pneumonia, septicemia, and heart failure represent the most common causes of *death*.

Table 21.2: Diagnostic clues to certain underlying etiologies

Psoriasis	• Excessive desquamation of silvery scales (Figs 21.2 and 21.3) • Nail changes like oil drop sign or nail pits may still be present due to slower turnover rate of nails • Face is often spared • Presence of arthritis
Pityriasis rubra pilaris (PRP)	• Distinct orange red color, appreciable in fairer skin • Prominent follicular papules may still be present in some areas (Fig. 21.5) • Thick yellow red thickening of palms/soles • Islands of sparing (*not* diagnostic; may also be seen in psoriasis, CTCL, eczematous disorders related erythroderma, pemphigus foliaceus)
Atopic eczema	• Prominent pruritus • Lichenification • Atopic erythroderma may occur at any age
Drug induced	• Sudden onset and rapidly progressing • Chronological correlation • *Supporting features:* Fever, peripheral eosinophilia, facial swelling, hepatitis, interstitial nephritis
Cutaneous T cell lymphoma (including mycosis fungoides and Sézary syndrome)	• Deep purple red hue • Intense pruritus • Marked skin infiltration; leonine facies • Prominent lymphadenopathy • Alopecia • Painful fissured keratoderma • Splenomegaly • Suggestive blood picture or lymph node histology
Norwegian scabies	• Thick crusting over body and palms and soles • Thickening of nails and thick underlying debris • Scabies in contacts
Lichen planus	• Individual violaceous papules may appear as erythroderma subsides • Lichenoid eruptions more likely to cause erythroderma than primary lichen planus
Pemphigus foliaceus	• Moist crusted lesions on face and upper trunk (Fig. 21.6) • Moist scales • Occasionally thin-walled bullae may be seen
Eczematous dermatoses	• Intense pruritus • Exacerbation of existing lesions precedes the generalization • Venous eczema is a common precedent in older age (Atopic: *see* above)
Parthenium dermatitis	• Occupation—farming commonly • Gender—mostly males • Previous history of summer exacerbation of skin eruptions • History of photoexacerbation often present • Patch testing (after subsidence)

Box 21.1: Common complications of erythroderma

Thermoregulation: Increased skin blood flow leads to higher skin temperature and heat loss. This can cause hypothermia and induce a higher compensatory basal metabolic activity.

Dehydration: Elevated transepidermal water loss (TEWL) and skin evaporation

Hypoproteinemia: Protein loss (because of the desquamation) and exudation
Protein loss increases by 25–30% in psoriatic cases and 10–15% in non-psoriatic cases

INVESTIGATIONS

Work up is directed towards reaching to a specific diagnosis and for management of the patient. Biopsy is the most important component for the former and may lead to a diagnosis in up to 57% cases according to some series. The best correlation is achieved with erythrodermic mycosis fungoides.

Though a detailed evaluative protocol is given in Table 21.3, in about **6–32%** of patients, no cause is found and these are labelled as

Table 21.3: Checklist of investigations for diagnosis and management

Investigation	Comments
Vitals	• Temperature, weight, pulse, respiratory rate charting • Fuid intake/output charting • Urine R/M
General Investiagtions	
Complete blood count	• **Hb:** Anemia due to malabsorption from gut, anemia of chronic disease, loss from skin • **High TLC:** Infection; leukemic condition if abnormal cells • **Eosinophilia:** Drug reactions, bullous pemphigoid
KFT, serum electrolytes	• Monitor loss of fluid and electrolytes • Renal dysfunction with severe drug reactions
LFT	• Derangement mostly with drug-induced cause • As a baseline for systemic drug therapy
Protein	• Hypoalbuminemia due to skin loss and malabsorption
Swab cultures from broken skin	• Loss of barrier predisposes to infections
Blood cultures	• Evidence of sepsis
Chest X-ray	• Pneumonia • Signs of CHF
Specific Investigations	
Sin scrapings	• Norwegian scabies
KOH mount	• Dermatophytoses
HIV serology	• With high index of suspicion; suggestive history; drug reactions
Antinuclear antibody, complement levels	• If doubt of a connective tissue disorder
Angiotensin-converting enzyme levels and serum calcium level	• Sarcoidosis
Skin biopsy	• Usually multiple biopsies required (in different stages and from different areas)

(Contd.)

Table 21.3: Checkilist of investigations for diagnosis and management (*Contd.*)

Investigation	Comments
	• Non-specific signs (hyperorthokeratosis, acanthosis, perivascular infiltrate) may mask diagnostic cutaneous changes • Biopsy any new suggestive lesion • Drug-induced: Often show a lichenoid interfacial dermatosis
Immunofluorescence	• When doubt of an immunobullous disorder or connective tissue disorder
Lymph node cytology/biopsy	• Reactive/dermatogenic commonly • May give clue to an underlying lymphoma
Patch testing	• After resolution of the acute phase and stoppage of immunosuppressive medications, to know the causative allergen
Serum and urine protein electrophoresis	• Multiple myeloma
Stool for occult blood, prostate examination, cervical smear, ultrasonography of the abdomen, chest radiograph, computed tomography scan, mammography, and sigmoidoscopy	• Malignancy screen • When no obvious cause/primary skin disease identified; resistance to standard treatments. • Imaging and endoscopies, guided by clinical findings.

primary or **idiopathic**. In patients with primary, idiopathic cases, laboratory abnormalities seen include leukocytosis, anemia, raised erythrocyte sedimentation rate, lymphocytosis, eosinophilia, and hypergammaglobulinemia with elevated IgE serum levels. Other findings are increased creatinine level, hyperuricemia, and hypoalbuminemia. Eosinophilia is not diagnostic. In Sezary syndrome, more than 20% of circulating Sézary cells is a diagnostic point, whereas less than 10% is a nonspecific finding. This lower count of Sézary cells can in fact be found in different benign dermatoses.

An approach to diagnosis is given in Flowchart 21.1.

TREATMENT

Specific therapy requires the proper diagnosis (Fig. 21.8) but all erythrodermas may initially be treated in a similar manner. The initial therapeutic strategy is control of symptoms and prevention of the complications of erythroderma. Specific treatment must be tailored to the underlying disease. Hospitalization or admission to a day skin treatment center should be considered, as an aggressive topical approach can be too complex and demanding for a home care plan. Elderly patients are at higher risk for significant medical complications.

General Care (Box 21.2)

1. Close monitoring of circulatory status and body temperature. Input output charting and temperature charting are essential.
2. A warm, humid environment must be provided.
3. Soaking in warm water followed by a bland emollient or petrolatum.
4. Careful use of topical steroids, as systemic absorption is greatly increased.
5. Sedating antihistamines like hydroxyzine 25–50 mg orally for control of itch and sedation. As antipruritic agents, mild topical steroids/emollients as well as wet wrap dressing can be used.
6. A high-protein diet with B vitamins, iron supplementation, and adequate nutrition is essential in view of the catabolic state.

Flowchart 21.1: Approach to diagnosis of erythroderma

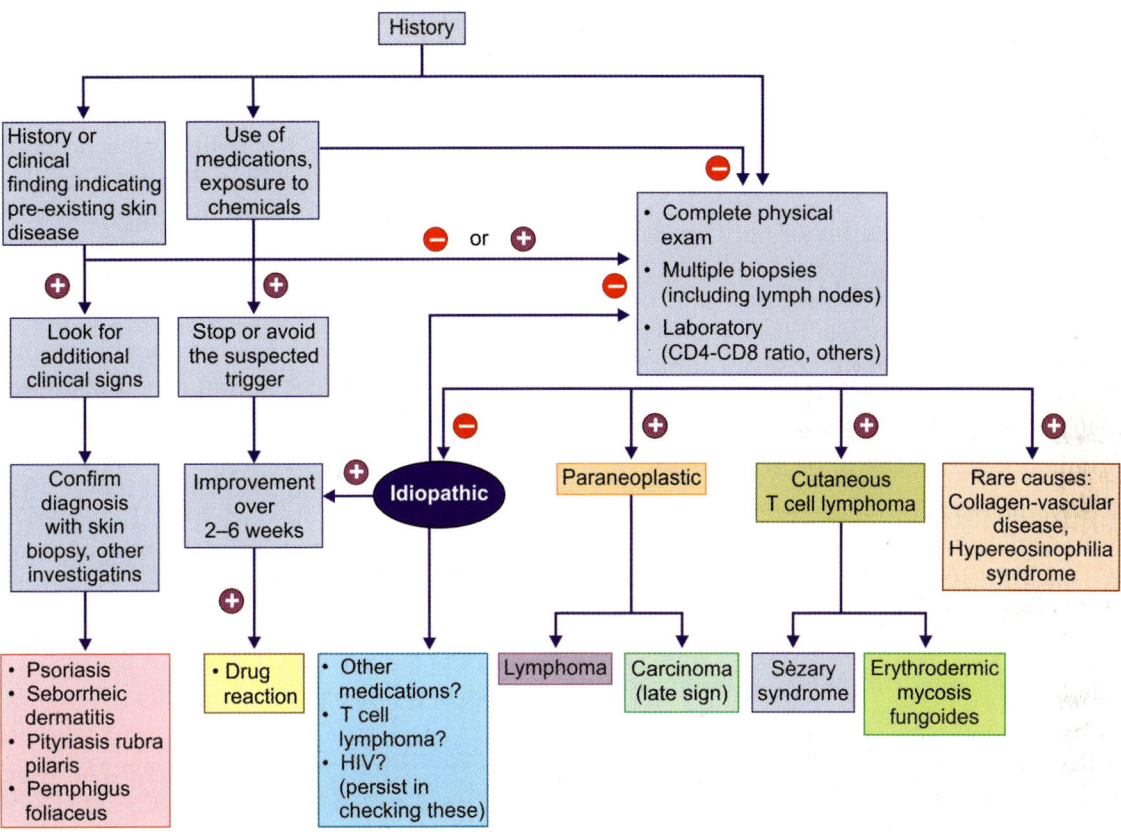

	Box 21.2: Overview of general measures	
General	• Hospitalization • Fluid intake monitoring • Electrolyte balance check • Temperature measuring • High-protein diet • Nutritional implementation • Stop any unnecessary drug	
Topical measures	• Lukewarm bath everyday • Wet dressing with topical steroids and emollients (triamcinolone acetonide cream, 0.025–1.0 %): 3 times a day	
Systemic	• *Antihistamine:* Hydroxyzine hydrochloride, 25–50 mg every 4–6 h • *Antibiotics:* If indicated; first- or second-generation cephalosporins or semisynthetic penicillins for 7–10 days, or macrolides, or clindamycin • *Steroids:* Prednisone 1 mg/kg/24 h, then gradually decreased • *Acitretin:* 0.3–0.75 mg/kg • *Cyclosporine:* 4 mg/kg/day slowly reduced after remission by 0.5 mg/kg every 2 weeks	

7. Discontinuation of all unnecessary systemic drugs is prudent, if drug-induced erythroderma is a possible diagnosis.

8. Oral, i.m., or i.v. sedative antihistamines are frequently needed.

9. In severe cases, systemic corticosteroids are the first-choice drugs.

Complete remission occurs in 1/3 of patients with idiopathic erythroderma, while 50 % of these patients demonstrate only partial remission. Patients where idiopathic erythroderma shows a chronic course are at high risk to evolve to cutaneous T cell lymphomas.

Specific Measures (Box 21.3)

1. Treatment of the underlying condition is essential, if the same is diagnosed on the basis of clinical findings and investigations.

2. Antibiotics are not necessary unless secondary infection is present.

3. Systemic **corticosteroids** may be employed in cases of refractory drug-induced or idiopathic, but not psoriatic, erythroderma. Initial dose of prednisone: 1 to 3 mg/kg/day is a reasonable start and should be *rapidly tapered* when clearing is achieved.

4. **Cyclosporine** has also been employed in refractory idiopathic patients. Initial dosage of 5 mg/kg/day with subsequent reduction to 1–3 mg/kg/day are appropriate.

5. **Psoriatic erythroderma:** Methotrexate, acitretin and anti-TNF biologics are the other commonly applied options.

6. In the treatment of **severe atopic dermatitis,** cyclosporine, methotrexate, azathioprine, and mycophenolate mofetil have been used with success.

7. For **PRP**, acitretin is the first line management with other options being cyclosporine, methotrexate and azathioprine.

8. **Dermatophytoses:** Erythroderma is seen in steroid modified cases (Fig. 21.9). Herein, the steroid suppression can be confirmed by testing the serum cortisol level. If the 8 am sample is <10 µg/dl, it is a good marker for immune suppression. In such cases, the systemic therapy may not work inspite of unnecessary updosing. Its our experience that after stopping topical steroids, for about 3–4 weeks, the results may be poor and hence, a longer duration of therapy is needed. It is established that applying 98 g of a super potent corticosteroid preparation over 2 weeks can suppress the HPA axis. It is recommended that patients should use no more than 50 g of a super potent steroid or 100 g of a potent steroid preparation per week and that prolonged usage at this high rate should be avoided. This is almost never complied with and in addition there is the use of parenteral and IM steroids by unlicensed practitioners. Thus, to tackle this situation, a **pulse regimen** of itraconazole has been used **(Majocchi granuloma)** 200 mg PO bid for 7 days, then off for 14 days (repeat 3 times total).

Erythroderma in Childhood

In children specially in neonates, the assistance of an ICU is essential as the infantile mortality is quite high (16 %), due to primary dermatosis or to the complications. Neonates have a higher risk of severe systemic infections, hypernatremic dehydration, hypoalbuminemia, hyperpyrexia, or hypothermia. These complications are more evident in collodion baby, severe lamellar ichthyosis, harlequin ichthyosis, Netherton syndrome, and Omenn syndrome. The skin fragility, fissures, cracks, erosions, or immunodeficiency of these conditions can lead to severe septicemic infections, resulting in high morbidity and mortality.

Apart from the measures listed above, as the hypermetabolic state can affect the normal growth, compensation for the same is essential and the energy intake should be increased by 10–30%. The physician should also pay attention to the prevention of infections. In general, topical emollients such as petrolatum

Box 21.3: Therapy for specific disorders

Psoriasis	*Methotrexate:* Initial dose 10–25 mg/week, maintenance dose 7.5–15 mg/week *Cyclosporine:* Initial mean dose 4 mg/kg/day, slowly reduced after remission by 0.5 mg/kg every 2 weeks *Acitretin:* 0.3–0.75 mg/kg *Phototherapy:* UVB, UVA, PUVA *Etanercept:* 50 mg subcutaneous injection twice a week, reduced 50 mg/week after 3 months *Infliximab:* 5 mg/kg i.v. at week 0, 2, 6, and later every 8 weeks Can be combined with methotrexate or acitretin *Adalimumab:* 80 mg at week 0, 40 mg at week 1, later 40 mg every 2 weeks
Atopic dermatitis	*Systemic steroids:* Prednisone 1 mg/kg/24 h, then gradually decreased *Antimicrobials:* If indicated, first- or second-generation cephalosporins or semisynthetic penicillins for 7–10 days, or macrolides, or clindamycin, etc. *Cyclosporine:* Initial mean dose 5 mg/kg/day, slowly reduced after remission by 0.5 mg/kg every 2 weeks *Phototherapy:* Broadband UVB (280–320 nm) Narrowband UVB (311–313 nm) UVA (320–400 nm), UVA1 (340–400 nm), PUVA *Azathioprine:* 100–200 mg/day, slowly reduced after remission *Methotrexate:* 10–25 mg/week, slowly reduced after remission *Mycophenolate mofetil:* 1–2 g/day, slowly reduced after remission Intravenous immunoglobulins: 2 g/kg/month for 3–6 months
Pityriasis rubra pilaris	*Acitretin:* 0.3–0.75 mg/kg/day, slowly reduced after remission *Methotrexate:* 10–25 mg/week, slowly reduced after remission *Systemic steroids:* Prednisone 1 mg/kg/24 h, then gradually decreased
Toxic epidermal necrolysis	*Supportive care: Most important* *Intravenous immunoglobulins:* High dose (up to 4 g/kg/day for 3–5 days) *Systemic steroids:* Prednisone 1 mg/kg/24 h, then gradually decreased *Cyclosporine:* 3–5 mg/kg/d *Plasmaperesis*
Scabies	*Topical permethrin 5%:* Once a day for 5 consecutive days *Oral ivermectin:* 200 µg/kg/day
Dermatophytoses	Most cases are due to steroid abuse. A baseline cortisol level is a good measure of HPA suppression. If so the immune respose may revert after about 4 weeks of stopping steroid use *Oral itraconazole:* 200 mg BD × 4–6 weeks *Itraconaozole pulse regimen:* 200 mg PO bid for 7 days, then off for 14 days (repeat 3 times total) *Oral-terbinafine:* 250 mg BD × 4–6 weeks *Topical:* Barrier cream (inflamed skin)—OD and azole cream HS Salicylic acid 6% what field ointment (lichenified skin—OD and azole cream HS)

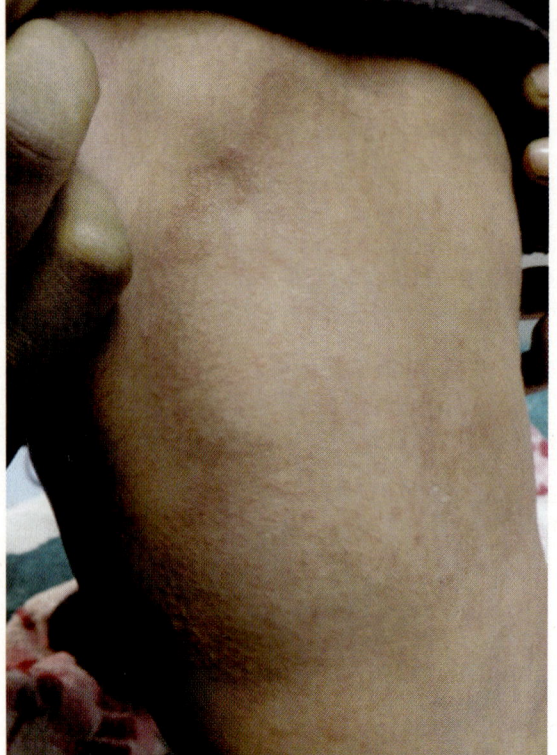

Fig. 21.9: A case of dermatophytosis in a neonate, possibly transmitted from the parents (Dr Konchok Dorjay)

or white soft paraffin and antifungals or topical steroids are recommended, with wet dressing, to maintain the barrier function of the stratum corneum.

Children affected due to staphylococcal scalded skin syndrome, infantile seborrheic dermatitis, or nutritional deficiencies can be completely cured. A short administration of systemic steroids (1 mg/kg/day) could be necessary in case of atopic dermatitis and drug-induced cases, while systemic metho-trexate or acitretin (0.5 mg/kg/day) could be helpful in psoriatic patients. Cases of ichthyosis may need retinoids.

Bibliography

1. Agarwal KK, Nath AK, Jaisankar TJ, D'Souza M. Parthenium dermatitis presenting as erythroderma. Contact Dermatitis. 2008 Sep;59(3):182–3.

2. Annalisa Patrizi and Michela Venturi. Erythroderma. Katsambas AD et al. (eds.), European Handbook of Dermatological Treatments, Springer-Verlag Berlin Heidelberg 2015.

3. Eczema. In. Sardana K, Mahajan S, Garg VK. Diagnosis and Management of Skin Disorders: An Evidence-Based Approach, 1/ e. Lippincott Williams and Wilkins, 2012 (reprint 2015).

4. Fast Facts: Eczema and Contact Dermatitis By John Berth-Jones, Eunice Tan and Howard I Malbach Published 2004.

5. Li J, Zheng HY. Erythroderma: A clinical and prognostic study. Dermatology 2012;225(2):154–62.

6. Mathew R, Sreedevan V. Erythroderma: A clinicopathological study of 370 cases from a tertiary care center in Kerala. Indian J Dermatol Venereol Leprol. 2017 Sep-Oct;83(5):625.

7. Mistry N, Gupta A, Alavi A, Sibbald RG. A review of the diagnosis and management of erythroderma (generalized red skin). Adv Skin Wound Care 2015 May;28(5):228–36.

8. Prakash BV, Sirisha NL, Satyanarayana VV, Sridevi L, Ramachandra BV. Aetiopathological and clinical study of erythroderma. J Indian Med Assoc 2009;107(2):100. 102–3.

9. Ragunatha S, Inamadar AC. Neonatal dermatological emergencies. Indian J Dermatol Venereol Leprol 2010;76(4):328–40.

10. Sardana K, Mahajan S, Sarkar R, Mendiratta V, Bhushan P, Koranne RV, Garg VK. The spectrum of skin disease among Indian children. Pediatr Dermatol. 2009 Jan-Feb;26(1):6–13.

11. Sarkar R, Garg VK. Erythroderma in children. Indian J Dermatol Venereol Leprol 2010; 76(4):341–7.

12. Thieme Clinical Companions Dermatology. Sterry, Dermatology© 2006 Thieme.

22

Prurigo Nodularis (Chronic Prurigo)

Kabir Sardana, Asit Mittal, Shivani Bansal

INTRODUCTION

Prurigo nodularis (PN) is a chronic relapsing, highly pruritic condition characterized by the presence of hyperkeratotic, excoriated, pruritic papules and nodules, with a tendency for symmetrical distribution. This condition is a difficult disease to treat and causes frustration to both the patient and the treating doctor. It has a high impact on the quality of life of the patient.

Incidence and prevalence of PN in the general population are unknown, because in epidemiological studies, PN is often listed under chronic itchy disorders (Iking A). In female patients, PN seems to be more prevalent, occurs at an earlier age, and is more severe than in male patients. Individuals with PN can be divided into *atopic* or *nonatopic*. In the setting of atopy, PN has an earlier age of onset and may be accompanied by cutaneous hypersensitivity to various environmental allergens.

ETIOPATHOGENESIS

The etiology is poorly understood. More than 50% of patients of prurigo nodularis suffer from atopic diathesis or atopic eczema. Inflammatory dermatoses such as cutaneous pemphigoid or lichen planus too can contribute to PN. The most common dermatological disorder associated is atopic dermatitis, described also as 'atopic prurigo' (Pugliarello S). Systemic diseases frequently associated are type 2 diabetes mellitus, thyroid disorders, chronic kidney disease, HCV infection, non-Hodgkin lymphoma and psychiatric disorders, particularly depression and anxiety (Winhoven SM). In some cases, no underlying disease is detected (idiopathic PN).

The pathogenesis of PN is still unknown; however, recent findings suggest that PN might be consequent to chronic itch induced by neuropathy (Yosipovitch G). A distinctive characteristic of neuropathic itch is the co-existence of other sensory symptoms such as paresthesia, hyperesthesia or hypoesthesia, as well as burning, tingling, stinging and heat and cold sensations. Nerve growth factor has been implicated in the pathogenesis of prurigo nodularis.

Calcitonin gene-related peptide and substance P immunoreactive nerves are markedly increased in prurigo nodularis when compared with normal skin.

Histological studies have identified various neural aspects that may play a role in the marked itching (Box 22.1).

A recent consensus has opined that PN showed a reduced intra-epidermal nerve fiber density (IENFD) in lesional skin and possibly scratching may contribute to reduced IENFD rather than an authentic endogenous neuropathy.

Box 22.1: Neural aspects specific to prurigo nodularis based on histological studies

- Epidermal and dermal nerve fibers are affected
- Mast cells: Dendritic appearance (normally round or elongated) with an enlarged cell body. They are usually degranulated
- Thickening of myelinated dermal nerves with neuroma formation (Pautrier neuroma)
- Subepidermal and dermal nerve fiber hyperplasia with degeneration and fragmentation of axons and Schwann cells
- Decrease of sensory C fibers in the nodules
- Hyperplasia of SP positive nerves

CLINICAL FEATURES

The term PN seems to restrict PN to cases where there is clinical presentation of nodules, but patients may also have papular or plaque type lesions.

It might be better to consider an umbrella term chronic prurigo which will encompass different morphologies including prurigo nodularis (Pereira MP) (Box 22.2).

The classic lesion in PN is a firm pruritic nodule that is hyperkeratotic. The lensions number from a few to hundreds, and range from a few millimeters to 2 cm in diameter (Fig. 22.1). There is a tendency for symmetrical distribution, with a predilection for extensor surfaces of the limbs; however, the trunk may be involved. The face and palms are seldom affected although no part of the body is exempt. Sparing of the upper mid-back, known as 'butterfly sign', is distinctive.

Prominent features include crusting and excoriations with post-inflammatory hyperpigmented and hypopigmented macules (Fig. 22.2). The skin between the lesions is usually normal but can be xerotic or lichenified. Occasionally the patient may violently scratch the lesions to precipitate bleeding (Fig. 22.3).

Box 22.2: Definition and diagnostic criteria of chronic prurigo (CPG)		
Parameter	*Term*	*Comment*
Definition	Chronic prurigo (CPG) is a distinct disease defined by the presence of chronic pruritus and multiple localized or generalized pruriginous lesions. CPG occurs due to a neuronal sensitization to itch and the development of an itch-scratch cycle. CPG can be of dermatological, systemic, neurologic, psychiatric/psychosomatic, multifactorial or undetermined origin.	
Diagnosis	Chronic prurigo (CPG)	• Umbrella term for all stages and manifestations of CPG; • 'Chronic' points to chronicity as an important part of the pathophysiology (peripheral and central neuronal sensitization)
State	Disease	Indicates an own state and distinction from the underlying etiology
Core symptoms (major criteria)	1. **Chronic pruritus** ($\geq$ 6 weeks) 2. **History and/or signs of repeated scratching** (e.g. excoriations, scars) 3. **Localized or generalized presence of multiple pruriginous* lesions**	• All core symptoms must be present to make a diagnosis of chronic prurigo. • Pruritus must be present and should be the initial sign. • Localized: An area such as the lower leg or lower arm. Initial presence of singular lesions does not fulfill the diagnostic criteria.

(Contd.)

Box 22.2: Definition and diagnostic criteria of chronic prurigo (CPG) (*Contd.*)

Parameter	Term	Comment
		*Definition of pruriginous lesion: Excoriated, scaling and/or crusted papules and/or nodules and/or plaques, often with a whitish or pink center and hyperpigmented border.
Range of manifestations	1. Papular type 2. Nodular type 3. Plaque type 4. Umbilicated type	Patients may present with one or more than one clinical manifestation of chronic prurigo. It is sufficient to diagnose the patients as chronic prurigo without mentioning the subtype.

Associated criteria (frame the disease in more detail)

1. **Signs**
   - Pruriginous lesions are distributed on areas of the skin accessible to scratching
   - Pruriginous lesions are usually symmetrically distributed
   - Normal or lichenified skin between pruriginous lesions
   - Other scratch-induced lesions may be associated, e.g. excoriations and scars
   - Face and palms are rarely affected
   - Pruriginous lesions are persistent

2. **Symptoms**
   - Pruritus precedes development of skin lesions
   - Pruritus might be accompanied by burning, stinging, pain and other sensations
   - Signs of chronicity: Continuous pruritus of high intensity, allokinesis, hyperkinesis, spreading of pruriginous skin lesions

3. **Function**
   - Impaired quality of life
   - Sleep loss due to disease
   - Days of absence from work
   - Obsessive-compulsive behavior

4. **Emotions**
   - Depression
   - Anxiety
   - Anger
   - Disgust
   - Shame
   - Helplessness

5. **Pathophysiology**
   - Neuronal sensitization towards itch induced by chronic pruritus and development of a chronic itch-scratch cycle
   - Etiology of chronic pruritus: Might be of dermatological, systemic, neurological, psychiatric/psychosomatic, multifactorial etiology, or idiopathic
   - Presence of other specific skin lesions may point to a concomitant skin disease

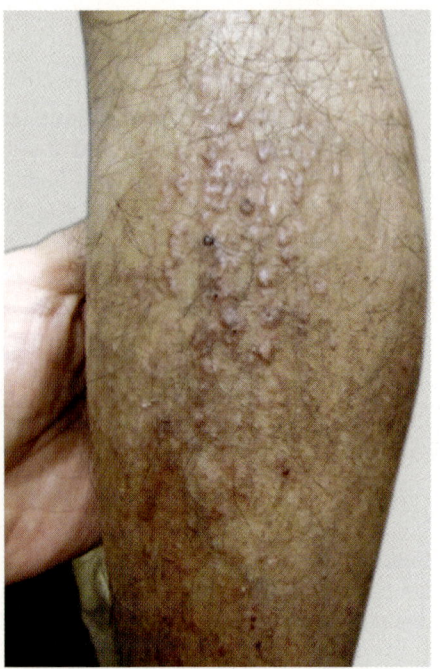

Fig. 22.1: Multiple hyperkeratotic nodules with some showing excoriation on the leg in a male patient

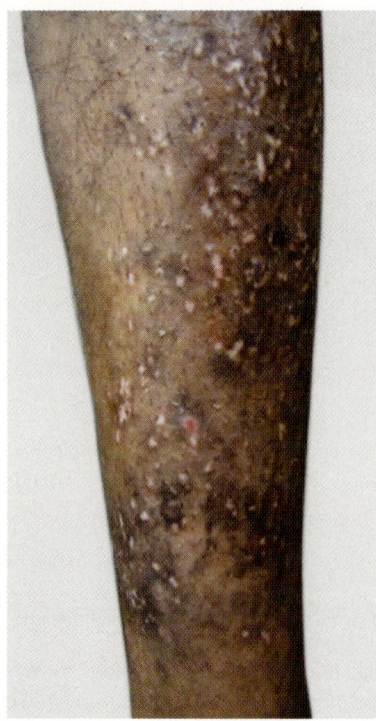

Fig. 22.2: This patient has visible and marked excoriations with associated hyper- and hypo-pigmentation

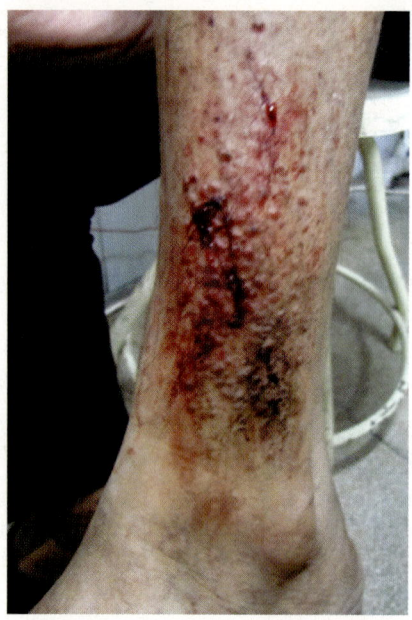

Fig. 22.3: A case of prurigo nodularis with violent bouts of scratching which overrides the pain. This patient was found to have an OCD for which he was initiated on pimozide 1 mg BD with a short-course of cyclosporine for prurigo

INVESTIGATIONS

An important first step in therapy is to identify any underlying associations and treat accordingly. Table 22.1 lists the suggested investigations for these underlying associations (Lee MR).

But another consensus has opined that with pruriginous lesions observed in CPG patients, the underlying etiology or trigger factors cannot be defined and there is no evidence that the initial underlying etiology has an influence on the clinics, severity or course of CPG. The itch-scratch cycle is a critical event promoting neuronal sensitization leading to CPG (Fig. 22.4). In other words, the presence of CPG should prompt a search for the underlying etiology of chronic pruritus but this can be considered just as trigger of CPG. Once established, CPG necessitates an own therapeutic approach and does not resolve if the underlying etiology is cured or treated (Fig. 22.4).

Table 22.1: Suggested investigations for associated disorders in prurigo nodularis (Sonja Ständer)	
Basic hematological work up	• Liver function test • Urea, creatinine, electrolytes • Parathyroid hormone level • Thyroid function test • Blood glucose
Advanced tests	• Hepatitis serology • HIV serology • Total serum IgE level
Skin directed tests	• Skin biopsy for histopathology • Direct immunofluorescence (bullous pemphigoid, epidermolysis bullosa acquisita) • Indirect immunofluorescence • Patch testing
Radiological tests	• Chest X-ray (rule out sarcoidosis, neoplasm, lymphoma, TB) • Ultrasound abdomen (rule out liver or kidney disease) • Magnetic resonance tomography of cervical spinal column, if patient has localized PN (e.g. on lower arms) • PN on the lower leg: Phlebological investigation to rule out chronic venous insufficiency

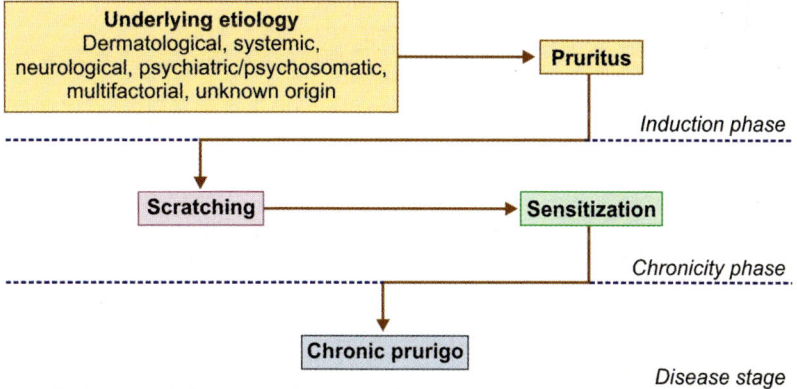

Fig. 22.4: Evolution of chronic prurigo. Different etiologies might trigger pruritus (induction phase), which leads to scratching. With time, this leads to sensitization processes (chronicity phase) and the development of papules, nodules, plaques and/or umbilicated lesions (disease stage). The clinical picture is depending on scratching but not on the initial etiology (Pereira MP)

TREATMENT

Treatment of PN is still a challenge, and it is frustrating for both dermatologists and patients because, in the majority of cases, the response is limited and unsatisfactory. Once the itch-scratch cycle 'takes over', it is extremely difficult to stop. There is no standardized therapy of PN, and evidence from RCT is limited.

Though stress plays a role, the notion that the disorder has a psychological basis is unfounded.

A detailed summary of treatment is given in Table 22.2.

Table 22.2: A summary of treatment options of prurigo nodularis based on best available evidence

	Topical	Systemic	Others
First line	• **Steroids (topical /IL)** Triamcinolone 7.5–20 mg every 3–4 weeks	**Antihistamines** Ketotifen: 1 mg/day for 4 weeks 10 mg montelukast/day and 240 mg fexofenadine twice daily	
Second line	**Capsaicin** (0.025–0.3%) four to six times daily	• **Gabapentin** 300 mg 3 times daily • **Pregabalin** 75 mg/day • **Naltrexone** 25–150 mg/day	• UVB phototherapy • Narrowband UVB • PUVA or bath PUVA • **Modified Goeckerman** scheme (UVB + LCD 2% + topical steroid)
Third line	• **Tacrolimus** • **Calcipotriol** • **Tacalcitol**	• **Thalidomide** 100 mg/d • **Cyclosporine** 3–5 mg per kg/day • **Methotrexate** 7.5–20 mg once weekly • **Lenalidomide** 5–10 mg/d • **Tacrolimus** 20 mg	
Research drug		**Aprepitant** 80 mg/day	

General Measures

Simple measures, such as clipping the fingernails and recommending the use of gloves or mittens, can be helpful. It is important to stress to the patient the requirement to apply emollients, as xerosis usually worsens the pruritus.

First-line Agents

Topical antipruritics, such as 1% menthol or phenol in a creamy base, may be used to reduce the itch. Oral antihistamines, such as promethazine hydrochloride 25–75 mg at night, or oral antidepressants, such as doxepin 10–75 mg at night, may be administered to reduce the pruritus.

Potent topical glucocorticoid creams or ointments, such as betamethasone dipropionate 0.5 mg/g, glucocorticoid creams under occlusion, and intralesional glucocorticoids, such as triamcinolone acetonide 10 mg/ml increasing to 40 mg/ml suspension, are often employed. Occlusive bandages are useful as they interrupt the itch-scratch cycle.

Second-line Agents

UV light exposure has been shown to lessen the pruritus and can be beneficial in the treatment of PN. The main effect of UV light treatment in PN is to break the cycle of itching and scratching. Cryotherapy is a useful therapeutic agent for the treatment of PN. It can also be combined with intralesional corticosteroids.

Recently, topical vitamin D_3 has been reported to be effective in the treatment of PN.

Vitamin D_3 downregulates cellular adhesion molecule expression by inhibiting TNF-α mRNA expression. Capsaicin has been shown to reduce pruritus and induce complete disappearance of lesions. When applied topically it induces itch and burning sensation as well as erythema. Topical capsaicin (0.025–0.3%) four to six times daily for periods of between 2 weeks and 10 months is effective.

Third-line Agents

Cyclosporine has demonstrated unequivocal improvement of PN as well as a reduction in the severity of pruritus. Cyclosporine inhibits lymphokine transcription and lymphocyte activation and proliferation. The dramatic response of this drug disproves the psychological notion of PN and in the atopiform form of PN has a near dramatic response. It is important to monitor blood pressue and kidney function during cyclosporine therapy. Oral and subcutaneous low dose weekly **methotrexate** (7.5 –20 mg) is another immunosuppressive agent, tried in cases of PN. With all these immunosuppressive therapies, associated risks and side effect must be first taken into account.

The first reported use of *thalidomide* in the treatment of PN was in 1975. Thalidomide inhibits polymorphonuclear leukocyte chemotaxis and selectively inhibits TNF-α production by enhancing degradation of TNF-α mRNA. It has been postulated that thalidomide causes central nervous system depression without causing incoordination, respiratory depression or narcosis.

Through its central sedative effect, it causes a decreased perception of peripheral stimuli. Thalidomide may have a direct peripheral action on the proliferated neural tissue in the lesions causing PN. There have been reported cases where oral thalidomide at **doses of 200 mg daily** demonstrated improvement of pruritus and flattening of lesions with no serious adverse events. However, fatigue, confusion and sensory neuropathy can sometimes be a problem with thalidomide therapy. Lenalinomide 5 mg per day, a second generation thalidomide analogue can also be an alternative.

Opioid receptor antagonist such as:

Naltrexone has been reported to have a high antipruritic effect in patients with PN. Opiates have been shown to evoke or potentiate itch, independently from their histamine-releasing effect. Combing μ opioid receptor antagonist and κ opioid receptor antagonist such as nalbuphine and butorphanol can have positive effect on PN.

Gabapentin, pregabalin and the neurokinin receptor 1 antagonist, *aprepitant,* seem also to be effective in the therapy of PN, but RCTs are still lacking (Fostini AC).

Antidepressants such as paroxetine, amitryptyline and mirtazapine too have been tried in severe PN.

Future therapies Neurokinin receptor 1 antagonists, aprepitant and serlopitant are currently been analysed for treatment of PN. Nalbuphine, a dual μ/κ opioid receptor antagonist is another agent with potential efficacy (Fostini AC).

Most patients with PN need to be approached with combination therapy, which includes suppression of multiple mediators, including cytokines and neuromediators.

Bibliography

1. Fostini AC, Girolomoni G, Tessari G. Prurigo nodularis: An update on etiopathogenesis and therapy. J Dermatolog Treat 2013 Dec;24(6):458–62.

2. Iking A, Grundmann S, Chatzigeorgakidis E, Phan NQ, Klein D, Ständer S. Prurigo as a symptom of atopic and non-atopic diseases: aetiological survey in a consecutive cohort of 108 patients. J Eur Acad Dermatol Venereol 2013;27:550–7.

3. Lee MR, Shumack S. Prurigo nodularis: A review. Australas J Dermatol 2005 Nov;46(4):211–18.

4. Pereira MP, Steinke S, Zeidler C, Forner C, Riepe C, Augustin M, Bobko S, Dalgard F, Elberling J, Garcovich S, Gieler U, Gonçalo M, Halvorsen JA, Leslie TA, Metz M, Reich A, ?avk E, Schneider G, Serra-Baldrich E, Ständer HF, Streit M, Wallengren J,

Weller K, Wollenberg A, Bruland P, Soto-Rey I, Storck M, Dugas M, Weisshaar E, Szepietowski JC, Legat FJ, Ständer S; EADV Task Force Pruritus group members. European academy of dermatology and venereology European prurigo project: expert consensus on the definition, classification and terminology of chronic prurigo. J Eur Acad Dermatol Venereol 2017 Aug 31. doi: 10.1111/jdv.14570.

5. Pugliarello S, Cozzi A, Gisondi P, Girolomoni G. Phenotypes of atopic dermatitis. J Dtsch Dermatol Ges 2011;9:12–20.

6. *Sonja Ständer, Malcolm Greaves. Pruritus, prurigo and lichen simplex. Rook's Textbook of Dermatology, Ninth Edition. Edited by Christopher Griffiths, Jonathan Barker, Tanya Bleiker, Robert Chalmers and Daniel Creamer. © 2016 John Wiley & Sons, Ltd. Published 2016 by John Wiley & Sons, Ltd.

7. Winhoven SM, Gawkrodger DJ. Nodular prurigo: metabolic diseases are a common association. Clin Exp Dermatol 2007;32:224–225.

8. Yosipovitch G, Samuel LS. Neuropathic and psychogenic itch. Dermatol Ther2008;21:32–41.

23

Miscellaneous Eczematous Conditions

Ananta Khurana

MEYERSON'S PHENOMENON/HALO DERMATITIS/HALO ECZEMA/MEYERSON NEVUS

The term classically describes a pruriginous, symmetric eczematous halo around a melanocytic nevus. The phenomenon may occur at any age. However, it has been observed most frequently in young adults. Thirty percent of reported cases in children occur in small congenital nevi. Pruritus is a common symptom and lesions are more common on the trunk and proximal extremities. Patients may present with multiple lesions, and this was observed in both of Meyerson's original cases. The phenomenon may occur as a collision dermatosis with atopic eczema or as an isolated phenomenon.

The original report by Meyerson (1971) had been of a papulosquamous halo dermatitis overlying pigmented nevi but the condition is now known to be associated with various other nevoid and acquired lesions, like melanoma, dermatofibroma, seborrheic keratosis, nevus sebaceous, keloids, congenital melanocytic nevi, mycoses fungoides, smooth muscle hamartoma, basal cell carcinoma, squamous cell carcinoma and portwine stain (Fig. 23.1). Thus, the term "Meyerson phenomenon" replaced "Meyerson nevus" in literature.

The dense dermal inflammatory infiltrate from the site of Meyerson phenomenon shows a predominance of CD4+ T cells. This differs from the irritant reaction sometimes seen in lesions such as seborrheic keratoses, which are characterised by a mixed infiltrate with neutrophils, lymphocytes, plasma cells and evidence of apoptosis in the central lesion. The Meyerson phenomenon is also a different reaction compared to Sutton's nevus as the inflammatory infiltrate in Sutton's naevus is predominately CD8+ T cells. In contrast with Sutton nevus, the Meyerson nevus persists after resolution of the halo of eczema. In the

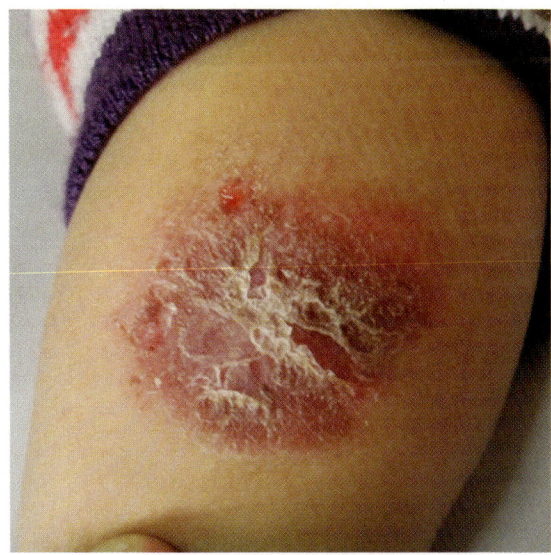

Fig. 23.1: Meyerson's phenomenon involving a portwine stain in a 6-month-old infant

case of melanocytic (usually compound) nevi, there is also an associated spongiotic dermatitis of the overlying epidermis.

Meyerson phenomenon has also been observed following treatment with interferon α-2b and ribavirin for hepatitis C. Up-regulation of intercellular adhesion molecule-1 (ICAM-1) on the endothelial cells and keratinocytes was found within the inflamed nevi, and their interaction with CD4+ lympho-cytes are proposed to be the cause in this scenario. UV radiation has been suggested as another cause trigerring the phenomenon.

The natural history of Meyerson pheno-menon is variable. When the inciting lesion is excised/treated, the inflammation resolves. Lesions left *in situ* may respond rapidly to topical corticosteroid use, or may persist for years before spontaneous resolution. The case depicted in Fig. 23.1 responded to potent topical steroids but would recur with stopping the same. Treatment with vascular lasers is an effective option for this case.

FOLLICULAR ECZEMA

This may present in the setting of atopic eczema or as an isolated entity, mainly in the pediatric age group. Follicular scaly papules develop in a discrete manner or in confluence forming discoid patches. There is generally a background of xerosis (Fig. 23.2). The lesions may develop anywhere on the body. This commonly encountered, but uncommonly described, entity needs to be differentiated from follicular predominant entities like keratosis pilaris, phrynoderma and lichen spinulosus.

Keratosis pilaris is a very common condi-tion presenting as small keratotic papules with perifollicular erythema, on the extensor aspects of arms and thighs, giving a rough feel to the involved region. Occasionally, the buttocks and lumbar region is also affected. Lichen spinulosus is an uncommon condition presenting with follicular papules, which may further coalesce into plaques, with a promi-nent pointed keratotic spine. The lesions are located over trunk, buttocks, neck, knees and elbows (Figs 23.3 and 23.4). Phrynoderma present with skin colored or hyperpigmented papules on the elbows and knees (or more extensively involving the buttocks and extensor limbs), in association with nutritional deficiencies.

Notably all the 3 differentials present in the pediatric age group, similar to follicular eczema. But, these are largely asymptomatic, while follicular eczema is a pruritic condition.

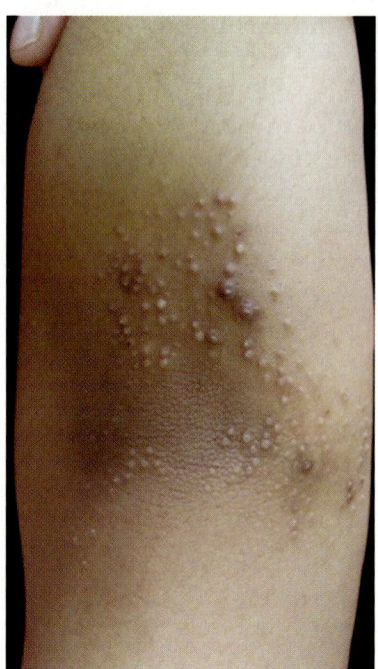

Fig. 23.3: Lichen spinulosus (spiny discrete follicular papules over the elbow of a 10-year-old girl)

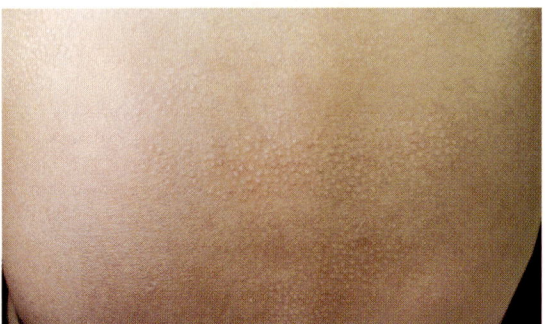

Fig. 23.2: Follicular eczematous changes over a background of xerosis on the back of a child

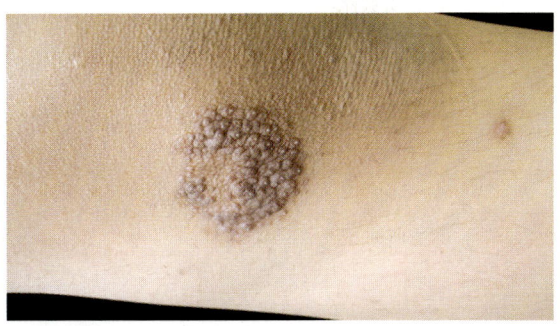

Fig. 23.4: Lichen spinulosus; spiny papules forming a plaque over the elbow

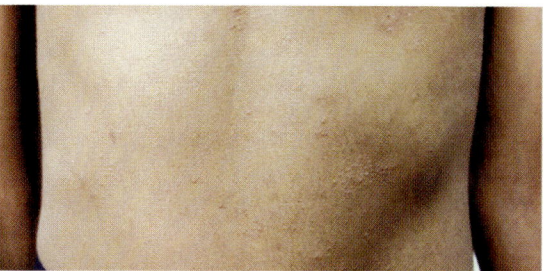

Fig. 23.5: Lichen scrofulosorum presenting as grouped follicular and extra-follicular papules over the trunk

The differentiation is important since keratolytics often used for the treatment of these may worsen the latter. Lichen scrofulosorum may also pose diagnostic difficulties in some cases (Figs 23.5 and 23.6).

Treatment

Application of emollients and mild steroids will clear the lesions (Fig. 23.7). Recurrences are usual in those with an underlying atopic diathesis.

TRAUMATIC ANSERINE FOLLICULOSIS (TAF)

This is an under-recognized, but not uncommon, entity presenting mostly in children. These occur closely set follicular papules (goose skin-like), on the chin, mostly corroborating with a habit of assuming a particular position causing pressure and friction at the site (Figs 23.8 and 23.9). Similar lesions known as "fiddler's neck" have been described on the jaw of violin players and follicular keratosis has been described over amputation stumps. TAF is usually seen in children and adolescents as their skin is delicate and more likely to be affected by friction and trauma. It is important to question both the child and parents for predisposing positions as children often refuse to accept the same. There is no gender predilection, although most initial cases were reported in females.

TAF was first reported by Goncalves in 1977, who also gave the condition this name.

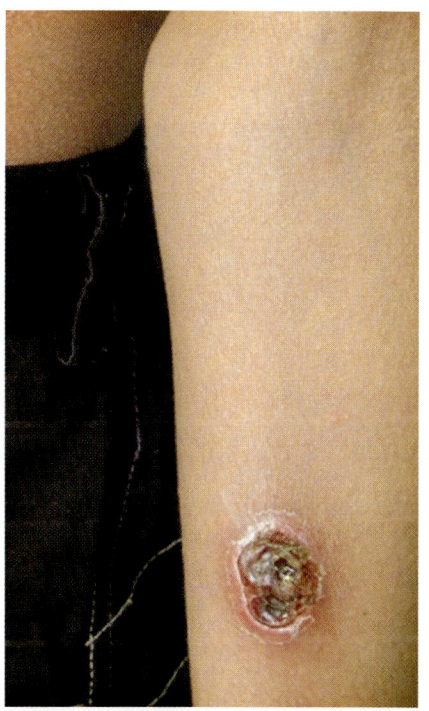

Fig. 23.6: The same patient (Fig. 23.5) demonstrated a highly positive Mantoux reaction with ulceration

Other names given to TAF are keratotic papular lesions of the chin and follicular keratosis of the chin. The etiology is proposed to be an abnormal follicular keratinization caused by local pressure and friction. Histopathology demonstrates cystic hair follicles containing keratotic material and a few fine vellus hairs. There is generally no inflammatory infiltrate.

Prognosis is excellent with total disappearance of the lesion after the patients stop

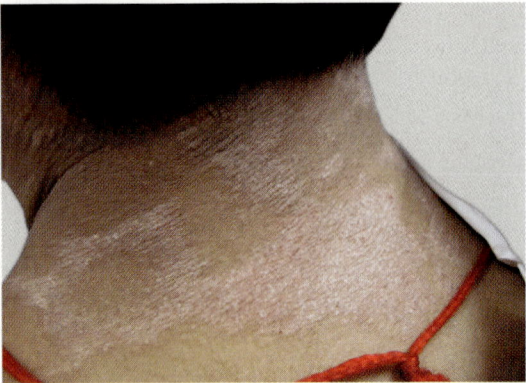

Fig. 23.7a: Follicular eczema; note the aggregated papules; the patient was on the "safe", slow, but in this, ineffective, homeopathic treatment

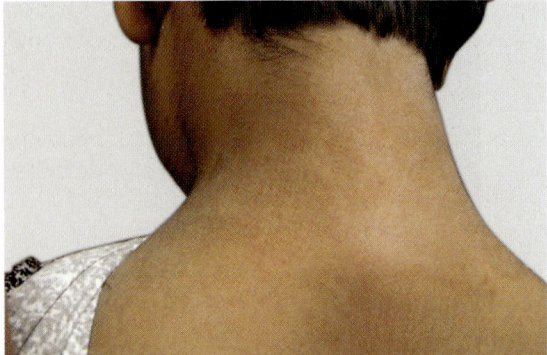

Fig 23.7b: Complete clearance with emollients and Class VI topical steroids (day 14)

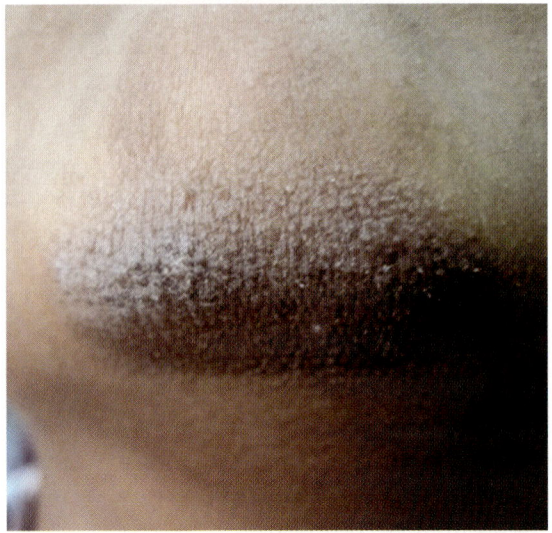

Fig. 23.8: Closely set follicular papules forming a plaque, on the chin of a 9-year-old boy

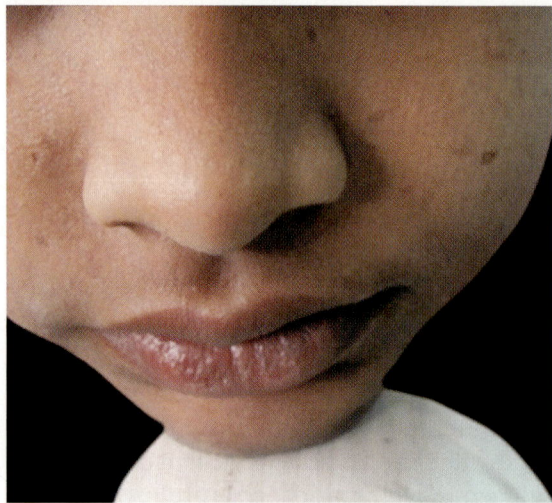

Fig. 23.9: Patient demonstrates his habitual posture while watching television

their habit of resting their chin on their hands or knee. Topical keratolytics hasten the resolution process.

POST-TRAUMATIC ECZEMA

Eczema developing as a Koebner's phenomenon is rare. The eruption may be the first manifestation of an endogenous dermatitis, or it may follow the onset of the dermatitis. It may also occur as an isolated phenomenon, which may be classified as idiopathic post-traumatic eczema. Cases have been reported following mechanical trauma, over saphenous vein graft donor site and over burn scars. Beukers *et al* described a case with recurrent dyshidrotic eczema at site of sharp instrumental trauma.

Mathias derived the following conclusions from his series of 13 cases:

1. Cutaneous trauma may precipitate eczema.
2. The implicated trauma is sufficient to cause obvious tissue damage accompanied by an inflammatory or regenerative response.
3. Eczema usually begins within a few weeks of acute injury at the site of the cutaneous trauma.
4. Eczema may occur as an isolated idiopathic reaction or as an isomorphic reaction either

preceding or following the appearance of an endogenous eczematous condition in nontraumatized skin.

5. Individual lesions of post-traumatic eczema may persist or recur for long periods of time.

6. The occurrence of post-traumatic eczema following occupational injury has important medicolegal implications.

REFERENCES

1. Beukers S, van der Valk PG. Idiopathic post-traumatic eczema. Contact Dermatitis. 2006 Mar;54(3):178.

2. Brenner S, Ilie B. Familial keratotic papular lesions on the chin. Int J Dermatol 1985; 24:320–321.

3. Conde-Taboada A, De La Torre C, Feal C, et al. Meyerson's naevi induced by interferon alfa plus ribavirin combination therapy in hepatitis C infection. Br J Dermatol 2005; 153:1070–2.

4. Gushi A, Hozumi H, Kanzaki T. A case of follicular keratosis of the chin. Nishinihon J Dermatol 2003; 65:95–96.

5. Ibbotson SH, Simpson NB, Fyfe NC, Lawrence CM. Follicular keratoses at amputation sites. Br J Dermatol 1994 Jun; 130(6):770–2.

6. Ingram JR. Eczematous Disorders. In Griffiths CEM, Barker J, Blelker T, Chalmers R, Creamer D, eds. Rook Textbook of Dermatology. 9th ed; Blackwell Publishing Ltd, UK.

7. Kanzaki T, Morita A, Takashima A. Follicular keratosis of the chin. J Am Acad Dermatol 1992; 26:134–5.

8. Loh J, Kenny P. Meyerson phenomenon. J Cutan Med Surg 2010; 14:30–2.

9. Mathias CG. Post-traumatic eczema. Dermatol Clin 1988 Jan; 6(1):35–42.

10. Mehta VR. Keratotic papular lesions on the chin in young females. J Cutan Pathol 1983; 10:376.

11. Meyerson LB. A peculiar papulosquamous eruption involving pigmented naevi. Arch. Dermatol 1971; 103:510–12.

12. Sardana K, Arora P, Mishra D. Follicular eczema: a commonly misdiagnosed dermatosis. Indian Pediatr 2012 Jul; 49(7):599.

Index

13